BELLEVUE

Also by David Oshinsky

Senator Joseph McCarthy and the American Labor Movement

A Conspiracy So Immense: The World of Joe McCarthy

Worse Than Slavery: Parchman Farm and the Ordeal of Jim Crow Justice

Polio: An American Story

*Capital Punishment on Trial: Furman v. Georgia and
the Death Penalty in Modern America*

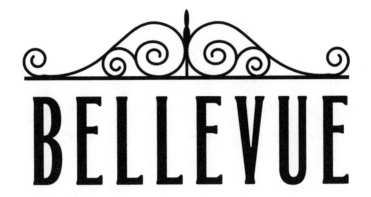

BELLEVUE

*Three Centuries of Medicine and Mayhem
at America's Most Storied Hospital*

David Oshinsky

DOUBLEDAY
New York   London   Toronto
Sydney   Auckland

All rights reserved. Published in the United States by Doubleday, a division of Penguin Random House LLC, New York, and distributed in Canada by Random House of Canada, a division of Penguin Random House Canada Limited, Toronto.

www.doubleday.com

DOUBLEDAY and the portrayal of an anchor with a dolphin are registered trademarks of Penguin Random House LLC.

Pages 370–371 constitute an extension of this copyright page.

Book design by Michael Collica
Jacket design by Michael J. Windsor
Jacket photograph: The Front Gates of Bellevue Hospital
(photo by Al Fenn / The LIFE Picture Collection / Getty Images)

Library of Congress Cataloging-in-Publication Data
Names: Oshinsky, David M., 1944– author.
Title: Bellevue : three centuries of medicine and mayhem at America's most storied hospital / David Oshinsky.
Description: First edition. | New York : Doubleday, [2016] | Includes bibliographical references and index.
Identifiers: LCCN 2016027568 (print) | LCCN 2016028334 (ebook) | ISBN 9780385523363 (hardcover : alk. paper) | ISBN 9780385540858 (ebook)
Subjects: | MESH: Bellevue Hospital. | Hospitals, Urban—history | History, Modern 1601– | New York City
Classification: LCC RA982.N5 (print) | LCC RA982.N5 (ebook) | NLM WX 28 AN7 | DDC 362.1109747/1—dc23
LC record available at https://lccn.loc.gov/2016027568

MANUFACTURED IN THE UNITED STATES OF AMERICA

1 3 5 7 9 10 8 6 4 2

First Edition

For my son Efrem,
who makes me joyful and proud

CONTENTS

BELLEVUE

INTRODUCTION

TAKEN TO BELLEVUE—it's a phrase nearly as old as New York City. First used in the eighteenth century to describe yellow fever victims packed off to a desolate pesthouse along the East River, it is so familiar today that newspapers don't bother to add the word "Hospital" to their headlines: "EBOLA DOCTOR TAKEN TO BELLEVUE," "WOMAN STRUCK BY BUZZSAW BLADE TAKEN TO BELLEVUE," "FAMOUS GRAFFITI ARTIST BUSTED FOR HITTING MAN WITH BEER MUG—TAKEN TO BELLEVUE."

It borders on ritual. "If a cop gets shot in Manhattan, his first choice is often Bellevue . . . If an investment banker goes into cardiac arrest, his limo driver knows where to take him," writes Eric Manheimer, the hospital's former medical director. The same holds true when a firefighter is injured, a prisoner takes sick, a worker falls from a scaffold, a homeless person lies dazed in the street—the destination, more likely than not, is Bellevue. Should a visiting pope or president require urgent medical attention, the hospital's superb emergency department awaits.

Bellevue closely mirrors an ever-changing New York. More than a hundred languages are translated at Bellevue, the most common being Spanish, Mandarin, Cantonese, Polish, Bengali, French, and Haitian Creole. Doctors and patients communicate on dual telephones through an interpreter trained in the nuances of regional dialects. The directional signs that guide visitors through the hospital are multilingual—the destinations now include a Muslim prayer room and a clinic for the survivors of political torture. Doctors and nurses have reported cases of a foreigner arriving at Kennedy Airport, hailing a cab, and uttering a single word: "Bellevue."

They come knowing they won't be turned away. Every immigrant group has availed itself of Bellevue's protective umbrella over the centuries; every disaster and epidemic has packed its spartan wards. "It was never the tidiest [place] in the world—how could it be, when its policy was always to accept those patients who with some justice could be called the dregs of humanity?" the gifted surgeon William A. Nolen observed. "At times it was so loaded with victims of typhus, cholera, and yellow fever that, within minutes of a patient's death, the body was in a coffin and a new patient was in the bed."

One could chart the severity of a New York winter by counting the pneumonia victims on the hospital's Chest Service, or measure the dangers of Prohibition liquor by totaling up the poisoned bodies in the morgue. If tuberculosis was running rampant through the city, then tuberculosis was what Bellevue treated. When AIDS arrived, when violent crime spiked, when addicts turned to crack cocaine, when released state mental patients became homeless, Bellevue usually saw it first.

Few hospitals are more deeply embedded in our popular culture. Tales of Bellevue as a receptacle for mangled crime victims, vicious psychopaths, and hopeless derelicts were always common fare, though the late-nineteenth-century circulation wars between William Randolph Hearst and Joseph Pulitzer churned out especially lurid exposés. The splashiest one—Nellie Bly's *Ten Days in a Mad-House*—had an indelible effect. From that point forward, the hospital became synonymous with bedlam, dwarfing its immense achievements in clinical care and medical research.

Hollywood found Bellevue irresistible. Much of Billy Wilder's *Lost Weekend,* the 1945 Academy Award winner for best picture, takes place there—the *New York Times* called it "a staggeringly ugly experience in the Bellevue alcoholic ward"—and the hospital makes a cameo appearance in the beloved *Miracle on 34th Street,* when the stubbornly proud Kris Kringle, caged in a tiny cell with barred windows, is deemed delusional and recommended for commitment. In search of the most forbidding hospital to film parts of *The Godfather,* Francis Ford Coppola quite naturally settled on Bellevue, whose morgue served in later scenes as Bonasera's Funeral Home.

It didn't help that Bellevue is a short ambulance ride from Greenwich Village. As such, its six-hundred-bed psychiatric building became a revolving door for legions of writers, artists, and musicians in various states of distress. William Burroughs spent time in Bellevue after cutting off a finger to impress his lover. Delmore Schwartz arrived in handcuffs following an attempt to strangle a hostile book reviewer. Eugene O'Neill visited the alcoholic ward often enough to be on a first-name basis with the staff. Sylvia Plath came after suffering a nervous breakdown, and saxophonist Charlie "Bird" Parker committed himself following two suicide attempts in 1954. (He died the following year.) Bassist Charles Mingus also signed in voluntarily, it was said, to escape a business dispute with the Mafia. He would later compose the jarring "Lock 'Em Up (Hellview of Bellevue)" to reflect the mania he found inside.

Poets and novelists such as Saul Bellow, Allen Ginsberg, and Richard Yates have memorialized Bellevue in their work. But the most detailed firsthand account remains unpublished. In 1960, Norman Mailer was committed to Bellevue for stabbing his wife during a drunken rage triggered, apparently, by her taunt that he couldn't shine Dostoyevsky's shoes. Mailer kept a private diary of his seventeen days under observation; clogged with detail, it reads like a narrative in search of a plot. Patients come and go—"spades" and "junkies," "Puerto Rican killers," and "teenage hoodlum homosexuals." Guards rule with fists and clubs. Straitjackets restrain the worst offenders. Two men return to Mailer's ward, close to unconscious. "Both had had shock [treatment], pipe to bite on, pillow under ass, hand on head. Wham. Drool from mouth." Mailer thought about weaving his Bellevue comrades into a piece of long-form journalism, but never did. "I said my goodbyes," the diary concludes, "feeling quite moved at leaving them."

Mailer was one of numerous celebrities observed by Bellevue psychiatrists following a violent criminal act. (Found competent to stand trial, he received a suspended sentence when his wife refused to press charges.) George Metesky, the "Mad Bomber" who set off explosives that terrorized the city in the 1950s, was committed there before spending the rest of his life in a state institution. When serial killer David Berkowitz, better known as "Son of Sam," sent a bizarre letter to the newspapers shortly before his capture, a team at Bellevue diligently parsed it for clues. The resulting profile described the author as a paranoid schizophrenic and likely loner who hated women, unleashing what one observer called "a flood of worthless tips."

John Lennon's assassin, Mark David Chapman, faced something quite different: a staff so uniformly hostile, so adoring of Lennon, that some of them questioned their own capacity to render a fair diagnosis. "When I first knew I was going to see him, I worried my anger toward him would interfere with my ability to do my job," Bellevue's chief psychologist recalled. "But he was such a pathetic character, I said 'hello' and he smiled—then he said, 'Oh, excuse me, I shouldn't be smiling.'" Meanwhile, Lennon's body lay wrapped in a sheet in the Bellevue morgue, a few buildings away.

Some illustrious patients arrived with no fanfare at all. The great songwriter Stephen Foster was taken to Bellevue in 1863 with a gaping hole in his skull; the prolific short-story writer O. Henry in 1910 with cirrhosis of the liver; the legendary bluesman known as Lead Belly in 1949 with a bone infection complicated by amyotrophic lateral sclerosis, Lou Gehrig's Disease. No private rooms or personal physicians or special amenities awaited them. They had come because they were destitute and desperately ill, and all three would die there while receiving emergency care. Their experiences—more than Mailer's or Chapman's—reflect the essence of Bellevue. In 2014, a recording mysteriously surfaced of a previously unknown Lead Belly song: "Bellevue Hospital Blues," written days before he died. It's the simple tribute of a man thankful for the attention he was shown.

Bellevue's hold on our popular imagination has come at a price. The relentless focus on its eccentricities has obscured its role as our quintessential public hospital—the flagship institution of America's largest city, where free hospital care is provided to the "medically indigent" as a right, not a privilege. In that role, Bellevue has borne witness to every imaginable disease and public health scare, every economic swing and

population surge, every medical breakthrough and controversy going back more than two centuries. Its history is fraught with conflict because it reflects the shifting political currents that have roiled the nation regarding its responsibilities to the poor. Calls for Bellevue's extinction are as old as the hospital itself. Its survival has never been assured.

A visitor to Bellevue in any era might see much the same thing: a well-schooled physician treating a charity patient against a background of bleakness and disrepair. It's a scene that dates back to the 1700s, when a prominent doctor, accompanied by a student apprentice or two, would wind his way through the decrepit, foul-smelling almshouse sick wards to offer diagnoses, prescribe medicines, and fix what could be fixed. The doctor volunteered his services for several reasons, including a Christian duty to the poor and the chance to hone his skills on bodies too powerless to resist.

Bellevue's early physicians were leaders of their craft (not yet a profession). They believed in the Miasma Theory, which blamed toxic clouds for the spread of disease, and considered bleeding and purging among the better methods for dealing with it. Most were enthusiastic grave robbers, participating in midnight raids that inflamed public opinion but provided the corpses needed for anatomical study. Some had studied in Europe, where clinical observation and laboratory research were changing the ways illness was understood.

New York in these years had only one medical school of note: the College of Physicians and Surgeons (P&S). But the city's explosive growth in the early nineteenth century led enterprising doctors to open two competing institutions: the Medical College of New York City (later NYU) in 1841, and Bellevue Hospital Medical College exactly two decades later. Their common denominator, aside from accepting every white male student able to pay the freight, was the lure of Bellevue as a clinical mecca for the study of sickness and disease. By the Civil War, it had become both the nation's largest hospital and its most important medical training ground.

The reason could be summed up in a single word: immigration. Bellevue's early history reflects the waves of Irish peasants fleeing starvation on "famine ships" bound for Canada, Boston, and New York.

Some carried deadly diseases that would devastate the slums and sweep through Bellevue itself, leaving numerous dead physicians and medical students in their wake. These outbreaks served a purpose, however: they brought reforms that eventually separated the "indigent sick" from the lunatics, paupers, orphans, and criminals who had once lived alongside them in a massive, multipurpose almshouse establishment. The former group stayed at Bellevue; the rest were shipped to newly constructed facilities on Blackwell's Island (now Roosevelt Island), a narrow spit of land in the East River. Though Bellevue would remain a bastion of the "low Irish" for generations, it had become a more manageable institution—a public hospital serving the acute health needs of New York's poor and working classes.

In medical circles, its reputation soared. It won plaudits during the Civil War for treating thousands of wounded Union soldiers and—more controversially—the anti-draft rioters who plundered large parts of New York City in the summer of 1863. It became the first American hospital to have a maternity ward, an emergency pavilion, and a medical school on-site; the first to organize an ambulance corps, a medical photography department, and a nursing school for women. (Its ill-fated men's nursing school, another first, would collapse amidst carefully buried charges of homosexuality.) In 1865, Bellevue doctors took the lead in writing the most important public health document of that era, *Sanitary Conditions of the City,* portraying New York as two distinct places—one prosperous, healthy, and native-born; the other desperate, diseased, and foreign-born. The response was dramatic. Within a year, New York City had its first official Board of Health in place.

Amazingly, Bellevue played a central role in the three great medical crises of the latter nineteenth century involving the American presidency. In 1865, twenty-three-year-old Charles Augustus Leale, a few months removed from Bellevue Hospital Medical College, was the first doctor to reach the gravely wounded Abraham Lincoln at Ford's Theatre. His central, if accidental, role in assisting Lincoln is still a matter of dispute. In 1881, Leale's Bellevue mentor, Dr. Frank Hamilton, was summoned to Washington to help save President James A. Garfield following the assassination attempt that eventually took Garfield's life. Some blamed Hamilton for the monumental blunders that marked

the president's treatment, with serious consequences for the practice of surgery. Then, in 1893, a team of five medical men, three from Bellevue, successfully removed a malignant growth from the mouth of President Grover Cleveland in a top secret operation performed on a luxury yacht off the coast of Long Island. Cleveland would go on to complete his term in the White House, the details carefully hidden from the public until after his death two decades later.

The years between Garfield's stunning demise and Cleveland's smooth recovery marked a changing of the medical guard. A new generation of clinicians and researchers came of age, wedded to the ways of modern science and contemptuous of the fading certainties of the past. Two of the most influential figures—William Welch, the father of modern pathology in America, and William Halsted, the era's most innovative surgeon—bonded as interns at Bellevue in the bitter struggle to bring antiseptic methods to the profession. Over time, Bellevue became a world leader in specialties ranging from forensics to psychiatry to infectious disease. Its faculty and graduates read like a "Who's Who" of modern American medicine: Hermann Biggs, a pioneer in the prevention of tuberculosis; Walter Reed and William Gorgas, who tamed the ravages of yellow fever; William Hallock Park, who brought the lifesaving diphtheria antitoxin to the United States; Joseph Goldberger, who discovered the cause of pellagra, a deadly nutritional disease; Thomas Francis, whose influenza research revolutionized the study of virus strains; André Cournand and Dickinson Richards, who perfected cardiac catheterization; Albert Sabin and Jonas Salk, who developed the two successful polio vaccines still in use today.

By the early 1900s, Bellevue seemed less a city hospital than a hospital city, with two thousand beds, a nursing school, the city morgue, a massive psychiatric pavilion, a special prison ward, top-flight laboratories, a maintenance force of four thousand, and a medical staff provided by the three best medical colleges in New York. A major facelift designed by the iconic architectural firm of McKim, Mead & White would remake the complex with mixed results, while the mass immigration of Italians and Jews to America dramatically reordered the patient profile. Bellevue remained what it had always been—a medical haven for the poor—though its admission rolls now showed many more Rossis and Goldbergs, and many fewer Rileys and O'Rourkes. Meanwhile, hospital officials took the revolutionary step of accepting numerous women and Jewish interns—partly to meet the growing patient load and partly because NYU Medical School, Bellevue's primary feeder, ignored the infamous "Jewish Quota" employed at Harvard, Yale, Columbia, Cornell, and most other medical colleges in the region.

Until this point, the American hospital had been the province of the lower classes. Those with the means to avoid one happily stayed away. There was nothing a hospital could do for the upper and middle classes that couldn't be done better at home. But advances in technology, sanitation, and nursing were changing that perception. At Bellevue, for example, the chance of dying from a postoperative infection following surgery in 1865 was almost one in two; by 1900, that figure had dropped below 10 percent. As hospitals became better at saving lives, a serious competition emerged for "paying patients"—those wanting the benefits of modern medicine without sacrificing personal comfort. Bellevue was not a serious option for these people unless a city ambulance plucked them unconscious from the gutter. But as "voluntary" hospitals began to convert some of their charity wards into private and semiprivate rooms, crowding in public hospitals became ever more intense.

The results were predictable. During the Great Influenza of 1918–19, Bellevue quickly ran out of beds, forcing the patient overflow to sleep on doors ripped from their hinges and piles of damp, fetid straw. Similar scenes appeared throughout the Great Depression, when a third of the city's workforce was unemployed. With far fewer New Yorkers able to afford a stay at a voluntary hospital, Bellevue bulged at the seams. Many of these patients were members of the "better classes" who had never set foot in a public hospital before.

And rarely would again. The return of prosperity following World War II revived the struggling voluntary hospitals, as group insurance plans like Blue Cross, often written into employment contracts, afforded the working classes access to amenities that a place like Bellevue couldn't possibly match, despite the excellence of its medical staff. Why put up with the indignities of peeling paint, miserable food, crowded wards, and perhaps a stabbing victim in the next bed when a semiprivate room in a well-appointed private facility could be had? The coming of Medicare and Medicaid in the 1960s—programs that funneled billions of tax dollars into the health care sector—further diminished public hospitals by giving poor and elderly patients greater freedom of choice.

In the 1960s, both Cornell and Columbia departed Bellevue, leaving NYU physicians to provide the medical care. The quality remained high; NYU had long been closest to the hospital because so many of its faculty and house staff were native New Yorkers from the working and middle classes who viscerally grasped Bellevue's importance to the city. In 1973, an enormous addition was opened—a partly finished twenty-five-story patient tower, two decades in the making—just as national economic stagnation took hold. The impact on New York City was dramatic. Vital public services, including free hospital care, were now in jeopardy. Crime and drug addiction flourished against a backdrop of white flight, a declining tax base, and the threat of municipal bankruptcy. For Bellevue this meant staff shortages and budget cuts in the midst of jam-packed emergency rooms and soaring psychiatric admissions. One crisis flowed into the next, the bottom reached in 1989 when a homeless psychopath raped and murdered a pregnant physician in her Bellevue office. The killer had not only been wearing stolen doctor's scrubs, complete with an identification badge and a stethoscope, he'd been brazenly squatting for weeks in a machinery room in the hospital, entirely overlooked.

Amidst the growing calls to close down or privatize the entire public system, a familiar truth reemerged: New York *needed* these hospitals, especially its flagship. When AIDS descended in the 1980s, Bellevue again became ground zero for an epidemic targeting those on the margins of public concern—in this case gay men and intravenous drug users. Many more AIDS patients would be treated (and die) there than at any other hospital in the United States. The story of AIDS at Bellevue is a complicated one, as we shall see, but nothing better defined the hospital's mission—its indispensable service to society's most vulnerable members—than its response to this seemingly endless medical nightmare.

Bellevue today remains a buttress against unforeseen crises that periodically arise—the successful treatment of New York's lone Ebola victim in 2014 being the latest example. And its resilience was displayed again in the heroic patient evacuation during Superstorm Sandy, which closed the hospital for the only time in its storied history. Bellevue reopened a few months later, its mission unchanged. The old ethnic groups have moved on—Irish, Jews, and Italians replaced by Hispanics, Haitians, Africans, South Asians, and Chinese. The patients it currently serves are every bit as poor and needy as the patients who preceded them in centuries past. And those with viable options almost always wind up going somewhere else. That's what makes Bellevue so comforting and so disquieting. It stands, for all its troubles, as a vital safety net, a place of caring and a place of last resort.

1

BEGINNINGS

At the southern tip of Fifth Avenue, in the heart of Greenwich Village, sits the leafy oasis known as Washington Square. A cherished landmark for New Yorkers, its iconic arch, imposing fountain, and flowered walkways provide no hint of its tumultuous past. At various times Washington Square has served as a military parade ground, a gallows, a haven for ex-slaves, and a magnet for artists, hustlers, street performers, and protesters of every stripe. After the American Revolution, it became a mass grave for the victims of epidemic disease.

All large cities have a "Potter's Field"—a cemetery for unclaimed corpses. The term comes from the New Testament: "And they took counsel and bought . . . the Potter's Field, to bury strangers in." New York established its Potter's Field in 1795 in response to a devastating yellow fever outbreak. Covering 9.5 acres, it created a furor because it abutted the country homes of New York's financial elite. "The field lies in the neighborhood of a number of Citizens who have at great expense erected dwellings . . . for the health and accommodation of their families during the summer season," read a letter of protest signed by Alexander Hamilton, among others. But Mayor Richard Varick stood firm, ruling that a medical catastrophe trumped the interests of a few dozen landowners, who included some of his closest friends.

It's estimated that twenty thousand people were buried in Washington Square between 1795 and 1826, when the Potter's Field was moved farther north to Fifth Avenue and 42nd Street, where Bryant Park stands today, and then to Hart Island, in the outer reaches of the Bronx. Most of the victims were recent immigrants who lived in squalid boardinghouses near the downtown wharves. Each summer and fall—yellow fever season—their bodies would be dumped into wagons and carted uptown. "The wheels of these chariots of death rolled heavily," a witness recalled, "the springs and timbers screeching and groaning as if chanting the requiem of friends departed."

Over the years, workers digging in Washington Square have routinely come upon human remains. But in 2009, a construction crew encountered something odd: a three-foot grave marker with the inscription still intact. "Here lies the body of James Jackson," it read, "who [left] this life the 22nd day of September 1799, aged 28 years, native of the county of Kildare, Ireland." The discovery raised a pointed question: Why would someone with the means for a headstone wind up in Potter's Field?

City records told the story. James Jackson had achieved some modest success in New York City as a grocer, leaving behind a wife, several children, and a personal estate valued at $262. He had also applied "to be a citizen of the United States." In normal times, a man of Jackson's standing would have been interred in a church cemetery. But New York was a city under siege in the 1790s, overwhelmed by yellow fever. In a desperate attempt to contain the disease, the dead bodies, believed by many to be contagious, were buried together in a single place. As a contemporary newspaper explained: "It is important to remark that no persons dead of fever are admitted to any other cemetery, which has not been the case heretofore." And that is how the body of James Jackson, the Irish grocer, came to rest in Washington Square.

But Jackson was fortunate in one respect: he almost certainly died at home. Dozens of others were brought to a place specially created for yellow fever victims who had nowhere else to go. Little more than a pesthouse—a way station, truth be told, on the path to eternity—it would earn a grisly reputation as New York City's dumping ground for the terminally ill and unwanted, taking its name from the deceivingly placid acreage on which it stood: "Bel-Vue."

—

A number of cities claim the honor of establishing the first hospital in North America. The problem is one of definition. Many of the almshouses in colonial America contained a small infirmary to care for the destitute. In 1752, however, Pennsylvania Hospital in Philadelphia opened its doors to medical patients alone. Founded by Dr. Thomas Bond, with a charter from the Pennsylvania legislature and the financial support of Benjamin Franklin, it was intended for "the reception and cure of the sick poor," not for those seeking food or shelter or a place to die. In this sense, Pennsylvania Hospital holds a very strong hand.

Some, however, consider Bellevue to be first. Citing records from the West India Company, when the Dutch ruled Manhattan Island, they trace Bellevue's existence to a small infirmary built in the 1660s for soldiers overcome by "bad smells and filth." Under British control, a permanent almshouse was constructed in 1736—a two-story wood-and-brick structure costing £80 for building materials and fifty gallons of rum for those who "laid the beams and raised the roof." It contained a workspace for the able-bodied, a room for the sick and the insane, and a prison in the cellar for the "unruly and obstinate," complete with a whipping post. Those found "to be Lousey or to have the Itch" were segregated "til perfectly Clean." This one-room infirmary, we are told, is "the seed from which grew the mighty oak of Bellevue."

Built on the site of today's City Hall Park, the almshouse became a vital public institution. Serving just nineteen paupers in 1736, it housed close to eight hundred of them by 1795, as New York's population soared. To stem the tide, city officials took to rounding up vagrants and prostitutes and paying their transportation out of town—but it barely made a dent. The almshouse commissioners demanded ever-larger budgets, blaming their costs on "the prodigious influx of indigent foreigners," mainly from Ireland. In the 1790s the city opened a larger almshouse financed by a municipal lottery, a common money-raising device. But its infirmary was soon overwhelmed by yellow fever, which brought dozens of sick and dying victims to its door. As panic spread, the Common Council leased a vacant property along the East River, far from the city center, to house the "wretched overflow."

The land they chose had a checkered past. Once prized for its lush gardens and freshwater breezes, it had first belonged to a prominent Dutch settler named Jacobus Kip, who built a house there in 1641—the Kip's Bay Estate—using bricks imported from Holland. In the 1700s, Kip's heirs had divided the land, selling one parcel to a local merchant who named it Bel-Vue for its rolling fields and river vistas. A grander home was soon constructed—one so impressive that it played host to both the fleeing General George Washington and his British pursuer, General William Howe, during the darkest moments of the Revolutionary War. Shortly thereafter, it passed into the hands of Lindley Murray, an eccentric scholar whose popular books about the English language had made him a spectacularly rich man. Murray wrote lovingly of a mansion "delightfully situated" on lush farmland overlooking "a grand expanse of water." In truth, he barely set foot there before sailing off to London—the proper place, he believed, for "the father of English grammar."

An advertisement soon appeared:

For SALE or to be LET. That beautiful COUNTRY SEAT called Bel-Vue, situated on the banks of the East River, about 3 miles from the city, and as its properties in point of health and other advantages are well known, it is unnecessary to describe them.

The price being steep, it didn't sell quickly. Five years passed before Henry Brockholst Livingston, a prominent New York attorney and future U.S. Supreme Court justice, paid £2,000 for the six-acre estate.

Livingston, it turned out, had no intention of living there, either. The property—referred to interchangeably as "Bel-Vue," "Belle-Vue," and, finally, "Bellevue"—passed from one renter to the next before the Common Council leased it in 1795 "to serve as a hospital for the accommodation and relief of such persons afflicted with contagious distempers"—or yellow fever. Described by nervous officials as "a proper distance from the inhabited part of this city," it was accessible by road and river, with a dock already in place. The plans called for hiring a steward, a matron, a resident physician, and "as many nurses as may be wanted." There would be "two men to transport the sick to Bellevue" in wagons and "a Boat with good oars-men" to ship in needed supplies. Port, brandy, and "assorted spirits" headed that list, with detailed instructions for the doctor. "Sherry wine, the most natural stimulus, should be given freely," he was told, and "beer, for those who are accustomed to its use, is a very valuable remedy."

New York City had seen its share of epidemic disease. From the Dutch settlement forward, infectious outbreaks were a common part of daily life. The first Europeans had praised New Amsterdam's "sweet and wholesome climate"—more forgiving than the brutal cold to the north in Boston, less treacherous than the fetid swampland to the south in Jamestown. But Manhattan's bustling harbor soon became a magnet for the world's microbes and maladies. Periodic eruptions of measles, influenza, scarlet fever, and "throat distemper" (diphtheria) killed untold numbers in the colonial era, especially children. Barely a decade went by in the 1700s without a serious outbreak of smallpox. New York recorded more than five hundred deaths from this disease in 1731, a staggering total in a city of barely ten thousand people. While the threat of smallpox would recede by the early 1800s—due mainly to the introduction of Edward Jenner's revolutionary vaccine—other diseases proved more difficult to contain. The most frightening one, by far, was yellow fever.

It seemed odd that a disease associated with the tropics would find a home this far north. Yellow fever—commonly known as "Yellow Jack" for the warning flags flown on infected ships—is transmitted by the bite of the female *Aedes aegypti* mosquito. In mild cases, the symptoms include a headache and moderate fever, similar to the flu. But the more severe ones can produce delirium, jaundice (lending skin a yellow tinge), and massive bleeding from the mouth, nose, and ears. Most early accounts of yellow fever refer to the victim's horrifying "black vomit," the discharge of blood-soaked material from the stomach. Case mortality in a serious epidemic can reach upward of 50 percent. The only good news is that the surviving victims are rewarded with immunity for life.

Yellow fever came to the Americas from Africa, carried by slave ships that docked in the West Indies. Water barrels on board provided an ideal breeding ground for the *Aedes aegypti*. Over time, as trade routes expanded, yellow fever reached North America's eastern ports. In the summer of 1793 it struck Philadelphia, the young nation's capital, with a fury that shook the national government to its core. By November, the streets were deserted and more than 10 percent of the city's fifty thousand residents were dead. Most of Congress was gone, along with President George Washington and Secretary of State Thomas Jefferson, who fled to their native Virginia. For Jefferson, a defender of rural values, the epidemic was a mixed blessing, with a powerful lesson attached. "The yellow fever will discourage the growth of great cities in our nation," he confidently wrote a friend, "& I view great cities as pestilential to the morals, the health and the liberties of man."

Jefferson was wrong, of course, though the enormous damage done to Philadelphia did dramatically slow its growth. Yellow fever reached New York City in the summer of 1795 on a brig from Haiti with a very sick crew. A port officer who boarded the infected vessel died a few days later, the first of many to come. While hardly matching the carnage of Philadelphia, the disease proved deadlier than anything the city had seen before.

What caused yellow fever was a matter of debate. Medical opinion in this era endorsed the so-called Miasma Theory, which blamed illnesses on chemical agents from decayed matter—corpses, rotting fruits and vegetables, swamp and sewer gases—that formed dangerous airborne clouds. Those who studied disease spent much of their time minutely analyzing atmospheric conditions: sunlight, humidity, temperature, rainfall, lightning, cloud cover, and wind direction. As late as 1888, Bellevue's specialist in childhood diseases insisted that diphtheria, a deadly bacterial infection, resulted mainly from inhaling the damp gases that rose from the sewers. (He also warned against the danger of kissing a cat.)

Yellow fever split the medical community into warring factions. One saw it as a contagious disease, much like smallpox or influenza, which could spread from person to person through the victim's breath or clothing—or corpse. How this occurred was still a mystery; one physician described the process as "effluvia arising directly from the body of a man under a particular disease, and exciting the same kinds of disease in the body of the person to whom they are applied." This camp viewed yellow fever as an *imported* illness, reaching New York harbor on West Indian ships. The solution, therefore, was to quarantine arriving vessels in order to isolate the carriers—an expensive process that severely restricted trade.

The competing group blamed local conditions for the disease, especially the "noxious smells and vapors" along the wharves. Person-to-person contact made little sense, these doctors argued, because they "continually touched the sick, lived in the midst of them, and breathed the same air" without personally contracting yellow fever. Their solution was to destroy the noxious miasma clouds by scrubbing the city clean; they saw no reason to quarantine its vital harbor.

On one point, however, both sides seemed to agree: *poor* New Yorkers were more susceptible to the disease. Contagious or not, yellow fever appeared most often in the flophouse waterfront districts catering to sailors, dockworkers, and recent arrivals. Valentine Seaman, a leading New York physician, drew a map of these yellow fever cases—a forerunner of John Snow's legendary cholera "Ghost Map"—to show the epidemic's concentrated path. Noting the large number of sickened Irish immigrants, Seaman thought this more than coincidental. Hard drinking and filth had weakened their constitutions, he believed, while their heavy "vegetable diet" had left them vulnerable to the rigors of American life. As further proof, New York officials claimed that only "five or six" native-born merchants and a lone minister—a questionable sort—had died in the epidemic. He was, the Episcopalian Seaman lamented, a Methodist.

The fact that shipborne mosquitoes thrived along the waterfront was not then a matter of concern. The very idea that a tiny vector like the *Aedes aegypti* could cause such an immense catastrophe was simply beyond scientific understanding. Still, what is striking about the writings of New Yorkers in the summer of 1795 is the constant *notice* of mosquitoes: swarming, biting, relentless, and inescapable. Valentine Seaman remarked that he had never seen as many people "covered with blisters from their venomous operations." His good friend, Dr. Elihu Hubbard Smith, recorded these words in his diary: "Thursday,

September 6—Passed a restless and perturbed night tormented with mosquitoes and incongruous dreams."

In 1793, the New York Common Council had appointed a special health committee "to prevent the infectious Distemper now raging at Philadelphia from being introduced into this city." As a leading member of that committee, Dr. Elihu Hubbard Smith understood the futility of the charge. One might prepare for the arrival of yellow fever, but there was no way (beyond fleeing the city) to avoid its deadly path. An epidemic was inevitable, if not this year, then the next, or the one after that. A tireless advocate for the poor, Smith had lobbied hard for a pesthouse to isolate and treat the victims. With the committee's approval, he recruited a man he barely knew to become its resident physician. In truth, there hadn't been much competition for the post, which combined low pay and long hours with dreadful working conditions. The minutes of the Health Committee meeting for August 24, 1795, read, simply: "Dr. Smith reported that he had procured a Young Gentleman to attend Bel-Vue—Doctor Alexander Anderson."

The epidemic was then at its peak. Scores were dead, and the harbor was quarantined. New York Hospital had recently opened its doors in lower Manhattan, but its board of directors, wary of catering to the city's unwashed masses, had refused most yellow fever cases. "In consequence of [this] rejection," a local editor fumed, "it has happened that men, like calves and other live stock, have been put upon carts [and taken to Bel-Vue] over the stony roughness of the pavement, and under the scorching noon-time sun!—a procedure which flared up indignation, as well as alarm, in the citizens who saw it."

Alexander Anderson arrived at Bel-Vue "in a state of confusion and perplexity"—his words lifted from a remarkable diary he kept during his brief medical career. The son of a printer, raised in quarters above his father's Wall Street shop, Anderson showed an early talent for engraving. But his deeply religious parents saw only one path for their son—a life devoted to God through medicine. The surest way to achieve this in eighteenth-century America was to do exactly what an aspiring blacksmith or carpenter might do: find a mentor willing to teach him the craft.

In New York City, a medical apprenticeship lasted four to six years. Anderson's parents sent fourteen-year-old Alexander to live with Dr. William Smith, a family friend. Much of the day was pure drudgery: feeding the horses, sweeping the office, and collecting overdue bills—the chore Anderson hated most. But the good hours were a clinical bonanza. The boy accompanied Dr. Smith on house calls, mixed his drugs and potions, and assisted with bleeding and tooth pulling while "reading all the medical books within reach."

At twenty, Anderson applied for a doctor's license, which required "an examination for the practice of physic." A committee of three physicians grilled him for an hour at a downtown tavern, where successful applicants were treated to a liquid celebration more taxing than the examination itself. Anderson received a "favorable report" from the committee and a suggestion that he mature a bit before hanging out his shingle.

Anderson chose Bel-Vue instead. The job of resident physician appealed to him because it was temporary, ending when the epidemic had run its course. Unsure of his future, yet determined to do the Lord's work, Anderson saw Bellevue as the ideal place to begin. "My present employment is much against the grain," he noted. "A sense of duty and acquiescence in the will of God are the chief motives which detain me here."

Anderson arrived at Bel-Vue to find six yellow fever patients and a patchwork staff. "[They] consist of Mr. Fisher, the steward and his wife, Old Daddy, the Gardner—an old negro, a black nurse and two white ones," he wrote that first evening. "I spent the afternoon in putting up medicines and arranging matters."

Things quickly got worse. Anderson's diary bears witness to the epidemic's grisly toll. "We lost three patients today," reads a typical entry. "I am sometimes tempted to resign my station, but, really, I am afraid that like Jonah, I shall meet a worse fate." And, "Another patient sent up in shocking condition. . . . Vomiting blood by mouthfuls; he died within two hour's time." More striking, though, was Anderson's tender, almost saintly demeanor in the face of overwhelming hardship and grief. At one point, he fired a nurse for dereliction of duty: "She is addicted to liquor, and our patients suffer neglect from her behavior, which is very rough and ill-suited to soothe the mind of a sick person."

At another, he berated the hearse drivers who "glory in a disregard to Feelings and Delicacy" when carting away the dead. Anderson held everyone accountable, including a cowardly peer. "Dr. Chickering's timidity surpris'd me," he wrote. "I could not prevail upon him to attend to two children labouring under the yellow fever."

The 1795 epidemic ended with the first autumn frosts. "Nearly 750 of [our] inhabitants fell to it," the Common Council reported. "There were admitted into the Hospital at Bel-Vue 238 patients. And 436 persons were buried at the Public Expense."

The experience left Anderson exhausted, but thankful to be alive. "I passed three months among yellow fever patients and witnessed above a hundred deaths," he wrote. "Although I was employed night and day and even assisted in opening four dead bodies, I escaped the infection, but suffered from depression of spirits."

His work at Bellevue complete, Anderson faced an uncertain future. Torn between his own desires ("I cannot help looking back to my engraving table and thinking it is a fitter station for me") and those of his mother ("If you give up medicine," she warned him, "you will have spent your six-year apprenticeship in vain"), he enrolled at Columbia's prestigious College of Physicians and Surgeons to get an academic degree. Anderson married, became a father, and opened a medical office in his home. His depression also returned. "I soon discovered that the practice was a different thing from the study of physic," he confessed. "The responsibility appeared too great for the state of my mind."

Forsaking medicine, Anderson opened a shop that sold children's books he personally engraved. But the business failed, leading to a nervous breakdown fueled by opium and wine. "I am really desperate for want of money," he wrote, "and every endeavor to pursue it seems in vain." In 1798, Anderson reluctantly returned to Bel-Vue as the resident physician. Yellow fever was back in New York City, even deadlier than before.

The world of the American physician in the late eighteenth century was primitive, to say the least. Edinburgh and London, along with Paris and Leyden, were then the major Western centers of medical training. To study there was an honor reserved for a handful of Americans, mostly young men from families of wealth and status who returned home to open lucrative practices in seaboard cities like Boston, Philadelphia, and New York.

British medicine in these years was divided into three categories: physicians, surgeons, and apothecaries. Physicians formed the elite. Centered in London, they defined their status through membership in the Royal College of Physicians, which required a degree from Oxford or Cambridge. The rules were strict, the numbers very small. A true physician used his head, not his hands. He observed the patient, judged the illness, and suggested a remedy. The Royal College frowned upon performing surgery or mixing drugs; such mundane tasks were left to lesser men. The physician advised the top ranks of British society on medical issues, and charged a hefty fee. Assuming the role of gentleman, he dressed the part, wearing academic robes and carrying a gold-tipped cane.

The surgeon played a distinctly inferior role. His was a craft, not a profession, often learned on a naval vessel or a battlefield. He went by different names—bone-setter and barber-surgeon were common—and performed the manual tasks expected of a general practitioner. In the era before anesthesia and antiseptic medicine, there was not much to recommend him—and a great deal to fear. A surgeon might successfully extract tonsils, pull a tooth, lance a boil, or close a wound; he knew the rudiments of bleeding with a lancet and evacuating the bowels. But only a desperate patient would contemplate something more. When it came to amputating a limb or retrieving a musket ball, the procedure was as likely to kill the victim as save him.

The apothecary formed the bottom rung of the hierarchy. He was the tradesman, and the most numerous by far. Under British law, an apothecary could sell the medicines he concocted, but couldn't charge for the advice he might render. Over time, the lines of separation among these groups inevitably blurred. Surgeons began to mix their own drugs, while apothecaries took on patients of their own. And below them was a growing mass of quacks and healers serving those too poor or isolated to look anywhere else.

American society, by contrast, was more provincial and democratic. It barely recognized medicine as a profession in this era, much less one with different levels of status and expertise. Most physicians had begun their careers as apprentices. But few of them had attended medical classes, and fewer still held a degree. Indeed, the United States could boast but four medical colleges in 1800—Columbia, Dartmouth, Harvard, and the University of Pennsylvania. Of the approximately five hundred men described as "medical practitioners" in eighteenth-century New York City and Long Island, twenty-five held medical degrees from Columbia, eleven from Edinburgh, and ten from other European colleges. The remaining 90 percent came to medicine in a multitude of ways: "apprenticed to Dr. Charlton," "studied with Dr. Cadwalader," "tutored by Dr. Wilson," "Barber, Seven Years War," "Examiner of Ships for Contagious Diseases," "Surgeon's Mate on Privateer," among them. In terms of intellect and training, Alexander Anderson stood head and shoulders above all but a fraction of his medical peers.

With most doctors located in the larger towns and cities, the average American went through life without ever seeing one. What passed for medical care in these years was performed mainly within the family. Women were expected to deliver babies, provide the nursing, and grow the "botanical remedies" of the day. When a serious illness struck, the typical family leaned on "networks of kin and community," wrote one historian, with deference afforded to older women "who had a reputation for skill with the sick."

To most Americans, the idea of *paying* for medical services seemed preposterous. The essentials, when unavailable within families, could easily be plucked from almanacs and medical tracts like John Wesley's *Primitive Physic,* which went through dozens of editions. Wesley urged his readers to use their common sense. "Physicians should be consulted when needed," the saying went, "but they should be needed very rarely."

In the 1760s, New York became the first colony to move against the "many ignorant and unskillful persons in physic and surgery" by requiring a formal examination of the candidate, not unlike the one that Alexander Anderson would pass in 1795. But popular fears of "elitism" following the American Revolution led most states to loosen the rules regarding would-be physicians. Even New York abandoned its examination in 1797; all it now required was proof of a successful apprenticeship with a "respectable preceptor," a term liberally applied.

In truth, doctoring was mostly a part-time occupation in this era, shared with farming, tavern owning, and the ministry. Those in medical practice routinely described themselves as "Barber and Wigmaker," "Pastor-Physician," and "Practitioner of Surgery and Physick at the Women's Shoe Store on Beaver Street." Legally, one needed a license to practice medicine in New York, but there was little fear of practicing without one. The end result of this egalitarianism was to draw even more quacks into the fold. "The law makes no account of the disastrous consequences of [such] ignorance," a leading New York doctor complained. "It punishes the larceny while it acquits the homicide."

The more educated American physicians had some knowledge of Western medical tradition, from the ancient teachings of Galen and Hippocrates to the modern writings of William Harvey on the circulation of blood. In 1800, that tradition endorsed the so-called doctrine of humors, the idea that sickness arose from an imbalance among the body's four primary fluids: blood, phlegm, yellow bile, and black bile. The number was crucial to the belief: it matched the four universal elements (earth, air, fire, and water); the four cosmos (earth, sky, sun, and sea); and the four seasons of the year. Good humors meant good health; bad humors brought on disease.

What caused the latter wasn't clear. Medical opinion mostly blamed poisons in the atmosphere for penetrating the body and contaminating its fluids. Sweating, vomiting, diarrhea—these were the common signs of illness, as the system fought to rid itself of dangerous invaders. A problem with yellow bile made one melancholic; too much phlegm made one phlegmatic. The physician's job was to restore the system's delicate equilibrium.

Blood was the primary fluid, the one to be most carefully controlled. Physicians had long been impressed by the body's ability to shed large quantities of blood with seemingly positive results. Hippocrates, for example, saw menstruation as a means "to purge women of bad humors." It followed, therefore, that the quantity of blood in the body was an essential measure. Too much of it was a bad thing, causing fevers, inflammation, and pain. "Bloodletting," wrote a student of the art, "was the single most continuously employed medical technique in human history. . . . Blood was taken from virtually every part of the body; hands, tongue, legs, and anus could be tapped."

Much of this work in America was done by barber-surgeons, whose red-and-white-striped poles became the telltale ornament of their craft—red for the blood, white for the tourniquet and bandages. Blood was drawn with a lancet, with leeches, or with a heated glass cup attached to the skin. Since there was no accurate way to measure body temperature or blood pressure at this time, the volume to be removed varied widely from one case to the next. It was quite common for the patient to lose consciousness during the ordeal; indeed, fainting was viewed as a positive sign, restoring calm to an overtaxed system.

A careful physician in 1800 would study a patient's humors much like a modern auto mechanic checks the fluids under the hood. Was the person flushed or constipated or coughing up phlegm? Was the urine clear or colored, thin or frothy? The doctor then set to work, armed with an array of concoctions to purge and cleanse the system. His medicine cabinet likely included laudanum, an addictive, opium-based painkiller used to relax overactive nerves; digitalis, a plant extract for the treatment of heart failure; and cinchona, or Peruvian bark, which worked miracles on some fever diseases, particularly malaria, because of the quinine it contained.

But the most popular weapon, by far, was calomel, or mercury chloride, a devastatingly effective cathartic. Hailed for inducing "volcanic vomiting and explosive evacuation of the bowels," this mineral compound became "a reflex for physicians" of the colonial era, despite causing hair loss, rotting teeth, and streams of foul-smelling drool. Doctors were expected to aggressively confront disease; those who wavered might be cast aside. "[We] must cure *quickly*," a physician complained, "*or give place to a rival*." Calomel became indispensable, its side effects a sure sign of its potency. If the patient recovered—and most do, whatever the treatment—the doctor got the credit.

Take, for example, an average calendar day of a New York City physician in the late eighteenth century:

Patient One: Bleeding, Bleeding Twice.

Patient Two: A Visit and a Calomel bolus.

Patient Three: Sewing Up Ye Boy's Lip [and] sundry dressings in the cure of it.

Patient Four: Rising in the night, a visit and dose of calomel ye child.

Patient Five: Mercurous wash, Calomel.

Patient Six: Purge for Child, Bleeding and Puke.

Patient Seven: Drawing a tooth.

Patient Eight: Draining a tooth.

The final treatment of George Washington in 1799 provides a more extreme example—the facts provided by his personal physicians. Suffering from a severe throat infection, the former president, then sixty-seven, "procured a bleeder in the neighbourhood, who took from his arm, in the night, twelve or fourteen ounces of blood." Feeling no better, Washington sent for his doctors. The first to arrive placed leeches in his throat, prescribed an enema, and then "two copious bleedings." Seeing no improvement, a second doctor ordered "ten grains of calomel . . . succeeded by repeated doses of emetic tartar," causing a massive discharge "from the bowels." Then the real bleeding began. Thirty-two ounces were drawn by lancet, while blisters were applied "to the extremities." (A person giving eight ounces of blood today must wait two months before donating again.) Washington finally told the doctors to stop. "Let me go quietly," he pleaded, and he did.

By the time Alexander Anderson returned to Bel-Vue in the summer of 1798, New York was in the midst of an unprecedented calamity. The body count from yellow fever already reached into the thousands. Witnesses described a city abandoned to coffin makers, gravediggers, and those too poor or too sick to flee. A number of dutiful physicians and medical students had stayed behind to help, including Anderson's Columbia classmate Walter Jonas Judah, the first native-born Jew to attend an American medical school. Judah had vowed to protect the members of Shearith Israel, New York's only Jewish congregation, though his duties quickly grew. He worked "tirelessly with the afflicted," it was said, prescribing treatments and paying for the medicines from "his own pocket." Judah died that September, at the age of twenty. He was buried in Chatham Square, New York's oldest Jewish cemetery. His tombstone, still visible today, reads:

In memory of
Walter J. Judah
student of physic who, worn down
by his exertions to alleviate the
sufferings of his fellow citizens
in that dreadful contagion
that visited the City of New York
in 1798, fell victim to the cause
of humanity . . .

Bel-Vue, meanwhile, was overwhelmed. A crude addition was erected to handle the fevered bodies deposited daily by horse cart and river barge. As the resident physician, Anderson employed the standard practices of the time. His guide was Dr. Benjamin Rush, the revered statesman-physician who had signed the Declaration of Independence and served as Washington's surgeon general in the Revolutionary War. For treating yellow fever, Rush employed copious bleeding and huge doses of calomel, which he termed "the Samson of drugs."

Anderson embraced Rush's "heroic" approach. His diary is filled with entries like: "Two young seamen arriv'd in a cart. The violence of their fever demanded blood-letting, which I performed immediately." But Anderson's tenure at Bellevue proved briefer than before. Vowing to "hold out while the Epidemic continues," he nonetheless resigned a few weeks later, victimized by yellow fever in an unimaginable way.

In July, his three-month-old son had contracted the disease. "I was up all night trying every method for [his] relief, but he died at 2 this morning," the diary read. "At day-break I took a walk [to find] a cabinet-maker. I knock'd him up, and bespoke a coffin." In early September, yellow fever claimed Anderson's brother, and then his father, leading him to depart Bel-Vue to watch over his surviving family members.

It did them no good. A few days later, Anderson's wife took sick and died. "The sight of [her], ghastly and emaciated, coughing up blood, struck me with horror," he wrote. "Those who knew her worth may imagine my feelings." In October Anderson's mother fell to yellow fever, completing the virtual destruction of his family. "I feel surpris'd at my own composure," he noted, "and am more disposed to impute it to despair than resignation."

On New Year's Eve 1798, Anderson reviewed the horror and tragedy of the previous months. "I have made more use of liquor than in all my life together," he admitted. But his religious faith had seen him through. "A tremendous scene have I witnessed," read his final entry. "Yet I have reason to thank the Great Author of my existence, and am still convinced that whatever is, is right." For twenty-two-year-old Alexander Anderson, being right meant taking responsibility for society's most fragile members. Forgotten today, he stands as Bellevue's first physician, serving a riverfront pesthouse in a murderous time.

Anderson soon abandoned the medical career his parents had forced upon him. He married again, fathered six more children, and returned to engraving, the work he loved, earning the distinguished title of "America's First Illustrator." But his brief autobiography, composed in 1848, is marked less by contentment than by gloom. "Constant employment has caused time to slip away," he wrote, "till I find myself in my seventy-third year. I have raised and supported a large family under rather discouraging circumstances, and what comes next is in the book of fate." Anderson died in his bed in 1870, at the age of ninety-five.

As yellow fever marked the life of this extraordinary physician-engraver, so, too, would it mark the place where he began and ended his medical career. In 1798, the Common Council bought the Bel-Vue Estate from Brockholst Livingston for £1,800, to be "opened only upon extraordinary occasions [for] those suffering the violent assaults of fever." It was used sparingly until 1811, when the cornerstone was laid for a new almshouse complex on the grounds. While few could deny the land's natural beauty, it had earned a frightful reputation as well. "Bel-Vue, a few miles from New York, on the East River [is now] considered by the people at large as *A House of Death*," wrote a popular pamphleteer. "So odious is the idea of being put there [as] to lessen one's chance of recovery."

Almshouse, pesthouse, death house—these are the indelible roots of Bellevue Hospital, thrust deep in the bedrock of America's fastest-growing city.

2

HOSACK'S VISION

New York City is no stranger to the mob. Its past is littered with explosions of public rage, from the Stamp Act Riots of 1765 to the Draft Riots of 1863 to the Hard Hat Riots of 1970, with endless turmoil in between. One of the most violent episodes occurred in 1788, when a crowd stormed the city jail bent on lynching several men held there in protective custody. These weren't traitors or murderers or disobedient slaves. They were, oddly enough, physicians and medical students accused of digging up corpses in the dark. The so-called Doctors' Riot ended with a full-scale military assault, leaving dozens wounded and several dead. Largely forgotten today, it would taint public perceptions of "medical men" and their practices for decades to come.

In 1750, two of these men, John Bard and Peter Middleton, performed the first dissection of a human cadaver in North America. The body, carefully chosen to avoid a public backlash, was that of a criminal hanged for a gruesome murder. But having established dissection as a teaching tool, Bard and Middleton had created a dilemma: Where would anatomists obtain a fresh supply of corpses? In New York City, as elsewhere, the local cemetery provided the answer.

Body snatching soon became a rite of passage for young doctors and medical students. Working on moonless nights, dressed entirely in black, they pilfered fresh remains from the city's most vulnerable graveyards—the one attached to the almshouse, for example, and those in which slaves and free Negroes were interred. Their raids aroused little interest until word got out that the corpse of a young white woman had been removed from the graveyard of Trinity Church, a hallowed resting ground. Other such "discoveries" followed, "raising a considerable clamor among the people," reported the *New York Packet*. "The interments not only of strangers and the blacks [have] been disturbed, but the corpses of some respectable persons [as well]." When letters of protest appeared, one of the grave robbers posted a mocking reply. "Through your excess of sympathy for the impassive bones of the dead, you have forgot the poor sufferings to which the living world is daily liable," he wrote, adding: "I take thee to be the most stupid of asses." It was signed, "A Student of Physic, Broadway, N.Y."

The address was revealing. In 1771, the city had received a royal charter to build a private hospital for "the reception of such patients as require medical treatment, surgical management, and maniacs." Located on Broadway, it had housed wounded British troops during the Revolutionary War and then been consumed by fire. It wouldn't reopen until 1791, under the name of New York Hospital, but a few rooms had been leased in the damaged structure for an anatomy class run by surgeons calling themselves the "Tribe of Dissectors."

The Doctors' Riot began on an April Sunday, when a group of children playing outside the Broadway building spotted a corpse dangling in a second-floor window. One of the boys ran to tell his father, a mason by trade, who was working nearby. Within minutes, a swarm of laborers had stormed the building, tools in hand. "In the anatomy room were found three fresh [corpses], one boiling in a kettle, two others cut up with certain parts of the two sexes hanging up in a most brutal position." The workers grabbed various body fragments—arms, legs, and heads—to show to the angry crowd gathered below. Then they dragged the terrified dissectors into the street.

A lynching seemed likely. "It is a wonder," a source remarked, that the young men "did not become anatomical specimens themselves." They were saved by the intervention of Mayor James Duane and the local sheriff, who bravely hustled the dissectors off to jail. As word spread, mobs ransacked their homes. A few days later, a crowd estimated at five thousand—the largest ever seen in the city—marched on the jail chanting, "Bring out your doctors! Bring out your doctors!" Blocking the way were the dons of New York society—Mayor Duane, Governor George Clinton, John Jay, Alexander Hamilton, and Baron Friedrich von Steuben—backed by a phalanx of state militia, bayonets fixed and gleaming.

Words proved useless. The crowd surged forward, hurling rocks and brickbats. John Jay and Baron von Steuben were badly bloodied before Governor Clinton gave the order to fire. Hit by several volleys at close range, the crowd fell back without reaching the jail. Estimates of those killed that afternoon ranged from three to well more than a dozen, because so many of the wounded were carried home to die.

The riot had erupted at a tense time in the city—the interval between the writing of the Federal Constitution and its successful ratification by the states. Some saw the lawlessness in New York as an example of what a strong government was meant to control; others thought the authorities had gone too far. What most everyone could agree on, however, was the arrogance of the grave robbers in pursuing their controversial goals. Such moral blindness, said a shaken physician, had "seriously interrupted the cordial feeling which has always existed between the medical community and the laity."

A few months later, the New York state legislature passed a law "to Prevent the Odious Practice of Digging Up and Removing for the Purposes of Dissection, Dead Bodies Interred in Cemeteries or Burial Places." The sentences ranged from a fine and imprisonment to "standing in the pillory [and] other corporal punishment (not extending to life or limb)." The law also provided that the bodies of executed criminals "shall be delivered to a surgeon for dissection, as such court shall direct." Though no doubt meant as an anti-crime measure—a warning to potential murderers and arsonists of punishment beyond death—it also affirmed the need for cadavers in medical research.

But this was hardly a solution. There simply weren't enough executed criminals to meet the demand for corpses, and the public was in no mood to supply any other kind. The dissection of unclaimed bodies wouldn't be legalized in New York state for another half century, a delay that only encouraged these dangerous nocturnal raids. The crime became so common that almost every prominent physician confessed to having taken part—none more boldly, or frequently, than David Hosack, the founder of "modern" Bellevue and the architect of public hospital care in New York City.

To elite members of New York society, brilliant, imperious David Hosack was the doctor of choice. His patients included Alexander Hamilton, DeWitt Clinton, steamboat inventor Robert Fulton, and Vice President Aaron Burr. In 1801, Hosack tended to Hamilton's oldest son, Philip, after a duel that took the young man's life, and then, three years later, to the elder Hamilton following his deadly duel with Burr on the very same New Jersey ground. His "sufferings during the whole of the day [were] almost intolerable. I had not the shadow of a hope for his recovery," wrote Hosack, who nevertheless charged Hamilton's estate $50 for services rendered during his good friend's "fatal illness." Hosack's annual income sometimes exceeded $10,000, an immense sum that included earnings from his medical practice and the tutoring fees he charged eager students who lined up at his door.

Hosack lived like royalty. He owned an elegant townhouse in lower Manhattan, which became a salon for literary greats like Washington Irving and William Cullen Bryant, and a country estate in the Hudson Valley, where he cultivated exotic plants and herbs. A founder of the New-York Historical Society, Hosack also created the nation's first botanical garden on the land where Rockefeller Center now stands. A granite slab there bears the inscription:

IN MEMORY OF DAVID HOSACK

1769–1835

BOTANIST, PHYSICIAN, MAN OF SCIENCE

AND CITIZEN OF THE WORLD . . .

Born and raised in New York City, Hosack entered Columbia College in 1786 to pursue a medical career. Determined to be a surgeon, he attached himself to the man whose anatomy class would ignite the infamous Doctors' Riot—Dr. Richard E. Bayley. Hosack wasn't present when the mob stormed the dissecting rooms that fateful Sunday, but learning of the trouble had rushed there to help. Caught in the crowd and "knocked down with a stone striking him in the head," he might have been killed had not a bystander carried him away. Hosack fled New York for the calm of Princeton, New Jersey, where he completed college before entering the University of Pennsylvania Medical School. Studying with the great Benjamin Rush, he wrote his dissertation on the mysterious plague known as "cholera," theorizing—incorrectly, it turned out—that "an acid" was "the most proximate cause of the disease."

The next stop was Europe. Hosack attended medical lectures and clinics in Edinburgh and London—a must for striving physicians—but came away unimpressed. Edinburgh had "passed its meridian," he thought, providing "polish" to a résumé but little more. Hosack had no interest in mimicking the cloistered world of the British physician. He hoped not only to examine patients, but to treat them as well. Returning to New York City in 1796, he became a professor of "materia medica" (in modern terms, pharmacology) at Columbia, while beginning a partnership with a prominent surgeon, Samuel Bard. In 1806, Hosack put his talents to work at a place quite familiar to the top medical men of his day. He became a visiting physician at the almshouse infirmary, the forerunner to Bellevue Hospital.

The job paid nothing. Men of Hosack's stature were expected to volunteer their services free of charge. Dr. Benjamin Rush had directed the almshouse infirmary in Philadelphia, while Dr. Joseph Warren, another Revolutionary War hero, had done so in Boston. Known for his well-heeled patients—"he is liberal, hospitable, and expensive," a friend wrote—Hosack had long tended to the poor. His good works included a birthing clinic for destitute women and a citywide campaign to vaccinate against smallpox. The almshouse infirmary seemed the logical next step.

There was more to this than simple charity, however. A visiting physician not only got to treat the sort of cases he would rarely see in private practice, he could also bring his student apprentices along with him, thereby increasing his fees. With its endless supply of compliant bodies, the almshouse remained the best place for experimenting with drugs and therapies and matters of the knife. Private patients were not inclined to be teaching exhibits for young men hoping to become doctors; almshouse patients were unlikely to resist.

Hosack urged his students to base their diagnoses on "long and habitual observation at the bedside of the sick," as opposed to blind loyalty to established norms. A botanist at heart, he favored mild remedies like chicken broth, lemonade, and medicinal baths over harsher methods like bleeding and purging. Once, following a rash of tetanus cases at the almshouse, he prescribed only "wine, spirits, and brandy"—affording the victims, if nothing else, a more peaceful demise.

Hosack rode to the almshouse twice each week in a polished mahogany carriage, complete with coachman and driver. And this led, quite innocently, to one of the more bizarre incidents of his career. In 1808, an almshouse resident named Lucy Williams accused Alexander Whistelo of fathering her child. "He carried me to a bad [place] and locked the door," Williams alleged. "I scuffled with him a long time, but . . . he [wore] me out." The story had an odd twist: Whistelo was Hosack's carriage driver.

Charges flew back and forth, with the almshouse commissioner demanding support for "this bastard child." Hosack responded by calling Lucy Williams a liar. The "proof," he claimed, was in the skin color. It would be impossible for Williams, a mulatto, and Whistelo, a full-blooded Negro, to produce an infant even "whiter" than the mother.

A public hearing was held, chaired by the mayor. With one exception, the parade of doctors called to testify supported Hosack's view of the case: the child's fair skin, the "want of crisp hair," and the absence of "primitive" features all defied "the general laws of nature." Whistelo could not have fathered the child.

The mayor, a good friend of Hosack's, posed a rhetorical question before reading the verdict. "Why would a woman choose to name a black father when she could name a white man?" He answered simply: "We do not know—some love the darkness rather than the light." Alexander Whistelo was exonerated. Lucy Williams and her child were returned to the almshouse, still wards of the city. David Hosack remained the visiting physician. The white father was never found.

—

New York was rapidly urbanizing in these years. The almshouse complex, a stone's throw from City Hall, held close to eight hundred dependents by 1800, more than twice the intended number. Visitors were shocked by the "haggard paupers and undisciplined children peering from [its] windows, hanging on the fences, and wandering in the park." The view from within was even worse. Among the witnesses was Ezra Stiles Ely, a young minister who kept a diary of his daily visits to comfort the sick and pray over the dead. Most entries included a description of the almshouse infirmary, where "the groans of agony" met "the stink of disease." Ely wrote of patients in rags, uncollected corpses, "bodies stowed as thick as they could lie." He claimed that "nine cases out of ten" were moral degenerates, and his diary is seeded with examples, from the foul breath of prostitutes to the blasphemy of drunks. "Not half an hour before he expired," Ely wrote of one, "he used his brief and dying [respite] to hurl wicked curses."

The destitute rarely leave a written record behind. It is the province of the literate to record how others lived and died, Ely being a prime example. In his diary, we meet "a half-starved blind man whose stomach has rejected almost everything"; "a young widow whose hands and feet having been frozen, are now in a state of progressive putrefaction"; "a woman of colour, dreadfully mangled by her husband"; a boy of fifteen "who slit his throat after being impressed on board a British ship of war"; "an aged sailor . . . of whom little remains but skin and bones"; and a demented ninety-six-year-old woman "who differs from an infant only in her form and the love of taking snuff." The list is long and depressing. "Their misery makes me sick at heart," Ely wrote, adding that many are "too near the grave to care."

Here, perhaps, lay the most obvious truth. Those who filled the almshouse infirmary were chronic patients—discarded and forgotten. Many had been there for months, some far longer. In a typical entry, Ely approached the bed of a young man in a coma. It had become a daily routine—a prayer uttered to no response. "He will open his eyes no more," the minister wrote, "until the resurrection."

—

A larger almshouse was sorely needed, far removed from respectable glances. And no spot seemed better suited than the old Bel-Vue Estate, the city-owned stretch of land along the East River that contained the municipal pesthouse where young Alexander Anderson had been the resident physician. In 1811, the Common Council negotiated a deal with the heirs of the Kip's Bay Estate to purchase "six [additional] acres, 1 road, 28 perches and eighty Seven Square feet of land adjacent to . . . Bellevue for the consideration of twenty two thousand four hundred and ninety four and 50/100 dollars." The goal was to fuse these two properties into one, providing a single complex for the diseased, desperate, criminal, and insane.

What followed was the largest and most expensive construction project in New York's history. To help raise money the city ran another lottery, the grand prize won, to the consternation of many ticket holders, by a free Negro. Meanwhile, the Common Council appropriated $45,792 to hire the "Stone Cutters, Carpenters, Blacksmiths, Masons and laborers" needed to lay the foundation and build a new dock. Throughout the spring of 1811, advertisements like this one appeared in the local press:

TO MASONS

Proposals Will Be Received at the Almshouse Until the First of May Next for Doing the Mason's Work of a Brick Workshop With Stone Cellar to be Two Hundred Feet in Length and Twenty-Five Feet in Width. Also, Proposals for the Workmanship of Two Brick, Hospitals With Stone Cellars, to be Each Seventy-Five Feet In Length and Twenty Five-Feet in Width. The Above Buildings are to be Built on the ground At Bellevue, a Plan, and a Particular Description of Them to be seen at the Almshouse.

Governor DeWitt Clinton laid the cornerstone in a boisterous celebration of civic pride. But then the War of 1812 intervened, and British warships blocked New York harbor. Stalled by various shortages, the complex took five years to complete. Opened in 1816, it housed the great bulk of New York City's welfare institutions: an orphanage, a morgue, a pesthouse, a prison, a lunatic asylum, and a huge four-story almshouse with an infirmary attached. Costing an incredible

$421,109, it sat behind an imposing stone wall and bore the name: Bellevue Establishment.

The structures were massive—the largest New York had ever seen. A sure sign of their importance was the decorative artifacts brought from Federal Hall, where George Washington had taken his first presidential oath of office in 1789: the embroidered wrought iron railings, the gold-plated weathervane, the very stone on which Washington had stood. "There is no eleemosynary establishment in the American Union equally splendid," marveled Yale's famously dour president Timothy Dwight.

At the dedication, a local minister urged the inmates to embrace their new surroundings. "Some of you, I am persuaded, indulge extreme anxiety on your removal so far from the city," he said of the isolated location. But fear not. Bellevue was a special place, designed "to wipe away your tears and supply all your necessities."

David Hosack had his doubts. He worried that New York City remained woefully unprepared for the medical crises that lay ahead. His words were cited in the newspapers, which added dire predictions of their own. Under intense pressure, city officials promised to build a much larger pesthouse on the Establishment grounds. Opened in 1826, the imposing brick structure stood on a bluff directly above the East River. There was talk of naming it "New York City Hospital," but complaints arose from the trustees of New York Hospital, who did not want their private facility confused with a lowly welfare institution. The Common Council agreed: "The Building lately erected . . . shall hereafter be . . . known by the name of Bellevue Hospital."

Still, Hosack wanted more. He dreamed not of a larger pesthouse, or a bigger almshouse infirmary, but of a true public hospital "fully commensurate with the increasing population of the city." When Hosack died in 1835, there seemed little chance of this. But he did live long enough to see the first of several crises that would help bring his grand vision to life.

In the first half of the nineteenth century, New York overtook Philadelphia as America's largest city. Yet its astonishing population growth— from 96,000 in 1810 to 942,000 by 1860—produced more worry than pride. New Yorkers had known their share of boom and bust, division and disorder. They had survived British occupation, economic panics, devastating riots, epidemics, and fire. But nothing had prepared them for the crush of human cargo now arriving daily on their shores. New York had become the world's leading port of entry for immigrants fleeing famine and persecution, or seeking a fresh start. Most stayed only briefly before heading west to farm, lay track, dig canals, mine coal, and pan for gold. Those who settled in New York were often too poor, or too exhausted, to go any farther. One port officer likened them to hogs "vile, offensive, and pestilential . . . literally wallowing in their own filth." By the Civil War, close to half the city's population would be foreign-born, with Ireland providing the lion's share, and Germany a distant second.

Until the early 1800s, New York hadn't extended much beyond the wharves and warehouses dotting lower Manhattan. "Shipping and trade were the chief occupations, and the artisans were largely independent workers," wrote a student of city life in the days before massive immigration and steam-powered factories. "Housing conditions were favorable; gardens and orchards were common; there were no tenements. Judging from what reports are available New York appears to have been a reasonably clean and tidy town."

This, perhaps, was an exaggeration. New York never resembled a scrubbed and orderly city; busy seaports rarely do. But as commerce and immigration expanded in the nineteenth century, New York became a different place. The completion of the Erie Canal, linking the city to the agricultural heartland, dramatically fed the growth. So, too, did the introduction of rail lines bringing grain and cotton for shipment abroad. California gold helped fuel the banks and stock market that turned Wall Street into America's financial center. Travelers to the city described a pulsing new energy—"a sea of masts" in the harbor, "streets jammed with carts, dray, and wheel barrows," buildings "rising everywhere."

New York had its share of shabby boardinghouses and fine brick mansions. But its mainstay had long been the "artisan dwelling," with a store or workshop on the ground floor and the family quarters above. Over time, a fair number of these merchants and tradesmen had moved away, selling their homes and shops to agents who converted them into multiple dwellings for the immigrant poor. By the early 1800s, the city's northward expansion had reached, and overwhelmed, a five-acre spring-fed body of water near Canal Street called the Collect, or Fresh Water Pond, known for its "great depth and unusual purity." Once a center for ice-skating and shoreline picnics, the Collect would become one of Manhattan's first ecologic casualties—a dumping ground for dead animals, rubbish, and factory waste. Too dangerous to drink, a place of "insufferable stench," it was filled with dirt and carved up for residential use. On this landfill rose the infamous slum known as Five Points.

Heavily Irish, Five Points contained a sprinkling of German immigrants and former African slaves. Most residents hailed from Counties Cork, Kerry, and Sligo—places of extreme poverty well before the devastating potato blight of the 1840s. A visitor to County Kerry described the tenant cottages there as the "most miserable I ever beheld." Those who reached New York naturally sought out Irish Catholic enclaves with the cheapest housing and the best chance for an unskilled job nearby. In Five Points, they found both.

This neighborhood, long since gone, is now part of American folklore. Moviegoers know it as the backdrop for Martin Scorsese's violent epic, *Gangs of New York*. In the nineteenth century, it appeared regularly in travel accounts of the United States. So celebrated was its reputation for squalor and mayhem that curious out-of-towners often toured its streets—an activity described as "slumming" in the press. Frontiersman Davy Crockett paid a visit to Five Points, as did presidential candidate Abraham Lincoln. "I saw more drunk folks, men and women, that day, than I ever saw before," said Crockett, no innocent himself. Charles Dickens inspected the neighborhood (with a police escort) during a trip to America in 1842. It was, he lamented, a "world of vice and misery. . . . All that is loathsome, drooping, and decayed is here."

It was true, of course, that Five Points contained a surplus of taverns and brothels, and that farm animals roamed its putrid alleys and yards. But many neighborhoods shared these problems, as New Yorkers well knew. By 1811, more than 1,300 groceries and 160 taverns were licensed to sell "strong drink" in the city, which had barely 100,000 people and not many Irish. Several years later, the diarist Edmund Blunt warned that "so long as immense numbers of swine are allowed to traverse the streets, so long as inhabitants think themselves justified in throwing out their garbage to them for food," the city would remain "proverbial for its filth." Others grimly agreed, noting thoroughfares covered in the waste of slaughterhouses, the droppings of horses, and the excrement from overflowing backyard privies.

What made Five Points unique, aside from its rural Irish flavor, was the incredible overcrowding. Families and boarders found themselves crammed into dwellings known as "rookeries" (the precursors of tenements), which rose to four and five stories. So many were built, one attached directly to the next, that Five Points soon rivaled the worst slums of London in terms of human density.

Its most infamous rookery, though not by much, was a converted brewery near the Collect landfill. An account of a visit there by a group of Protestant clergy is worth quoting—less for its accuracy, perhaps, than for the contempt it heaped upon the tenants. Entering a basement room, the group counted twenty-six people. "A man can hardly stand erect in it," the leader wrote. "The smoke and stench of the room was so suffocating that it could not be long endured, and the announcement that [some children] had the measles to boot, started most of our party in a precipitous retreat from the premises.

"Miserable beings!" he concluded. "Life is at best an unpleasant necessity, but to them it must be an awful punishment."

In 1832, cholera came to Five Points. It arrived during a lull in the city's ongoing struggle against epidemic disease. Smallpox had receded a bit, thanks to the growing popularity of vaccination. And yellow fever had mysteriously disappeared from New York and other Northern seaports, moving southward to terrorize cities like Memphis and New Orleans. As for cholera, little was known. It had only reached Europe in the 1820s, moving along Asian trade routes by caravan and boat. An intestinal disease, cholera spreads when food and water are contaminated with the excrement of infected victims. The bacterium responsible, *Vibrio cholerae,* causes the body to expel huge quantities of liquid through vomiting and explosive diarrhea. What makes cholera so terrifying is the damage it can do within hours of entering the system. There is no incubation period, no time to prepare. The victim can be fine in the morning and dead by nightfall.

Cholera in the United States is a distant memory, though it remains a serious threat in the developing world. Effective sewage systems, chlorinated water, powerful drugs, better hygiene—all played a role in its demise. Should a case of cholera appear, the patient would be pumped full of fluids and given an antibiotic to kill the microscopic invaders. Of course, none of this was known in 1832. Some saw dirt and dampness as the culprit, others swore off shellfish, unripe fruit, green vegetables, even milk. But most medical thinking still blamed miasmas—noxious atmospheric clouds—for spreading deadly epidemic disease.

Like yellow fever, cholera seemed to favor recent immigrants, with the Irish at greatest risk. A Bellevue Hospital physician explained why. "As a class of people," he wrote, they were "exceedingly dirty," "exhausted by drunkenness and debauchery," and "crowded together in the worst portions of the city." In truth, Five Points did suffer higher rates of cholera for reasons all too clear. First, there was no means of escape. The people were too poor to pack up and leave when an epidemic occurred, unlike wealthier New Yorkers who fled the city in droves. (One observer compared the exodus of "well-filled stage coaches" in 1832 to the stampede from Pompeii "when the red lava flowed.") Second, these immigrants had no choice but to use whatever water was at hand. In Five Points, that meant a series of shallow wells polluted by the fecal waste from backyard privies. Rich folk could drink from purer sources. Some even paid to have fresh water carted in from lakes and springs north of the city—not because they feared contamination, but because it tasted better. That simple preference likely saved their lives.

New York hadn't seen an epidemic of this size since yellow fever several decades before. In June 1832, the Bellevue Establishment held 145 "general patients" and 97 "maniacs." By summer's end, it would admit more than 2,000 cholera cases and record 600 deaths. The victims, described by one doctor as "low Irish," were young and single, for the most part, and recently arrived. "O'Neill was seized with the malignant cholera and died the next day," read a typical case history. "He was very intemperate, had been drunk all week, and had fallen, while intoxicated, into the North [Hudson] River."

Indeed, what is striking about these cases is the head-scratching that occurred in the rare instances in which a victim didn't fit the Irish stereotype. "Mr. Fitzgerald was by trade a tailor and a temperate man," wrote a perplexed Bellevue physician. "His wife was also a neat housekeeper, so that in this case neither of the most common causes of cholera, viz, dirt and intemperance, were present." That the couple lived in Five Points—"the resort of all that is vicious and dissoluble"—seemed the best explanation.

The resident physician at Bellevue Hospital in 1832 was Isaac Wood, a member of New York City's medical elite. A graduate of Queens College (Rutgers) Medical School, and a fearless body snatcher in his younger days, Wood now confronted a problem that few Westerners had ever seen, much less treated. Clueless as to the cause of cholera, or its remedy, Wood relied on the standard remedies for treating epidemic victims: bleeding and purging. For a disease like smallpox or yellow fever, such methods were bad enough; for cholera, which involved an extreme loss of bodily fluids, they bordered on torture.

Wood did see a silver lining, though. An epidemic of this size would allow him to increase his medical staff and perhaps find a cure for the disease. There were no rules regarding the "informed consent" of the patient in nineteenth-century America, and no constraints beyond a physician's conscience and imagination. Free to follow their hunches, Wood and his assistants tried a variety of treatments. To increase "physical stimulation," patients received "hot bricks to the feet and body," "severe shocks of electricity," and the "intense friction applied by the rubbing of two stout men." One patient, eight months pregnant, was given heavy doses of calomel, killing her baby. She then became part of an experiment in which a vial of tobacco juice was injected into her arm at a temperature of 112 degrees. "Vomiting followed, with deep convulsive inspirations," her doctor noted. "She felt sleepy but did not sleep; about 5 o'clock death closed the scene."

Tobacco was believed to have purgative qualities, causing "excitement of the bowels." Some at Bellevue thought it an ideal cleansing agent—instantly powerful, while doing no real harm. "The patient has only then to recover from the tobacco," it was argued, "and he is comparatively well." Early on, the substance was credited with saving numerous cholera victims, including "an idiot, aged 14," whose "unceasing vomiting" had been eased with "a tobacco infusion by mouth." "I am already satisfied that there is no remedy which we have yet tried that can compare with it," a physician declared.

The problem, it turned out, was that no one beyond Bellevue could replicate these results. "Tobacco has been administered in nine cases—seven were positively injured," reported the director of a nearby pesthouse. "The other two were for a short time revived, but soon collapsed again, and finally died."

By autumn, cholera had killed 3,500 in a city of 200,000 people. Statistics showed foreign-born deaths at 2,486, or 71 percent of the total, at a time when immigrants, just starting to pour into New York, comprised barely 10 percent of its population. This meant that close to 15 percent of the city's foreign-born perished in the 1832 cholera epidemic, as opposed to less than one percent of the native-born.

At Bellevue, Dr. Wood found himself "stepping over the dead and dying." The bodies were piled into carts and hauled away for burial in mass graves sprinkled with lime. That summer, Wood himself became a casualty. Barely surviving his own bout with cholera, he left Bellevue to regain his health. There is no record of the treatment Wood received—it would take him five years to fully recover—though he appeared to swear off tobacco shortly thereafter. "I believe," he said, "it is detrimental to many persons, and in various ways."

Cholera would return in the coming decades, devastating immigrant neighborhoods and swamping Bellevue's morgue. In 1849, it killed 5,071 New Yorkers, including 3,250 foreign-born. But over time, in laboratories across Europe, cholera's secrets would be exposed. In 1854, the British physician John Snow proved that the disease was transmitted not by noxious fumes in the atmosphere, but rather by a specific agent in the water. His diligence in tracing the victims of a single London epidemic—the so-called Ghost Map—would become the model for future studies of infectious disease. Exactly thirty years later, in

1884, the German researcher Robert Koch identified the specific agent as the comma-shaped microorganism *Vibrio cholerae,* a discovery that helped demolish the Miasma Theory for good.

Some New Yorkers saw cholera as a blessing in disguise. "Those sickened must be cured or die off," wrote an unforgiving official, "& being chiefly of the very scum of the city, the quicker [their] dispatch the sooner the malady will cease." For him and his allies, the answer lay in restricting the flow of immigrants to America and quarantining those who did reach its shores.

Others disagreed. The Irish were here to stay, they thought, and not likely to change on their own. Cursing their filth and intemperance, while a natural response, did little to prevent epidemics that put the entire city at risk. A more practical approach was to focus less on the moral failings of these immigrants, which city officials couldn't effectively control, and more on the environmental causes of disease, which they could. If foul vapors and general filth were the cause of cholera and other epidemic diseases, then why not whitewash the tenements and close down the stinking wells?

Epidemics can be tricky as agents of change. They arrive with frightening force, do their awful damage, and leave as mysteriously as they come. It's easy to view them as freaks of nature, or divine occurrences, impossible to control. In the case of cholera, however, some valuable lessons would be learned. It was no accident, for example, that Five Points got its first major street cleaning in 1832, exposing the paving stones that lay beneath piles of sludge. Three years later, New Yorkers approved the construction of a forty-one-mile-long aqueduct to bring clean water from the Croton River, north of the city, to holding reservoirs on 42nd Street, where the main branch of the public library stands today, and the Upper West Side, in what is now Central Park. The project, costing $11.5 million and employing four thousand workers, allowed the city to slowly phase out its hodgepodge of contaminated local wells. In 1849, following another deadly cholera outbreak, an ordinance was passed banning swine from New York's most populated neighborhoods. "Overcoming sometimes violent resistance by impoverished owners, the police flushed five to six thousand pigs out of cellars and garrets and drove an estimated twenty thousand swine north to the upper wards."

Cholera also exposed the flaws of the Bellevue Establishment. Opened to great acclaim in 1816, it had quickly become an attraction for social reformers like Alexis de Tocqueville, who remained oddly silent about the conditions he saw there but scathing in his review of the banquet thrown to honor him. (The planning, Tocqueville wrote his sister, "represented the infancy of the art: the vegetables and fish before the meat; the oysters for dessert. In a word, complete barbarism.") What others noted, however, was the ever-growing crush of bodies, which periodic epidemics made worse. Was it wise to mix so many people, with so many different problems, within the same set of walls?

David Hosack had predicted as much: the Bellevue Establishment had failed. Medical care remained captive to the dreary world of the almshouse and the pesthouse, foreclosing better options for the poor. Until things changed—until that link was broken—a true public hospital for New York City seemed all but impossible.

3

THE GREAT EPIDEMIC

In antebellum New York, much like today, wealth played a key role in one's health care. The rich paid handsomely for the privilege; the poor relied on the charity of others. Yet what neither side fully grasped were the slender distinctions that separated the "best" from the "worst" medical treatment of this era—a time of painfully slow progress in the field. Money may have provided the illusion of proper care, but it did nothing to protect a child from diphtheria, a mother from puerperal fever, or a father from tuberculosis. The medical profession simply lacked the tools to be effective. As the physician-philosopher Lawrence Henderson aptly put it, "a random patient, with a random disease, consulting a doctor at random had no better than a fifty-fifty chance of profiting from the encounter."

The same went for hospitals. Americans saw little need for them in the early 1800s because what occurred there could be done more safely and comfortably at home. Lacking anesthesia, antisepsis, and X-rays, among other modern essentials, the hospital resembled a poorhouse with a vaguely medical bent. No institutions except the military and the penitentiary seemed as perilous to human health. Even in London, where the tradition of hospital care was far stronger than in the United States, "the probability of a sick man dying [in] one," reported a medical board in the mid-nineteenth century, was "many times greater than had he stayed away."

For wealthy New Yorkers, the alternative was private care: a prominent physician, often under contract, would be summoned whenever a family member or a valued servant took ill. "One visited nice persons in their homes; they did not ordinarily come to one's office," wrote a student of the New York medical scene. "It was considered, indeed, a matter of good planning to visit frequently enough to oversee the progress of a case, but not so frequently as to give the impression that one was padding the bill."

Those who served New York's best families were a breed apart. Most had graduated from a medical school, studied abroad in Edinburgh or Paris, and apprenticed with a well-known physician—a David Hosack, perhaps—before entering private practice. In the 1830s and 1840s, these men had created a number of groups to promote the latest advances from "the best schools of Europe and America." At each month's meeting of the exclusive New York Medical and Surgical Society, papers would be read on topics ranging from smallpox vaccination to a daring breakthrough in pain control: "the inhalation of ether." But all too often the speakers rehashed an assortment of old bromides—the Miasma Theory, for example, or the finer points of bleeding and purging. One told of curing a case of scarlet fever with "wine whey." Another explained how he had dislodged a coin from a child's esophagus. "The treatment," he said, "was to stand him on his head till it fell out."

With status, of course, came financial reward. Commanding handsome fees, elite doctors never lacked for clients. One of the legendary tales of this era involved a conversation between John Wakefield Francis, an illustrious New York physician, and a wealthy merchant who had hired him on retainer. "Doctor, I got your bill the other day," said the merchant, "but I don't remember any of us being sick this year." "Very likely not," Francis retorted, "but I stopped several times at the gate and inquired of the servants how all of you were."

These were the exceptions, of course. Most New Yorkers saw a lower order of "physician," with each visit paid in cash and, hopefully, on the spot. "People labor under the delusion that doctor's fees, especially in New York City, are very extravagant," a newspaper reported, adding: "This is a mistake." One medical journal complained that the average doctor earned less in his lifetime than a greedy financier made in "a single day on the exchange."

The main problem, it appeared, was competition. For those seeking private care, the New York City Directory listed 506 "medical doctors" in 1836, excluding herbalists, homeopaths, phrenologists, faith healers, and patent medicine men. Many of these "doctors" touted a diploma of some sort—and a specialty as well. "Dodge, Jonathan, M.D.," read a typical advertisement. "Operative Surgeon and Mechanical Dentist, original and only manufacturer and inserter of premium and incorruptible teeth."

For the poorest New Yorkers, even a Dr. Dodge was beyond reach. Many relied on the home remedies and patent medicines familiar to all groups, but aimed especially at the "lower classes." For 25 cents, Dr. Fubarsch's "Vegetabilische Lebenspillen" offered relief from fever, worms, and hemorrhoids. For 50 cents, Van Pelt's "Indian Vegetable Salve" promised to make carbuncles and breast lumps disappear. For a dollar, one could purchase "Ladies Silver Pills," described, rather delicately, as "the rich man's friend and the poor man's need."

There were other options. Virtually all societies distinguish between the "worthy" and "unworthy" poor. In nineteenth-century America, the "worthy" poor were those who innocently lacked the means to care for themselves: widows and children; an injured farmer or tradesman; the blind, disabled, elderly, and insane. The "unworthy," by contrast, were those who created unseemly obstacles to their own success: drunks and prostitutes; beggars, gamblers, and the chronically unemployed.

Medical care reflected this divide. A prime example was the "Dispensary System," imported from London in the late 1700s. Similar to the outpatient clinics of today, the dispensary flourished in American cities as a working-class alternative to the almshouse infirmary—the early Bellevue model—that smacked of failure and despair. In 1828, the *New York Evening Post* praised the Northern Dispensary, which had just opened in Greenwich Village, for providing medical care to "the honest workmen . . . who [otherwise] must either receive assistance from the charity of neighbors, or be removed to the hospital or perish."

How did a dispensary separate the worthy poor from the unworthy? A common device was to solicit donations from wealthy patrons, who could then recommend several patients (often a servant or a factory worker). No one would be treated without a "signed certificate" from a patron, and even that was no guarantee. Those deemed unfit or incurable could still be turned away.

Most dispensary cases were routine: a cough, a cut to be closed, a tooth to be pulled. The Northern Dispensary listed a patient in 1836 who complained of a head cold—a neighborhood writer named Edgar Allan Poe. Some stopped in to be vaccinated, especially when smallpox was around; others were drawn by the free potions of the apothecary, often bringing "a bottle or tea-cup to receive and hold the medicine." Given the rather mundane range of ailments, the mortality rate was low. Reviewing its first year, the Northern Dispensary claimed that 860 patients had been "cured," 24 had died, and 17 had been "discharged as disorderly."

The dispensary served a variety of needs. Employers viewed them as good for their workforce, while health officials saw them as buffers against epidemic disease. But no one benefited more from these clinics than recent medical school graduates and physician-apprentices. Dispensary doctors were grossly underpaid, and some feared that the low wages would "lure only the young, unpracticed, and needy members of the profession." But that was precisely the point. Competition was fierce for these jobs because they offered a path to a more lucrative career. The trustees of the New York Dispensary, the city's largest, admitted as much when they described their facility as "a practical school for physicians." By 1860, New York's five major dispensaries were treating over 100,000 patients each year, making them the main source of clinical instruction for new doctors—and medical care for the "worthy poor."

Some, however, watched these rising numbers with alarm. Free medical care not only meant fewer paying patients for doctors serving the working classes, it also raised fears about the moral impact of such largesse. The dispensaries "are nothing less than a promiscuous charity," a local physician complained. "They are the first stepping-stones to pauperism."

In fact, such complaints had particular targets. For years, dispensary doctors had fretted over their increasingly Irish Catholic clientele. They were so numerous and repulsive, drunk and surly, said one, as to drive away the "deserving American poor."

—

There were times when the combination of poverty, ill health, and circumstance made a hospital stay inevitable. It might be a stranger to the city, a seriously injured worker, a chronic disease sufferer—someone needing more care than a family or dispensary could provide. In 1850, New York City had two major "hospitals." One was voluntary, the other public. One was privately endowed, the other relied on public funds. One accepted the worthy poor; the other turned no one away.

New York Hospital opened its doors in 1791, "a handsome structure set amid shaded lawns," a few short blocks, yet a world away, from the almshouse where Bellevue was born. Financed by the city's leading merchant families, New York Hospital was never meant as a refuge for the down-and-out. Indeed its founding physicians, John Bard and Peter Middleton—the first dissectors—viewed it as the very antithesis of the Bellevue Establishment, which Middleton described as "a public receptacle for poor invalids" and "a reproach to the community." Such a place, he fumed, was "undeserving of the name Hospital."

The contrasts were stark. "From the beginning," wrote the historian of the institution, "New York Hospital had drawn a line between the diseases it would handle and those—mainly chronic and incurable—it would not." That line was rarely crossed. New York Hospital made this clear in the 1790s when it refused to accept the victims of yellow fever, and again in the 1830s when many cholera cases were turned away. The "do not admit" list also included drunks, vagrants, and those with smallpox, "the itch," and "contagious distempers." A compromise of sorts was reached regarding venereal disease: men could be admitted, but women—i.e., prostitutes—could not. The hospital treated mostly short-term patients—those with a good chance of recovering quickly from their ills. "Persons [of] Decrepitude . . . are considered as fitter Objects for an Almshouse than for this Hospital," its charter read. In a word, Bellevue.

There were three patient categories at NYH: those receiving free care; those paying a small weekly charge; and merchant seamen supported by the federal government. The largest category—free care—consisted of the worthy poor: those of a "better grade." Rules abounded.

Patients were expected to be "submissive," to attend Sabbath services, and to read the Bibles placed in every ward. Cursing, gambling, and stealing were grounds for expulsion. Wards were segregated by sex and race, though black patients were rare because attending physicians did not like treating them. No doubt issuing such decrees proved easier than enforcing them, especially where "maniacs" and hard-drinking merchant seamen were concerned. But New York Hospital had the means to resolve these issues—first by constructing a separate insane asylum, known as Bloomingdale, in the northern reaches of Manhattan; then by moving the merchant seamen into their own "Marine House" with iron bars on the windows.

New York Hospital also differed from the Bellevue Establishment in physical design. One had been built as a refuge for the sick, the other a warehouse for the destitute. One had a welcoming facade; the other resembled a walled-in fortress. One had spacious wards with large windows to scatter "unhealthy emanations" and "noxious physical matter." The other stacked its patients like cordwood. "Imagine a lunatic asylum, hospital, house of correction, smallpox victims and every series of vagrant huddled together [and] crammed with dead and dying," a report observed. That was Bellevue—circa 1837.

New York Hospital claimed to welcome all types of worthy poor. "Animated by the Principles of Christianity," its charter declared, "[we] uniformly disclaim any influence of contracted Attachments to any national, civil, or religious Distinctions." But immigrants often felt uncomfortable there. While the charity wards did see an increase in foreign-born patients in the 1830s, relations could be tense. A Protestant minister at New York Hospital described the Irish he met as "hardened infidels" and "despisers of the Bible." During a severe typhus epidemic in 1851, the hospital agreed to admit its share of cases. But the decision set off a firestorm among the donors, who thought the victims, mostly Irish, belonged at Bellevue. Within days, the offer was rescinded "for the protection of other patients."

No medical facility in this era of limited hygiene was immune to waves of bacterial disease. New York Hospital would be racked by outbreaks of pyaemia (blood poisoning), trachoma (eye inflammations), erysipelas (a severe skin rash), puerperal fever (a deadly infection following childbirth), and surgical gangrene. These maladies, known collectively as "hospitalism," reflected the dangers inherent in all such institutions. But here, too, New York Hospital enjoyed advantages that a public institution couldn't match. Better funded, more selective, and less congested, its patient mortality was consistently lower than Bellevue's, where the annual death rate sometimes topped an alarming 20 percent.

In the 1840s, a ray of hope appeared. A new almshouse complex opened on Blackwell's Island in the East River, dramatically thinning the droves of paupers and lunatics at Bellevue. It didn't do much good. The mass transfers to Blackwell's Island coincided with a flood of impoverished refugees from Europe, leaving Bellevue more crowded than before. "Our city is particularly burdened with them," a bitter official wrote of these new arrivals. "The opportunities for relief [here] are too easily obtained and certainly too eagerly sought."

By 1850, fully one quarter of New York City's population was on some form of public assistance, and three quarters of the recipients were foreign-born. The vast majority of prison commitments now read, "Nativity, Ireland," as did admissions to the almshouse. At the new lunatic asylum on Blackwell's, the figures for 1850 were: Ireland, 199; USA 97; Germany 53; England 29. A few doctors there took a sympathetic approach, jotting notations such as "privation on shipboard" and "arriving in a strange land" alongside the Irish names. Many of the cases were young, single women overcome with loneliness and despair. Most would be released from Blackwell's Island in a matter of months, though the asylum superintendent saw little hope for their future. The Irish, he explained, owed their "exceptionally bad habits" to a "low order of intelligence" resulting from "imperfectly developed brains." When "such persons become insane," he added, "I am inclined to think the prognosis is peculiarly unfavorable."

But it was the Bellevue Establishment where the crush of new arrivals hit hardest. In 1846, Bellevue Hospital—the city pesthouse—had admitted 3,600 patients, with 2,200 listed as Irish. A year later, the numbers surged to 6,541 patients, including 4,863 Irish. A deadly epidemic had again reached New York City, with unmistakably immigrant roots.

It went by several names: Irish Fever, Ship Fever, and Jail Fever. But physicians called it typhus—from the Greek *typhos*, meaning hazy—for the dizzying state it produced. Typhus is a bacterial disease that thrives in close, filthy quarters. Spread by a body louse, it is best known for decimating Napoleon's army during the Russian campaign of 1812, and for the millions of soldiers and civilians it killed in Europe during both world wars. Perhaps the oddest thing about typhus is how rarely it has appeared in the United States. There is no record of a serious outbreak during the American Revolution or the Civil War, despite abysmal troop conditions. Research suggests that the environment here proved inhospitable to the vector—the body louse. In truth, nobody knows.

There had been occasional typhus outbreaks in New York City during the early 1800s, concentrated in the immigrant slums. Then came the devastating potato blight in Ireland. "The potato was the staff of life," wrote one historian, "the staple consumed at every meal and burned for fuel." At least a million Irish died in the years between 1846 and 1852, spurring the exodus to North America. Each day an armada of so-called famine ships departed Liverpool for Canada and the eastern port cities of the United States. Passengers spent the ocean voyage packed like cattle in quarters with little food or clean water, no spare clothing, and barely a breeze. Fires, storms, and icebergs were among the dangers, but the big killer was disease. One immigration official described conditions on board as "no better than that of a slaver or a coolie ship," adding: "Ten deaths among one hundred passengers was nothing extraordinary; twenty percent was not unheard of; and there were cases of 400 out of 1,200 passengers being buried before the ships left port."

The main debarkation point was New York City, which received an average of three hundred Irish immigrants a day in the famine years, with many choosing to settle. Each passenger had been checked for obvious diseases before leaving Europe, and "foreign" ships entering New York harbor were met by a health inspector. While evidence of sickness could mean quarantining everyone on board, in most cases only the visibly ill were singled out and ferried to the New York Marine Hospital on Staten Island called the Quarantine. In 1846, this eighty-bed facility admitted 900 patients; a year later, the figure was 8,000 and climbing. Of the 730 deaths recorded there in 1848—the highest total ever—433 were from typhus.

Staten Island seemed ideal for the Quarantine—a sparsely settled expanse of farmers and oystermen whose concerns about "dangerous foreigners" were casually brushed aside. That proved a mistake. In 1858, a mob of locals stormed the Quarantine, and burned it to the ground. Fortunately, the patients had been "removed before ignition."

Because the telltale signs of typhus—rash and fever—are not immediately apparent, many future victims escaped detection on board. Once off the boats, they headed for the tenements of Five Points and other slums, carrying lice in their clothing and body hair. What made typhus different from smallpox or yellow fever or even cholera was its limited geographic range. A fixture of the poorest neighborhoods, it caused little panic in the city as a whole. There were no mosquitoes, or contagious victims, or contaminated wells, to spread the danger much beyond the miserable quarters of the immigrant poor.

Many typhus victims died where they lay, but hundreds more wound up at Bellevue Hospital. Beds were shared and "pest tents" were pitched on the lawn. A more ideal setting for typhus transmission could hardly be imagined. The patient death rate at Bellevue soon topped 40 percent, and for the staff it was even higher. So many resident physicians fell to typhus that medical students were asked to fill the void. To scroll through the fatalities in 1847–48 is akin to reading the names on a war memorial:

Gorham Beals, M.D. . . . died in New York City, January 9, 1848; cause: typhus fever, contracted while on duty in the hospital.

William Cahoon, M.D. . . . died in 1848: cause: typhus fever, contracted while on duty in the hospital.

John Fraime, Jr., M.D. . . . died in New York City in 1847; cause: typhus fever, contracted while on duty in the hospital.

Elihu Hedges, student of medicine, died in 1848; cause: typhus fever, contracted while on duty in the hospital.

Henry Porter, M.D. . . . died in 1847; cause: typhus fever,
  contracted while on duty in the hospital.
David Seligman, student of medicine. . . . died in 1848;
  cause: typhus fever, contracted while on duty in the
  hospital.
Augustus Van Buren, M.D. . . . died in 1847; cause: typhus
  fever, contracted while on duty in the hospital.
Sidney B. Worth, student of medicine. . . . died in 1848; cause:
  typhus fever, contracted while on duty in the hospital.

The typhus outbreak of 1847–48, known at Bellevue as the "Great
Epidemic," would be recalled with bitterness and pride. The house officers and medical students who died there were well-connected young
men seeking clinical experience before entering private practice. They
had remained at their posts through the worst of it, some rising from
their deathbeds to train others to carry on. But hard feelings lingered:
typhus, after all, was a reminder of what Bellevue had always been, and
seemed destined to remain—a dumping ground for those deemed too
ill to be anywhere else.

What could be worse than admitting hopeless patients and then
being blamed for having such a high mortality rate? "At least two-
fifths of those who die at our hospital [come] in a dying state," a Bellevue doctor fumed. "During the past year, three have died at the very
door . . . ten more within two or three hours after admission, and forty
within the first week." The doctor then singled out the worst offender.
"Very many are sent from New York Hospital, where they have been . . .
pronounced incurable and dismissed for us to take charge during the
remainder of their lives."

There was truth to this. New York Hospital had a long history of
dumping its sickest patients, a pattern that would continue well into
the twentieth century. In this instance, however, it did treat some
victims from the "famine ships" because of growing public pressure.
Interestingly, just 10 percent of its typhus patients would die there, and
only one of its doctors contracted the disease. He returned to duty
three months later.

—

Typhus would not soon disappear. Each year that passed without a doctor's death at Bellevue seemed cause for genuine relief. "It is a subject worthy of congratulation," read the hospital's annual report in 1852, "that we can [speak] without the melancholy necessity of paying an obituary tribute to . . . members of the House Staff who have fallen victim to the typhus fever." But it returned with a vengeance a decade later, killing "nine of twenty-two employees" who contracted it, and "six of fifteen physicians." Conventional wisdom still blamed the disease on foul vapors from decomposed matter, which led a young visiting physician named Alonzo Clark to pose a logical question: If typhus arose from harmful miasmas—whether inside a coffin ship, a tenement, or a hospital ward—shouldn't its treatment be linked to commonsense remedies such as less crowding, cleaner surroundings, and purer air? Bellevue might not be able to match New York Hospital in these matters, but surely it could do better.

Clark ordered his own typhus ward to be whitewashed, the windows flung open, and the doors removed from their hinges. He also replaced the heroic therapies of bleeding and purging with gentler measures designed to spur a "natural recovery." His aim, aside from dissipating the bad air, was to quietly stimulate the body rather than harshly deplete it. Like David Hosack, Clark employed alcohol as his main elixir, though in larger amounts. As legend has it, every typhus patient under Clark's supervision recovered. From this point forward, the treatment for typhus at Bellevue would include oceans of spirits—"the brandy bottle replacing the lancet"—along with bone-chilling blasts of East River air.

The Great Epidemic proved a watershed event. It was one thing for a hospital to lose paupers to disease; quite another when the victims included much of the medical staff. "A thorough change in the mode of governing the establishment was needed," a physician recalled, "and it came at a time when the epidemic occurrences of typhus fever raised the existing evils . . . to a culminating height."

What followed was thorough, indeed. Under intense fire, city officials in 1852 turned over the administration of Bellevue Hospital to a ten-member Board of Governors dominated by physicians and social reformers. Day-to-day operations would now be handled by a professional warden, whose duties ranged from policing the wards to taking "personal charge of all wines and spirituous liquors required for hospital purposes." Patient care would be supervised by four distinguished "consulting" physicians and surgeons, with a dozen "attending physicians and surgeons" a rung below. All would visit Bellevue on a regular basis, "granting their services gratuitously." The job descriptions seemed distinctly unappealing—great responsibility with no apparent compensation. In fact, these positions would be deeply coveted by the city's medical elite as a sign of professional status and Christian duty. And each man could bring "three of his students gratis to see the practice of the house"—an accommodation for lucrative tutoring on the side.

At the bottom of the ladder were five recent medical school graduates who would live at Bellevue and earn a nominal $130 for a six-month term. Known as the house staff, they were to visit the wards each morning and evening accompanied by five current medical students who performed routine procedures like "bleeding, cupping, leeching, and dressing wounds" (a sign that the old ways of heroic medicine had not been fully abandoned). On paper, at least, the house staff would be chosen by competitive examination. "All are received upon common footing; all are [tested] by the same committee. . . . They must stand on their merits alone, incited by the hope of entering Bellevue Hospital."

Most revealing were the new guidelines regarding patient selection. "No person shall be admitted whose case is judged to be incurable," read a key sentence in the new *Rules and Regulations for the Government of Bellevue*, "nor shall any who [are] judged insane or who shall have the smallpox or measles, or any malignant or contagious fever, to be received." Such patients would be sent to the new East River facilities on Blackwell's Island, freeing Bellevue from its notorious almshouse–pesthouse past.

Here, at last, were the outlines of dramatic change. General and acute care would become top priorities. Chronic and contagious cases would no longer clog the wards, except in extraordinary circumstances. Those suspected of insanity would be examined first at Bellevue—but then either released or shipped to Blackwell's Island for incarceration. One thing that wouldn't change, however, was the credo of the institution. Bellevue would accept "only patients who were unable to pay for their board and maintenance"—those, in short, with nowhere else to turn.

"Who shall take care of our sick?" This vital question, posed by anxious Catholic Church leaders in New York, had become an increasingly popular refrain. The mass exodus from Europe had overwhelmed the city's meager health services, leaving immigrant communities, for the most part, to fend for themselves. One might use the dispensary system for minor ailments, or a charity birthing clinic if a bed were available. There were separate spaces now for lunatics and epidemic victims—but not much more. New York City claimed but two general hospitals in 1850, and neither held much appeal for the immigrant poor. One was seen as too judgmental and aloof; the other too chaotic and grim. And neither was acceptable to the Roman Catholic Church.

The reason was clear enough. Hospitals in this era had a Protestant, evangelical bent. They were considered places of redemption—ideal for wooing vulnerable patients back to Christ. "Many are brought in wholly ignorant of the first truths of the Gospel, arrested in a life of sin," a nurse explained. "[But] the fear of dying overwhelms them, and they are thankful and willing to listen to words of instruction and prayer."

While New York Hospital was less appealing to the city's Catholic clergy, Bellevue posed the greater spiritual threat. For one thing, it kept a Protestant chaplain on the payroll at city expense. He "leaves no room unvisited," the warden noted, delivering Bibles to the patients and leading them in prayer. For another, Bellevue treated far more Catholics and stood several miles from the downtown immigrant strongholds, isolating patients from family and friends. For church leaders, the real worry at Bellevue wasn't the high mortality rate, but the conversion of fearful Catholics into Protestants. Bellevue, said one suspicious Jesuit, was like "a royal hunting ground."

No one took this threat more seriously than John Hughes, America's first Roman Catholic archbishop. A native of Ireland, known as "Dagger John" for affixing a "stiletto-like cross" to his signature, Hughes was determined to protect his growing immigrant flock. Headquartered in

Manhattan, he would become the model for future "brick and board" prelates, constructing an impressive defense line of churches, convents, schools, and cemeteries throughout his diocese. The situation at Bellevue particularly galled him, because Catholic priests weren't welcome there unless specifically requested by a patient—a humbling affront.

In 1849, the Sisters of Charity opened a thirty-bed hospital in a rented house on East 13th Street, led by the archbishop's biological sister, Ellen Hughes. The order was "just about the finest thing the immigrant Church had for the sake of public relations," wrote Dagger John's biographer. Founded by Elizabeth Seaton, it had courageously treated the poor during the great New York cholera epidemic of 1832, when most religious leaders were seen running for their lives. The new hospital, named St. Vincent's for the canonized seventeenth-century French priest, was intended for "the Catholic indigent sick." Conditions were spare: the original building lacked gaslight, indoor toilets, and running water. Those with means were charged $3 a week for "board, washing, nursing, and medical attendance." Those with no money were declared charity cases. The Sisters slept on the floor of the front parlor, next to the mortuary on the porch.

The beds, however, were always full. In 1855, the Sisters moved to larger quarters on West Ninth Street and Seventh Avenue, with an eye toward further expansion. Money was raised the Catholic way—through block parties, raffles, and the trusty collection box. Lot by lot, dollar by dollar, the Sisters methodically bought the land they needed. "Building in New York," wrote their frugal treasurer, "is very expensive."

The city's first Catholic hospital, St. Vincent's was unique in other ways. While serving an Irish immigrant clientele not unlike Bellevue's, it relied on private funding to survive. Among its lasting (if premature) innovations was a small space, set apart from the charity wards, that offered "well-furnished private apartments" for those requiring "special accommodations." Who might these people be? A New York City guidebook, published in 1872, provided some examples: "To clergymen or other persons stopping at hotels or to strangers of means, overtaken suddenly with disease, these rooms offer peculiar advantages, combining the comfort of a home with the advice and treatment of the Hospital."

St. Vincent's had little trouble recruiting a medical staff. As one of only three general hospitals in Manhattan, it provided a vital outlet for doctors looking to hone their clinical skills. But what kept St. Vincent's afloat in its difficult early years was the devotion of its nuns. Even the most rabid bigots showed a grudging respect for the Sisters of Charity. They "serve for life with no expense to the Institution save board," marveled an anti-Catholic journalist. "[Their] self-imposed penury . . . life-long toil and sleepless vigilance [to] the Mother Church, notwithstanding all their errors of faith and practice, present a sublime anomaly in the history of the world, and are eminently worthy of imitation."

And imitation, it turned out, is precisely what occurred. The mid-nineteenth century saw a dramatic surge in voluntary hospitals throughout New York City. The example of St. Vincent's spread to other ethnic groups, including German Americans who comprised New York's second-largest foreign-born community. Always a presence in the American colonies, Germans had come in waves to the United States in the 1840s and 1850s to escape political and economic turmoil at home. More than a million Germans entered the country in these decades, most through New York City, with the great bulk moving on to the farms and cities of the Midwest and Great Plains. Still, about one in ten settled where they landed, making New York the third-largest German-speaking city in the world, behind only Vienna and Berlin.

Many of these newcomers lived in *Kleindeutschland,* or Little Germany, a Lower East Side enclave seen, through native eyes, as the German equivalent of Five Points. In truth, *Kleindeutschland* was more diverse, with Protestants, Catholics, and Jews, Bavarians, Prussians, and Saxons living side by side. And, while every bit as cramped as other immigrant neighborhoods, it wasn't quite as poor. Many Germans had been forced from the land, like the Irish, but those who settled in New York came with skills better suited for an expanding urban economy. According to the New York State Census of 1855, Irish immigrants constituted a majority of the city's laborers, teamsters, dockworkers, and domestic servants. For Germans, by contrast, it was bakers, tailors, cabinetmakers, and grocers.

On any given Sunday, it was said, *Kleindeutchland*'s beer halls and wine gardens did a brisker business than its churches. But German Catholics in New York City faced a special problem: their diocese was a solid Irish preserve. When they demanded their own priests, speaking their own language, Archbishop Hughes acquiesced. When they built their own churches, he didn't blink. The strategy, said one diocese official, was simply to "ignore their existence." As a result, a German Catholic could no more fathom the idea of going to St. Vincent's than he could of going to Bellevue. One hardly seemed better than the other.

The German migration had included a large number of physicians—so large, in fact, that by 1850 fully one third of New York City's medical community had been born and trained in Germany. Before long, a dispensary appeared, offering "medical advice to inhabitants of New York City who speak the German language, our indigent sick [being] ignorant of the English tongue." No references were required, no religion was preferred, and care was provided free of charge. "The institution is open every day with the exception of Sundays and holidays," read its first brochure. "The hour of 12–1 is set aside for children and women, and the hour 1–2 is for all other patients."

Medical journals lauded the doctors who worked there, calling them some "of the best in the city," while noting their "modes of treatment not in use in American institutions"—a reference to the homeopathic methods popular among German physicians. Growing steadily, the dispensary took on the name "German Hospital" and moved from *Kleindeutschland* to Manhattan's Upper East Side in 1868, along with much of the upwardly mobile German American community. Over time, homeopathy would give way to more traditional practices, though the doctors and nurses still spoke German to the patients—and to each other—well into the twentieth century.

That largely ended, however, with the hyper-patriotism of World War I. A ferocious backlash led orchestras nationwide to stop playing the music of Bach, Beethoven, and Wagner. Several state governments banned the teaching of German in schools, and cities took to scrubbing German names from thoroughfares and public buildings. In Chicago, Hamburg Street became Shakespeare Street and the Bismarck Hotel became the Randolph Hotel. New York City proved no exception. In 1918, the trustees of German Hospital reluctantly agreed to rename their institution for the land on which it stood: Lenox Hill.

While Jews had been a small part of the great German migration, their numbers were large enough to swell New York's Jewish population, once dominated by Spanish and Portuguese refugees, from two thousand in 1846 to more than forty thousand by 1860. Like other groups, Jews had typically boarded their indigent sick with families in the community. Sending a *landsman,* or fellow Jew, to a place like Bellevue or even New York Hospital was unthinkable. Stories had long circulated about Protestant clergy who specialized in deathbed conversions. (In the Jewish rendering, a young transient named Kahn becomes violently ill, is carted off to Bellevue, and must beg to be "buried among *Yehudim.*") The new German Dispensary was an improvement, though hardly ideal. Jews spoke many languages. They celebrated a different Sabbath and worried that gentiles would mock their religious rites, "their *tefillin* and *zizit.*" The time had come to build a special house for their indigent sick, as instructed by the Talmud.

An attorney named Sampson Simson took the lead. A graduate of Columbia College and a protégé of Aaron Burr's, Simson donated the land on West 28th Street, between Seventh and Eighth Avenues, and coaxed sizable gifts from others—the largest one, $20,000, coming from Judah Touro, a New Orleans businessman best known for preserving North America's first Jewish cemetery in Newport, Rhode Island. Another $7,000 was raised through a novel device—the fundraising dinner—held at Niblo's, the city's premier restaurant and saloon. "There were over 800 persons present and the entertainment was faultless," the *New York Times* reported, complimenting "the Israelite women" for "cooperating in so noble a cause."

Naming the institution was simple. Inscribed boldly above the entrance were the words JEWS' HOSPITAL, with the Hebrew name BET HOLIM written alongside. But recognizing the donors proved more difficult. Their names were already well known to the community. Was it appropriate to list them on the hospital walls as well? Some community leaders thought not. Further attention bordered on the unseemly, they believed, undermining the true intent of charity and needlessly humbling the poor.

The hospital board felt otherwise. Listing the contributors, it agreed, was both a reward for a good deed and an incentive for others. When Jews' Hospital opened in 1855, four marble tablets bore the names of each donor, with a fifth one honoring the recently departed Judah Touro, "whose liberal bequeath to this institution," it read, "is hereby acknowledged . . . in the erection of this memorial." A tradition had begun.

The new hospital admitted only Jews, except "in cases of accident or emergency," and required payment from those who could afford it. But records showed that fewer than 10 percent of the patients contributed to their own support. Much like St. Vincent's, Jews' Hospital attracted recent immigrants, unattached and desperately poor. The male patients were mostly itinerant peddlers, wrote an attending physician, "cast upon our shores without profession or trade." And many female patients worked as domestics in the homes of other Jews, "coerced into service as a means of subsistence."

Jews who died at Jews' Hospital—or *any* New York hospital—were buried in a Jewish cemetery, rarely in Potter's Field. Indeed, one of the enduring stories of the Bellevue morgue involves an attendant who tricked the Hebrew Free Burial Association into taking the unclaimed body of an Irishman by stuffing copies of a Jewish newspaper into the dead man's coat. "Somewhere in a Jewish cemetery today," it is said, "rests this son of Erin, and quite comfortably, no doubt, beneath the Star of David."

The most controversial issue facing Jews' Hospital in these early years concerned the performance of autopsies. Were they permissible under religious law? The issue grew so heated that the chief rabbi of the British Empire was asked to intervene. His opinion—that autopsies be permitted in cases where knowing the cause of death might aid the living—became the standard in most Jewish institutions.

When the Civil War began in 1861, Jews' Hospital opened a special ward to treat wounded Union soldiers. Two years later, in the midst of the violent draft riots that tore through New York City, it admitted dozens of badly wounded victims, almost all of them gentiles. By war's end, Jews' Hospital had changed its strictly sectarian ways, allowing it to receive funding from the state. It would be renamed Mount Sinai Hospital in 1866.

The coming years would see a host of these facilities, each with a special clientele. Presbyterian Hospital would cater to Presbyterians, St. Luke's Hospital to Episcopalians, St. Francis Hospital to German Catholics, and Columbus Hospital to "poor Italians unable to make themselves understood." In a prescient speech on the state of medical care, circa 1857, Dr. B. W. McCready noted that New York had just begun a process started centuries ago in cities like London and Paris. "Here our rich men have not yet had time to die and endow hospitals," he explained, singling out Jews' and St. Vincent's as models for what hopefully lay ahead.

Like David Hosack, however, the prestigious McCready wanted more. A great metropolis required a great public hospital, he said, and Bellevue's time had come. "May the beauty and salubrity of its site . . . be equally preeminent in the successful cultivation of medical science and in the relief of human suffering." New York City, he conceded, was in desperate need of both.

The 1850s had seen dramatic changes at Bellevue. The Great Epidemic, the waves of immigrants, the growth of Blackwell's Island, the emergence of voluntary hospitals—all played a role in its reinvention. Standing on the nearly abandoned Establishment grounds, Bellevue Hospital now occupied the main building where the old almshouse had stood. Physical improvements followed. In 1853, the Common Council allotted Bellevue $60,000 to build a new morgue. The remains of Protestant patients would still be sent to Potter's Field in the Bronx, but the bodies of Catholics, in response to heavy pressure from Archbishop Hughes, would be ferried to the new 350-acre Calvary Cemetery in Queens—the "City of the Celtic Dead"—where a free burial awaited. Two years later, a four-hundred-seat, glass-domed operating theater was added to Bellevue at a cost of $100,000, sparking rumors of a medical school to come.

But perceptions changed slowly. Hospitals were still viewed as places to be avoided by the "better" classes, and Bellevue, now the largest in the United States, remained the ideal magnet for lurid stories and exposés, often with good cause. Rats were abundant in New York City at the time—as, alas, they are today—and Bellevue, abutting the East River with its maze of pilings and wharfs, was especially vulnerable. One visitor, an observant sort, counted forty of them in a single bathtub. "Myriads swarm at the water side after nightfall, crawl through the sewers and enter the hospital," the *New York Times* reported, quoting parts of a sensational affidavit from a Bellevue physician, despite warning its readers that the details were "unfit for publication."

"At six Monday morning," the affidavit began, "I was called . . . to see Mary Connor, an unmarried woman, aged 31 years. I immediately examined, and found [a] child beneath the hips of the mother, in a lifeless condition, and mutilated, apparently by rats. The nose . . . upper lip and a portion of the cheeks seemed to be eaten off. The toes of the left foot and a portion of the foot were eaten off, or apparently so. The lacerated portions were covered with sand and dirt."

The *Times* did note the doctor's opinion that the infant had died of natural causes before "the gnawing was done." (An investigation by the coroner would support this contention.) But the newspaper offered a warning as well: "The vermin have full possession of the building," it said, and any plan to remove them short of gutting the structure "will be more than amazing."

Such was the confused and turbulent state of Bellevue Hospital—at once promising and repulsive. It had come a long way since its days as an almshouse appendage and a pesthouse for victims of epidemic disease. Progress had been erratic over the years, yet a new Bellevue had emerged. David Hosack's grand vision was finally at hand. New York City could now boast of a true public hospital, standing alone.

4

TEACHING MEDICINE

In 1847, with the Great Epidemic at its peak, a city alderman accused Dr. Meredith Reese, Bellevue's lead physician, of "pocketing an unlawful fee for the sale of dead bodies from [his] institution." Though a special committee would exonerate Reese, calling the charge against him "entirely unfounded," the incident stoked memories of the infamous Doctors' Riot of 1788. Almost sixty years had passed since that bloody confrontation, but little had changed. New York's medical schools still relied on grave robbers to meet their "anatomical needs." The bodies still came from the city's poorest burial grounds, which remained the easiest to rob. And the demand for corpses still outpaced the supply, leading to fears that medical training in New York might grind to a halt. "It is well known," said a local physician, that "more than 600 young men . . . have had their studies arrested by a [dearth of cadavers.]"

The shortage fell hardest on the city's two established medical schools—the College of Physicians and Surgeons at Columbia and the Medical College of New York University—while jeopardizing hopes for a third one at Bellevue Hospital. Fresh cadavers were an essential teaching tool; without them, students had to rely on illustrations and wax figures. Even the most devoted anatomists knew that grave robbing had to stop: it produced too few corpses and put the robbers at great risk. What was needed, they believed, was a way to increase the cadaver supply by portraying dissection as a public good. Didn't better medical training benefit everyone in society, rich and poor alike? "For the sake of living humanity," a local physician pleaded, "permit your colleges to dissect the dead!"

Exactly *which* dead spurred a bitter debate. It was one thing to claim that dissection served a larger purpose, quite another to determine whose remains would wind up on a slab in an anatomy class. Taking the lead was New York University's John Draper, a British-born physician with well-known anti-Irish views. For years, Draper had lobbied the state legislature to increase the supply of fresh corpses to medical schools. Taking the moral high ground, he titled his 1854 proposal "An Act to Promote Medical Science and Protect Burial Grounds." Others called it "the Bone Bill."

At the time, New York state law allowed but one category for legal dissection: executed criminals. Draper's proposal added corpses from prisons and almshouses not picked up within twenty-four hours—a sizable pool. The wording was blunt: "All vagrants dying, unclaimed, and without friends, are to be given to the institutions in which medicine and surgery are taught for dissection: the debris to be buried in the public cemetery." The beauty of the bill, Draper argued, was that it satisfied the needs of medical education without resorting to grave robbing. Cemeteries would once again be safe havens. The respectable dead could finally rest in peace.

There was moral posturing as well. Those supporting the Bone Bill believed that prisoners and paupers owed a final debt to society. "By offering up their bodies to the advancement of a humane science," a state legislator declared, "they will make some returns to those whom they have burdened by their wants, or injured by their crimes." The twenty-four-hour grace period allowed grieving friends and relatives to claim those deserving a proper burial, leaving only the unworthy behind. The clear intention was to send only the lowest of the low to medical schools for dissection—those "whose vices have worn out the patience of their friends."

The Bone Bill had its opponents. Some raised ethical objections. "We cannot help but think that the necessities of medical science have been greatly overrated," wrote the editors of *Harper's New Monthly*. "Better that the causes of some bodily diseases remain concealed than that the knowledge of them be obtained at the sacrifice of some of the best feelings of the soul." But the loudest protests came from the neighborhoods most affected by the bill. How, in God's name, could anyone see "the bodies of men as of no greater import than the bodies of dogs?" thundered Five Points assemblyman Peter Maguire. On St. Patrick's Day, thousands marched in Manhattan behind a green silk banner reading, "WE PROTECT THE SICK AND BURY THE DEAD."

Passed by just one vote in 1854, the Bone Bill proved quite effective in securing its goals. Grave robbing would drop sharply in the coming years, and medical schools got their precious cadavers. As the 1855 catalogue of the College of Physicians and Surgeons put it: "Thanks to the enlightened liberality of the legislature, the supply of anatomical subjects has not only been ample but without the difficulties and dangers of [the past]."

A banner class was expected.

In the first decade of the nineteenth century, fewer than four hundred students received a medical degree in the United States. Between 1850 and 1859, that number reached 17,213, matching the nation's enormous growth. Most American cities now claimed a medical school, and some rural towns did as well. But not everyone called this progress. The nation's first medical schools, attached to well-established colleges like Harvard, Columbia, Dartmouth, and the University of Pennsylvania, had expected their applicants to have a modest classical education—a familiarity, at least, with Greek and Latin and natural philosophy (physics). Those days were long gone. The new "proprietary" medical schools required little more of a student than the ability to pay the tuition and fees. Typically some local doctors would rent a building, offer a series of lectures, collect their money, and hand out degrees. There was no professional oversight because most legislatures had already done away with the licensing of physicians on the grounds that it denied ordinary citizens the right to choose their favored vocation. As the state of Maine reported: "the field is now open to all."

Profit was the driving force. The goal was to pack in as many bodies as the buildings could hold. Few college graduates applied, preferring the loftier careers in the law and clergy. Once "accepted," the medical student took two terms worth of lectures—the subjects varying with the size of the faculty. In a medical school with five "professors," the student sat through five eye-glazing presentations each weekday; the term, lasting about four months, was repeated verbatim the following year for "mental retention." There was no laboratory work (beyond basic anatomy) and no chance to examine a patient. To graduate, one passed a simple examination, paid a commencement fee, and sometimes wrote a thesis (which a modern observer compared to "the term paper of a college sophomore").

Why would a young man pay money for this when he could simply hang out a shingle after apprenticing with a local physician? One reason was that a medical education probably did help those who had faithfully attended the lectures and participated in the dissections. A medical degree also attracted well-to-do patients in cities like Boston, Philadelphia, and New York, where credentials mattered more.

The College of Physicians and Surgeons (P&S) traced its roots back to the eighteenth century, with close ties to Columbia College, New York Hospital, and the city's medical elite. Nothing better reflected its lofty status than its move, in 1856, to a brick and brownstone building on the corner of 23rd Street and Fourth Avenue, with ample classroom space, a surgical amphitheater, and a dissecting space with twenty-five tables. Its brochure boasted of rooms warmed by a hot air furnace, lighted by gas, and blessed with pure Croton water. Built for the princely sum of $90,000, it was financed entirely by the professors who taught there.

That they could afford to do this was telling. P&S had long recruited faculty members with the biggest medical reputations. Those fortunate enough to teach there generally stayed until retirement or death. The position guaranteed both a steady income from student tuition and a private practice attracting New York's upper crust. Not surprisingly, the number of faculty positions remained rock solid—frozen at around seven or eight—despite a steady climb in enrollments. Exclusivity had its rewards.

No faculty member added greater distinction in these years than Dr. Valentine Mott, who would go on to found NYU Medical College and become an indispensable part of Bellevue's future. Historians of American medicine regard Mott as the premier surgeon of his time. Contemporaries went even further. "The boy was father to the man," an admirer wrote worshipfully of Mott's upbringing. "Docile, obedient, pure in mind, cautious in speech, neat in dress, erect in person, walking as one who reverences God, and who respects the rights and feelings of his fellows: in a word, a perfect gentleman."

Born in 1785, the son of a Quaker physician from Long Island, Mott had apprenticed with Dr. Valentine Seaman, a leading New York City surgeon, before traveling to England for further study. Superbly trained, with an impeccable pedigree, he returned home to become a professor of surgery at P&S. At a time when European medical opinion scoffed at the skills of American "knife-men," Mott remained the conspicuous exception. He was among the first surgeons to amputate successfully at the hip. He performed hundreds of lithotomies, extracting "the largest [gall] stone ever removed from the living body," a friend wrote, "its weight being seventeen ounces and two drachms." Mott revolutionized vascular surgery by placing ligatures within inches of the heart. "He cut firmly and boldly," it was said, "yet with a certain gentleness, too." And he was perfectly ambidextrous, working fluidly with either hand. In the words of Sir Astley Cooper, England's leading surgeon: "Valentine Mott has performed more of the great operations than any man living."

Among Mott's favorites was a procedure he devised to relieve the "exquisite suffering" of a man whose testicles "had been drawn up by a gradual contraction of the surrounding muscle." (When dealing with "malignancies," Mott, by his own count, had removed "over a bushel of testicles, some of them weighing more than a pound.") The case at hand had baffled numerous "surgeons of eminence" because the patient, while forced to find a "more harmless" line of work, still enjoyed "a reasonable amount of pleasure" in the bedroom. Upon examination, Mott "decided to cut down, divide the spermatic nerve and remove a larger portion of the cremaster muscle." This caused the testicles to descend and the pain to disappear. The result, it was said, "unfolded new truths . . . in alleviating the afflicted."

Much of his success came before the introduction of anesthesia. "In

Mott's early days," a colleague recalled, "stout arms held down the writhing man; firm violence was requisite to keep quiet the shrieking child [whose] trachea must be cut to save her life. What nerve, what firmness, what determination were the attributes of him."

Mott loved the operating theater, and he didn't come cheap. For private patients, he charged as much as $1,000 for a complicated procedure—an immense sum at that time—and never lacked for business. For charity patients, he charged nothing; their role was to provide the raw material needed for clinical instruction. When lecturing his students, Mott stressed two basic rules: Never perform an operation that you, the surgeon, would refuse to undergo yourself. And never attempt a procedure on the living without first practicing it on the dead.

Not everyone bowed to his genius. The cranky New York diarist George Templeton Strong described Mott as something of a fraud. Strong's uncle had suffered from a painful facial neuralgia that Mott apparently promised to relieve. There followed a "very severe operation" that failed the patient but produced a sizable bill. "The Hercules that finally vanquished the Hydra—that all Dr. Mott's science wasn't up to—was a preparation of rather quackish origin," Strong explained, "an ointment prepared by rubbing down five grains of aconitine [an extremely toxic plant] and applying it twice a day. . . . It effected an immediate cure."

Failures, though, seemed few and far between. A more typical Mott story, told and retold by his many students over the years, involved a memorable performance in the dissection of a cadaver. "The scalpel slipped and a portion of [Mott's] own finger was cut off and fell on the table," a witness recalled. "Perhaps now he who had . . . never flinched when those around him were groaning under operations might become unnerved . . . dismiss the class . . . and retire to his room."

Not so, Dr. Mott. "Putting his finger in his mouth, he sucked the wound, then wrapped it in his handkerchief, shrugged his shoulders . . . and went on lecturing till the gong sounded. I had my eye on that piece of surgical flesh . . . but being detained to assist in bandaging the Professor's finger, a brother doctor slipped into the lecture-room and secured the prize. He now can boast of Dr. Mott in alcohol."

Mott seemed the closest thing to a celebrity doctor that early-

nineteenth-century America could produce. A physically imposing man—"fully six feet with broad shoulders, and a fine muscular
development"—he lived with his wife and children at One Gramercy
Park, a four-story Italianate mansion known as the finest dwelling in
New York. The Motts entertained "in a style of magnificence which we
have not witnessed for a long time," wrote a guest at one of their galas
for visiting royalty. The doctor's net worth hovered somewhere around
a million dollars, feeding juicy gossip in the press. "He daily rose at
7 o'clock, breakfasted at 8, and dined at 5," a friend noted, "rarely taking anything in the interval, except perhaps, a glass of water. . . . At
9 o'clock he went into his office, and except when interrupted by his
college lectures or a call to attend some urgent case, remained at home
until 1 o'clock." Afternoons were filled with surgical operations and visits to his patients. "His horse and carriage were always in perfect order
and never driven beyond a slow, dignified pace. . . . His evenings were
always spent in his library, reading, writing, or conversing with friends."

In 1835, "overcome by the fatigues of his pursuits," Mott fled New
York City to travel the world. His published thoughts, popular at the
time, are best left to the ages. "He is humorous only about the smell
of vagrant Greeks, the large-sized bed-bugs on the plains of Marathon,
and the obesity of women in Asia Minor," a critic observed. Stopping in
Constantinople, Mott removed a growth from the head of reigning sul-
tan Abdul Medjid, earning a knighthood and, one suspects, a hefty fee.

While in Europe, Mott had corresponded with friends about starting a medical school at New York University, an institution chartered
only a decade before. Mott knew that his name would be solid gold.
His plan mimicked the arrangement between Columbia College and
P&S: the medical school would offer a degree through the university
but otherwise be self-sufficient. And, as with P&S, the students and
faculty would have full access to the clinical riches of the Bellevue
Establishment—an arrangement, negotiated by Mott himself, that virtually guaranteed the school's survival. In 1841, Mott and five other
physicians bought an impressive granite building on lower Broadway.
The group included Surgery (Mott); Chemistry (John Draper); Anatomy (Granville Pattison); Materia Medica (Martyn Paine); Theory
and Practice of Medicine (John Revere); and Diseases of Women and
Children (Gunning S. Bedford).

Though few doubted the need for a second medical school in America's largest city, the rank commercialism of the project raised some eyebrows. Mott and his colleagues planned to admit just about any white male student able to afford the costs. Rigorous standards jeopardized the public's health by excluding those who would go on to be doctors anyway, they explained. Better to have some schooling than none at all.

The enormous entering class of 271 included almost everyone who applied. Only blacks, women, and complete illiterates were rejected. Who, save the utterly ignorant, would prefer "this rotten and disgraceful concern" to the "dignified and meritorious" College of Physicians and Surgeons? a critic sniped. "Heaven only knows what is to become of all the Doctors ground, or rather bolted, out of the innumerable [diploma] mills from Maine to Texas."

Tuition was $105 per term, plus a $5 "matriculation" fee, a $10 "broken" fee (for damaged equipment), and a $20 "anatomical" fee (for fresh cadavers). With four terms required to graduate, plus a $30 "graduation" fee, the total for each student ran to $550, a hefty sum. According to the ledger books, the faculty split close to $40,000 a year after expenses.

Handpicked by Mott, the faculty was eclectic, to say the least. John Draper, the Bone Bill man, preached the virtues of modern science, while Martyn Paine, a traditionalist, taught the old ways of calomel and the lancet. (To pass one of Paine's examinations, it was said, required but a single answer to every question: "The treatment is blood-letting, sir.") John Revere, the youngest son of colonial patriot Paul Revere, was among Mott's closest friends. A gifted writer—his *Treatise on Medicine* was a standard text in that era—Revere would die from typhus in 1847 while tending to one of his students.

Gunning Bedford, a visionary of sorts, had a gift for attracting publicity, much of it bad. Honored today for opening one of the first obstetrical clinics in the United States, he was best known in the 1840s as a crusader against abortion. Bedford aimed to replace the midwife with a physician trained in both the medical and moral aspects of childbirth—someone who saw the fetus as fully equal to the mother. He thus opposed all procedures that endangered the infant, the most common being the craniotomy, which reduced the skull in order to fit it through the birth canal; and he regularly employed cesarean section, explaining that it saved babies in distress (though it put the mother at greater risk of deadly infection).

Critics portrayed Bedford as a fanatic and a fraud. His unfortunate habit of lifting the writings of others—what we call plagiarism today— was well noted in the press, which mocked him as "a Psychological and Literary Phenomenon!" Yet his advantages were clear. Immigrants were pouring into New York, and Archbishop John Hughes, a friend of Bedford's, had declared that Catholics, whenever possible, must patronize doctors who satisfied the teachings of the Church. Bedford provided a bridge between the new medical school and the city's foreign-born population. His Obstetric Clinique would soon be treating ten thousand patients each year.

Even more controversial was Mott's choice of the eccentric Granville Sharp Pattison, whose most notable talent, aside from teaching anatomy, lay in creating ill will almost everywhere he went. Born in Scotland, Pattison had held and lost a string of medical posts before coming to the United States—the reasons ranging from an indictment for grave robbing to an affair with a senior colleague's wife. Taking a position at Philadelphia's Jefferson Medical College, he fought a duel with General Thomas Cadwalader, a local hero, over a family insult, leaving the general with an arm withered for life. A notorious reveler, Pattison gulped down mercury—the common "cure" for syphilis—in copious doses. What brought him to Mott's attention were his undeniable pedagogic skills. "As a lecturer on anatomy," a student recalled, "he almost made the dead body before him speak."

At first, Pattison and Mott worked well together—so well that the newspapers took to covering their exploits. In the summer of 1841, the pair performed an amputation at Mott's Surgical Clinique in Bellevue Hospital, where several hundred doctors and students gathered each Saturday afternoon to watch the master at work. Done in an era before anesthesia or antisepsis, the operation required incredible speed to keep the patient from dying of shock. On the table this day was a fifteen-year-old boy with a horribly infected upper leg. "One professor [Mott] felt for the femoral artery, (and) had the leg held up . . . to ensure the saving of blood," the *New York Herald* reported. A tourniquet was placed on the artery, with the body secured by the boy's father and an assistant. "A little wine was given to the lad," who appeared "pale but resolute."

Then it began. Pattison took a "long, glimmering knife, felt for the bone," and opened the flesh. "Tears ran down the father's cheeks—the blood gushed by the pint—the sight was sickening—the screams were terrific—the operator calm."

Out came the saw. The screams grew louder, and several spectators fled the room. "The father turned pale as death—the boy's eyes fastened on the instrument with glazed agony—grate—crush—once—twice—and the useless limb from the toes to the center of the thigh was quietly dropped into the tub under the table." With that, the father "fell senseless to the floor."

Two months later, the boy was said to be doing well. "When he was placed on the operating table he seemed [to be] sinking from the effects of hectic fever," Pattison reported. "He is now in vigorous health—the stump has healed beautifully—and the lad is a living illustration of the blessings of scientific skill."

Pattison and Mott soon took to feuding. The reasons are unclear—some blamed Mott's princely share of the tuition money—but the two drifted icily apart. In 1853, Mott retired from NYU to accept the post of "consulting surgeon" at Bellevue. The move spurred talk about creating a third medical school there, placing pedagogy *within* a hospital—something America had not yet seen. Meanwhile, enrollments at the NYU Medical College dropped off, owing, most agreed, to "the withdrawal of Dr. Valentine Mott . . . then the foremost surgeon of the country [and] a magnetic attraction to the school."

Calls for a medical college at Bellevue had been circulating since the late 1840s, when the hospital separated from the almshouse. Physicians and medical students from across the city now flocked to attend the Saturday clinics and demonstrations in its glass-domed operating theater. Contained within Bellevue was "every disease mankind is heir to," a doctor marveled. "I have seen Lascars and Chinamen, Indian mixed breeds, Spaniards from South America, lying side by side with natives of every nation in Europe, and of every state in the Union."

Few doubted that Bellevue would soon get a medical school. The hard question was: Exactly what kind? Americans had grown weary of the excruciating treatments of orthodox medicine, often centuries old, which rarely seemed to work. This had led to a search for alternatives, some imported from Europe, others homegrown. In the early 1800s, a self-trained New Hampshire physician named Samuel Thomson became immensely popular by promoting the "vegetables of our own country" as the cure for most ailments. Thomson had a bone to pick with traditional medicine, having seen his mother copiously bled and purged by local doctors following their diagnosis of "galloping consumption." "They galloped her out of the world in about nine weeks," Thomson recalled, adding: "Much of what is at this day called medicine, is deadly poison."

Thomson went by a simple slogan: Heat is Life; Cold is Death. A healthy body generated warmth through the food it consumed, much like a furnace burning firewood. Problems arose, however, when the digestive system became clogged. "This causes the body to lose its heat," Thomson explained. "Then the appetite fails; the bones ache, and the man is sick in every part of the whole frame."

Thomson relied on spicy botanicals—hot peppers, cayenne, and lobelia, a plant commonly known as "puke weed"—to cleanse the system. In doing so, he tapped into the public's growing dread of bleeding and purging, especially with violent mineral laxatives like calomel. Commonsense medicine came from "studying patients, not books," he liked to say, from "experience, not reading."

The appeal lay partly in the milder remedy. An enema of pukeweed was a bed of roses compared to the lancet or mercury-laden drugs. But even more important to Thomson's success was the nation's changing political landscape. "Thomsonianism" took root in the expanding democratic culture of Jacksonian America, with its suspicion of entrenched elites. Many state legislatures in this era abolished all restrictions on who could become a doctor or a lawyer in order to discourage "monopolies." Thomson insisted that ordinary people, using common sense, could effectively heal themselves. His goal, he stressed, was "to make every man his own physician."

While Thomsonianism declined rapidly following its founder's death in 1843, it did signal a revolution at hand. Alternatives to traditional medicine were flourishing, the most popular being homeopathy, brought to American shores by the disciples of a German doctor named Samuel Hahnemann. Like Thomson, Hahnemann believed in herbal cures. Unlike Thomson, Hahnemann held a college medical degree and had taught at the prestigious University of Leipzig. His goal was not to turn every man into his own physician, but rather to turn every physician into a homeopath. In the United States, at least, he seemed to be gaining ground.

Hahnemann viewed bleeding, purging, and even surgery as barbaric relics of the past. Careful study had convinced him of two things: First, a drug that produced specific symptoms in someone who was well could cure the very same symptoms in someone who was ill—a process he called *similia similibus curantur.* Thus, a certain herb or bark that caused a fever or a high pulse rate in a normal patient could also relieve that fever or high pulse rate in a sick patient. Furthermore, these drugs worked better when given in minute doses—the logic being that highly diluted solutions served to replace the patient's stronger symptoms with weaker ones, giving the body a better chance to respond.

Hahnemann forged a different base of support. Where Samuel Thomson's followers were mostly rural and poorly educated, Hahnemann's included the likes of Henry Wadsworth Longfellow and Harriet Beecher Stowe. One observer wryly described it as "the radicalism of the barnyard" versus "the quackery of the drawing room."

By the late 1840s, homeopathy claimed somewhere between 5 to 10 percent of New York City's doctors, the numbers rising steadily with German immigration. This led traditional native-born physicians to create organizations like the American Medical Association to separate "regular from irregular practitioners." A showdown was inevitable. In 1857, a number of Hahnemann's prominent followers, including Horace Greeley, editor of the *New York Tribune,* demanded that the wards at Bellevue Hospital, a public facility, be split evenly between "homoeopaths" and "allopaths" (the term for those who practiced regular medicine). The pressure grew so intense that Bellevue's Medical Board agreed to study the matter—a move quite unthinkable just a decade before.

The rebels sensed victory. "Five of the [board members] are homeopaths," boasted a Hahnemann supporter, "and one more vote is alone required to give [us] half the wards in the largest hospital in the country." It wasn't to be. The rebels' error, it appeared, lay in interpreting the rejection of bleeding and purging by many physicians as an endorsement of Hahnemann's approach, which wasn't remotely the case. What most of them wanted, said a local doctor, was a path "between the two extremes, neither verging towards meddlesome interference on the one hand, nor imbecile neglect on the other." In short, a middle ground.

And that seemed the majority view at Bellevue as well. Most physicians there now rejected the "heroic medicine" of the past while still considering Hahnemann a quack. Typhus, tetanus, peritonitis—it hardly mattered. The lancet, leeches, and gut-wrenching mercury purges were on their way out; opium, quinine, and whiskey were already in. "Blood-letting, as clinical observation has shown, is not a curative measure," a Bellevue study announced. "King alcohol appears to reign supreme."

On the advice of Valentine Mott and other Bellevue dons, the Medical Board formed a "select committee" of three members, two of them firmly in the "allopath" camp. Their "majority report" mocked Hahnemann as a dangerous fraud, akin to the English monarchs who once claimed healing powers through "the royal touch." Bellevue had come too far for such nonsense, they wrote. Surrendering half the wards to charlatans would reverse the momentum that had turned it from a wretched almshouse into "a well-appointed hospital crowded with grateful patients."

There was more. Bellevue's stature depended in large part on the clinical opportunities it provided. "No one who visits can fail to be struck with the throng of students and medical men who crowd its ample theatre, and the eagerness with which they listen to the instruction," the report went on. "[This] high standing has given it a national reputation in the medical profession, and rendered it an object of inquiry and compliment abroad."

The message was clear: those who controlled the hospital might soon be running a medical school as well. And with that came the duty to train would-be physicians in a responsible manner, ignoring the "foolery" of Samuel Hahnemann and his misguided legions.

—

The pieces were in place. The Bone Bill had dramatically aided medical education in New York state, and the homeopaths had been routed. With close to one thousand beds spread across thirty-four different wards, Bellevue offered clinical riches on a massive scale. From Boston, meanwhile, came word of a breakthrough—a miracle, really—that would revolutionize medicine and hospital care as few things had before.

In Harvard's Countway Medical Library hangs a massive canvas of a surgeon standing over a young man who appears to be asleep. The surgeon, holding a scalpel to the patient's neck, is surrounded by a group of curious colleagues; behind them are rows of spectators in neatly angled seats. Painted over a full decade by Robert Cutler Hinckley, *The First Operation Under Ether* ranks among the most famous scenes in medical history.

The procedure took place in an operating theater in Massachusetts General Hospital on October 16, 1846. The origins of surgical anesthesia—who perfected it; who cheated whom out of fortune and glory—are still in dispute. One historian recently described the tangle as "fishy enough to populate an aquarium." But most agree that this brief demonstration in Boston marked anesthesia's successful debut. It was here that a local dentist named William T. G. Morton put a tube to the lips of Gilbert Abbott, "a consumptive young man with a vascular tumour [on] his jaw," and told him to breathe in the vapors. It took about four minutes for the sulfuric ether to do its job. With Abbott seemingly unconscious, Morton turned to Dr. John Collins Warren, the surgeon standing beside him, and said, "Sir, your patient is ready."

The operation took twenty-five minutes. Anticipating the screams that normally followed the first incision, Dr. Warren was astonished to hear none. When Abbott awoke, his tumor cut away, he claimed to have felt nothing beyond a bit of roughness on his neck. Warren then turned to the audience and uttered what some insist are the five most famous words in American surgery: "Gentlemen, this is no humbug."

Pain was one of the two biggest obstacles to major surgery—the other being postoperative infection. By the 1840s, a well-informed surgeon knew enough about human anatomy to prevent serious blood loss through the binding, or ligation, of surrounding arteries and vessels. But the operation itself caused such intense suffering that it had to be done lightning-quick, with several men to hold the patient down.

In the days before anesthesia, Dr. Warren recalled, the surgeon would actually quiz the patient on the operating table before proceeding. "'Will you have your leg off, or will you not have it off?' If the patient lost courage and said, 'No,' he had decided not to have the leg amputated, he was at once carried back to his bed in the ward. If, however, he said, 'Yes,' he was immediately taken firmly in hand by a number of strong assistants and the operation went on regardless of whatever he might say thereafter. If his courage failed him after this crucial moment, it was too late and no attention was paid to his cries of protest."

The best that could be done, aside from merciful speed, was to dose the patient with laudanum or whiskey and then stuff his ears with cotton to muffle the sound of the instruments slicing through flesh and bone. Surgeons confessed to vomiting before each procedure; one compared his work to "a hanging." "There is not an individual who does not shudder at the idea of an operation, however skillful the surgeon or urgent the case," wrote another, "knowing the great pain that the patient must endure."

Anesthesia would have its critics. Some saw physical suffering as a punishment from God, not to be tampered with; others worried about the dangers of inhaling a foreign gas. Samuel Hahnemann viewed pain as both a vital diagnostic tool and a natural part of healing. "Better let the patient suffer a while," he wrote, "than complicate the troubles and retard the final recovery, or risk the patient's life."

But these were minority opinions, to be sure. The news from Boston that day was electric. No longer would pain "make all men cowards," wrote an ecstatic Valentine Mott. Patients would lose their fear of the knife, allowing surgeons to perform operations "which the most bold and adventurous of [us] would not have had the temerity to touch." For those like Hahnemann who opposed anesthesia, Mott had a message: "Away with the stupid fanaticism that would inculcate the patient endurance of suffering when it could be relieved."

The impact was dramatic. Before anesthesia, demonstrations in the operating theater had been so ghastly that guidelines were needed to keep order. At Bellevue, surgeons were told: "it is better to lecture *before* or *after* cutting human flesh, and not while the agonized patient is writhing under prolonged torture, or held still while gaping wounds are coldly commented on." It did little good. A Bellevue intern wrote that "the first operation I witnessed without anesthesia was so disquieting . . . that I was nearly driven from the profession"—and he wasn't alone. Numerous young men, including Charles Darwin, quit their medical studies for fear of inflicting such pain on others. "To behold the keen shining knife . . . to hear the saw working its way through the bone produced an impression I can never forget," one of them recalled. "I could not look upon the operation, but covered my eyes to keep myself from fainting."

As Mott predicted, the "calculus of suffering" was forever changed. At Bellevue, the number of major operations slowly increased, as did the quality of those who performed them. Joining Mott was a group destined to lead the field: Lewis A. Sayre in orthopedic surgery; Frank H. Hamilton in fractures and battlefield wounds; and Stephen Smith in general surgery and public health. All—save Mott, now well into his seventies—would be founding members of the Bellevue Hospital Medical College.

Their announcement came early in 1861, promoting a new school on the Bellevue grounds. Quite naturally, it stressed the connection between a medical college and a hospital with "immense" clinical resources. Students at Bellevue would travel seamlessly between their classes and the wards. Births and operations would be studied in real time. Anatomy would be taught in "commodious" dissecting rooms with "abundant material"—thanks to the Bone Bill of 1854. "The day is not far distant," the circular boasted, "when Bellevue will rank, not only as the first hospital in our country, but as one of the most important schools of medical education in the world."

There were no firm standards for admission beyond a three-year apprenticeship with "a responsible practitioner of medicine," which was rarely enforced. The curriculum included four terms of lectures, clinics in obstetrics and surgery, and dissection classes in the morgue. Graduation required an exam "in each of the departments of instruction" and "an acceptable thesis in the handwriting of the candidate." Forty percent of the entering class lived outside New York state, many coming from New England and a handful from foreign countries— a testament, it appeared, to the promise of a hospital-linked medical college.

That appeal, however, was not immediately realized. Students griped that there were too many boring lectures and too few bedside visits. And bitter feelings surfaced about *the habitual neglect of punctuality* among faculty members more interested in their "ordinary professional business" than in their teaching duties. Given the "liberal compensation" involved, the students clearly expected more. The end result was a vague faculty resolution regarding "dereliction of duty." But no penalties were enforced.

Bellevue's entering class was entirely white and male, reflecting the race and gender boundaries of the time. At Harvard Medical College a few years before, a tepid attempt by several faculty members to enroll a woman and three blacks had led to a full-scale campus revolt. Calling the move "socially repulsive," the students successfully threatened to resign en masse and "complete our medical studies elsewhere."

Until the Civil War, only one woman had ever earned a degree alongside men at an American medical school. In 1848, the dean of Geneva Medical College in upstate New York was asked by a physician friend to admit a brilliant candidate named Elizabeth Blackwell. A devoted feminist, born in England, Blackwell had been rejected everywhere else she had applied—one administrator telling her, "You cannot expect us to furnish you with a stick to break our heads with." Fearing a backlash, the Geneva dean agreed to let the students decide the issue by *unanimous* vote. The students, thinking it a joke, gave their boisterous consent.

When Blackwell arrived on campus two weeks later, "a hush fell upon the class," a witness recalled, "as if each member had been stricken with paralysis." Though Blackwell would graduate with honors, the reaction to her medical degree was severe. "It is much to be regretted," read a typical complaint, "that she has been led to aspire to . . . duties which by the order of nature and the common consent of the world devolve upon men." Geneva barred female students thereafter.

Women seeking to become physicians often attended female homeopathic colleges. Manhattan housed two of them by the 1860s, but with few available resources they encouraged their students to audit medical lectures at Bellevue, which were open to anyone who bought a ticket. In 1864, the *New York Times* published a story that surprised no one familiar with medical school culture: female visitors, it said, had been repeatedly insulted at Bellevue and dreaded going there.

The story sparked a flurry of letters. Some blamed an "ill-bred" clique of male students for making "gross remarks too shocking to the moral senses to even be repeated." Others, however, thought the boorish antics of the men less provocative than the misguided ambitions of the women. "The profession of medicine," said one, "is too high for them to aspire to."

A letter-writer calling herself "Mother of the Old School" worried that coeducation hurt both sexes by limiting what properly could be taught. Was it really possible to discuss intimate body parts and procedures in mixed company? "One of [our] ablest and most celebrated physicians has told me that in lecturing at Bellevue his cheek has blushed to find women as his auditors. With such feelings [he] cannot give true scope to his subject, his manliness is insulted [and he] must be obliged to study his language and clothe his sentences in a way least offensive to the [female] ear. Ought medical lecturers be thus annoyed and trammeled?"

The *Times* fully agreed. Certain occasions were ill-suited for mixed company, it thought, and this clearly was one. "For our part, we think it is incompatible with devotion to study . . . to have the sexes mingling in attendance at [one] of the great hospitals and medical schools of this city."

The issue would not soon disappear. While some Bellevue faculty tolerated female auditors, others tried to drive them away. In 1872, a furor erupted when a professor of surgery, preparing "a cancerous penis" for amputation, supposedly grabbed hold of the organ, stretched it playfully for maximum amusement, and remarked: "Gentlemen, this is an old penis. I would rather amputate a younger one as it would prevent more mischief." Then, counting aloud to three, he lopped off the cancerous part and tossed it "some distance" to the floor. As word of the incident spread, there were calls to fire the professor and replace him with "gentlemen who have not forgotten that their mothers, wives, and sisters are women."

Nothing came of it. Bellevue would remain the reluctant host for a generation of female auditors with nowhere else to turn. In 1916, looking back fifty years to her time as a medical student in New York City, Dr. Anna Manning Comfort recalled the dread she felt upon entering Bellevue's massive walls. "There were 500 men students. We were jeered and catcalled," she wrote, "and the 'old war horses,' the doctors joined the younger men. All the work at the hospital was made as repulsively unpleasant for us as possible."

Each visit brought a fresh insult. "If I wore square-toed shoes and swung my arms they said I was too mannish, and if I carried a parasol and wore a ribbon in my hair they said I was too feminine." Manning Comfort stuck it out as many of her classmates dropped away. Five decades had done little to dim the memories. Life for women students at Bellevue, she noted, was "beyond belief."

5

A HOSPITAL IN WAR

Bellevue Hospital Medical College opened its doors on April 11, 1861. The following day, Confederate gunners rained down cannon fire on Fort Sumter, in Charleston harbor, and the Civil War began.

No Northern metropolis was more divided by this conflict than New York. The city's financial elite—its bankers, speculators, and merchants—had extremely close ties to the Southern economy. Much of the credit needed by planters to buy slaves and harvest cotton came from Wall Street, and much of that cotton (or "white gold") was shipped to British factories through the port of New York. By the 1850s, wealthy Southerners were a fixture in the city, shopping with abandon and filling the best restaurants and hotels. Even the downtown theaters catered to their tastes, with romps about "happy-go-lucky" plantation life. "[Our] city," wrote the *New York Times* with modest exaggeration, "belongs almost as much to the South as to the North."

New York City was a Democratic Party stronghold with a powerful immigrant working-class base. In the 1860 presidential election, Republican candidate Abraham Lincoln had carried New York State while losing badly in the city. The key issue was race. Recent immigrants in particular feared the consequences of emancipation, which they believed would lead thousands of newly freed slaves to flood Northern cities in search of jobs and housing. Sooner or later, warned the New York *Daily News,* "we shall find negroes among us thicker than blackberries swarming everywhere." On the eve of the war, Democratic mayor Fernando Wood, a Southern sympathizer, actually floated the idea of turning New York into an independent entity—"a free city"—if the South seceded. Crazy or not, it raised the troubling question of whether Northern resolve was strong enough to preserve the Union. "The crucial test of this is New York City," wrote one local newspaper, "the spot most tainted by Southern poison."

The answer came quickly. Fort Sumter ended loose talk of pacifying the South. The idea of "a free city" died a merciful death as New Yorkers closed ranks behind the Union. "Flags from almost every building," Wall Street lawyer George Templeton Strong noted in his diary. "The city seems to have gone suddenly wild and crazy." When President Lincoln called for 75,000 volunteers to put down the "rebellion," New York's recruiting centers overflowed. Regiments formed overnight, led by immigrant units like the First German Rifles, the Garibaldi Guard, and the Irish Brigade. Black volunteers, however, were turned away.

With doctors in high demand, men of all ranks and ages at Bellevue rushed to enlist—on both sides. Three dozen interns would leave during the war to serve the Union cause, while fifteen would join the Confederacy—men like Moses John De Rosset, an "assistant surgeon of artillery" in Stonewall Jackson's command, and Isham Randolph Page, a "surgeon of artillery" in Robert E. Lee's Army of Northern Virginia. Students and interns supporting the Union received a "certificate of completion" from Bellevue for their military service. Those supporting the Rebels did not.

Each Union regiment, about one thousand strong, was assigned a surgeon and an assistant. Early on, these positions were filled mostly by hometown doctors who had never seen, much less performed, a serious operation. The Bellevue volunteers were a clear cut above, having dealt with knifings, shootings, and bone-crushing accidents. They'd also trained alongside top-flight surgeons like Frank H. Hamilton, who had just offered his own services to New York's 31st Regiment, which was expected to lead the fight.

At forty-seven, with a large family to support, Hamilton was not the typical volunteer. "Of medium stature, slightly built in appearance, with a mercurial temperament," he'd enlisted to be close to his oldest sons, who were already at the front. "I believed the war would not last but a few months," Hamilton recalled, "and I wished to be near my dear children in case they were wounded. In all this, my dear wife consented."

There was another reason, of course. As the nation's foremost military surgeon, Hamilton was expected to serve. Indeed, he'd been preparing two hundred Bellevue students "for the field" when the war broke out. A surgeon's job began with an examination of the recruits, Hamilton told them. Be alert for maladies that could cripple a regiment, he warned, listing hernias, severe limps, missing digits, rheumatism, chronic coughing, and strabismus, the medical term for "cross-eyed." And watch out for troublemakers, especially those "excited by liquor."

Severe limps and hernias would be the least of Hamilton's problems. In July 1861 his regiment was dispatched to Manassas, Virginia, along a creek known as Bull Run, to confront the Rebels in the first major battle of the war. Hamilton set up shop "in a snug wooden house, occupied by Negroes, as if we were in Bellevue," he wrote later. "The operating table was ready, the bed arranged, and the instruments, sponges, bandages, cordials, &c., in order." As the wounded fell, they were to be brought to the house in stretchers borne by "the drummer boys and a few volunteer aides, who together composed my ambulance corps." That, at least, was the plan.

The day went badly for Union forces. Poorly trained and led, they proved no match for Stonewall Jackson's infantry and Jeb Stuart's Black Horse Cavalry. Within hours, Hamilton was forced to abandon his position and move farther to the rear. His operating room became a tavern, then a private home, and finally a church. Supplies ran out. His stretcher-bearers fled. Hamilton performed two amputations that day, one below the knee, the other above the elbow joint. "Both of them, I confess, were done very badly," he recalled, "but I could, at the time, and under the circumstances, do no better. My back seemed broken and my hands were stiff with blood. We [soon] had no sponges and scarcely more water than was necessary to quench the thirst of the wounded men."

The Union retreat soon became a rout, with fleeing soldiers leaving the dead and injured behind. Though Hamilton would be captured twice by Confederate forces in future engagements—once in Tennessee and again in Kentucky—the panic at Bull Run would remain his most haunting wartime memory. "I could not tell them I was about to leave them," he said of the wounded, "and [trust] I did no wrong. I could be of no more service to them . . . and presumed they would be in the hands of a civilized and humane enemy who could care for them better than we could."

As with most desperate presumptions, it turned out to be wrong.

Like Dr. Hamilton, most Northerners had expected a quick and easy fight. Their adversary seemed badly overmatched. The North had more troops, more capital, more factories—indeed, more resources of almost every kind. "A Short War Probable," the *New York Times* had boasted. "We are opposed by troops who, whatever may be their personal courage or endurance, are vastly inferior in soldierly qualities to those of the North. . . . It is discipline that wins, and this is the last quality of which Southern soldiers are capable."

Bull Run demolished this fantasy. For the next eighteen months, Confederate troops easily beat back the Union's ponderous attempt to encircle Richmond, the South's wartime capital, inflicting heavy losses. Yet the fighting had proved an early bonanza for the North's large cities, none more so than New York. To finance the war, the Treasury Department had borrowed heavily from Wall Street to award military contracts to the city's factories, foundries, shipyards, and slaughterhouses. New Yorkers, wrote the admiring *Journal of Commerce,* have "learned how to prosper without the South."

A surreal quality took hold in the city. Shoppers who flocked to Macy's Department Store on 14th Street, or the more fashionable Lord & Taylor, couldn't help but pass the survivors of Bull Run and a dozen other battles, many without limbs, some with their faces shot away, others ravaged by disease. It was impossible to walk the streets without seeing a soldier's widow dressed in black or a military hearse go by. Or to pick up a newspaper without scanning the names, row upon row, of the missing and the dead.

Dark stories circulated, some of them true. New York's J. Pierpont

Morgan took advantage of the conflict to sell defective weapons to the army, while Brooks Brothers produced such shoddy uniforms for the local regiments that public rage forced the clothier to replace them free of charge. More troubling, though, was the growing chasm between the city's rich and poor. While the war boom created many jobs, severe inflation had caused a drop in working-class spending power. Meanwhile, the number of millionaires in New York jumped from a dozen to more than three hundred, with the top one percent of the pyramid accounting for close to 60 percent of the city's wealth. The resentment over poor soldiers fighting and dying in the midst of such avarice grew with each new luxury paraded by the rich. In terms of class conflict, a fuse had been lit.

The war dramatically transformed daily life at Bellevue—depleting its medical staff, on the one hand, while adding severely injured troops, on the other. In most cases, these soldiers would be treated first by the regimental surgeon, then at a facility behind the lines, and finally at a hospital near the patient's home. "The major event in my world has been the arrival of 400 sick and wounded soldiers from the James River," Dr. Titus Coan, a Bellevue physician, wrote his family in 1862. "We look every day for another transport from the seat of war with a new load for us." He added: "I think that our loss is much greater than is popularly supposed."

The numbers grew so large that General George McClellan, the top Union commander, visited Bellevue several times. "He spoke with each man," the physician noted, "asking such questions as 'What's the matter with you? What's your regiment? How is your wound? Does it give you much pain? Are you getting along pretty well?'" His concerns seemed heartfelt, a staffer observed. "He inquires with as much interest as their fathers would & they love him more than ever."

As physicians and medical students left for the front, Bellevue filled the void with inexperienced "contract doctors" hired by the government at $100 for a three-month stint. "I am house surgeon of the second surgical division [at Bellevue] and have besides the Lying-In Department, with 60–70 mothers and babies to take care of," Coan, just twenty-five, proudly wrote his family. "I have sole management unless I call in the visiting physician in cases of extreme gravity." Coan wasn't complaining: wartime Bellevue offered him a rare chance for growth and advancement. "This," he admitted, "is the ideal place for learning medicine."

John Vance Lauderdale, another "contract doctor," got to perform major surgery at Bellevue because so much of the staff was away. "I was just in blood to my elbows," the twenty-nine-year-old Lauderdale told his sister. "The scalpel was handed to me and an unfortunate man was relieved of a horribly lacerated leg." The patient was "doing well," Lauderdale boasted, adding: "It is *very* seldom that house staff are allowed to do anything of this sort."

There was less room now for Bellevue's former clientele. As the wounded poured in, hundreds of "noncritical" patients were packed off to Blackwell's Island. This process helped the bottom line, since the government paid a weekly stipend for each soldier and spent freely to outfit the recovery floors. "A stroll of inspection in and about Bellevue is not now what it was short years ago," a visitor observed, "when rats ran riot through the wards seeking whom they might devour, occasionally concentrating on a pauper baby for a midnight lunch."

Yet even with several thousand soldiers arriving at Bellevue during the war, the number of admissions actually declined. One reason, it appeared, was that the group most likely to burden the local jails, asylums, and hospitals had joined the army and left town. In the words of one relieved city official, "this reduction may be accounted for by the enlistment of men who have heretofore been driven to crime, or fallen into habits of inebriation and folly"—a clear stab at the Irish. "In regard to the female portion," he added, regretfully, "the war continues to keep up an increased supply."

There was more to these numbers, though, than the exodus of immigrant "riff-raff" from the city. Slow but steady changes had been occurring at Bellevue as it progressed from an almshouse appendage to a public hospital. By 1860, its patient base had moved beyond "the worst fed and worst nurtured" to include a fair share of the city's working classes. Bellevue would retain its primary mission, receiving "only patients who are unable to pay for their care." But its rules now required the superintendent to weed out those "who feign sickness to enjoy the comforts of a hospital."

The Bellevue ledgers of the 1860s give some sense of this change. One study of close to seven hundred nonsurgical patients showed the majority to be young, unmarried Irish immigrants holding down jobs as laborers and domestics. The most common illnesses included phthisis (tuberculosis), pneumonia, diarrhea, and acute alcoholism. About half of these patients would be discharged within two weeks, regardless of the diagnosis. Unlike the almshouse days, almost no one turned a stop at Bellevue into an indefinite stay.

Titus Coan's ledgers showed much the same thing. A number of Coan's admissions included drifters plucked from the city streets— men like "Thomas Rigney, 36, Irish: Went on a spree . . . Sick to stomach . . . Hands trembling . . . Face and eyes have peculiar expression." But for each Thomas Rigney one finds three or four entries like that of "John Crane, 45, Irish, manual laborer, never sick before, fell from a stone cart, broke right femur." And "Nicholas Duff, 13, run over by a coal-cart, fracturing his jaw, brain injury." And "Ellen Cummings, Irish, 52, domestic, had cramp in her leg and fell, fracturing right tibia." And "Michael Edwards, 19, Irish, cut off finger with an axe while chopping wood." In Coan's minute scribble can be traced Bellevue's evolution from a warehouse for the decrepit to a hospital for the working poor.

There would be curious exceptions, of course—the society woman badly mangled in a carriage accident, or the mysteriously poisoned financier needing his stomach pumped. And there'd be occasions, even then, of someone famous arriving in a state of unconsciousness and disarray. In the winter of 1863, a thirty-eight-year-old man was rushed to Bellevue from a Bowery flophouse with "injuries accidentally received." He had come in a police wagon following a fall that split open his head. He would die there three days later, with a few coins in his pocket.

No one recognized the patient at first, despite the odd notations on his chart. Under the column listing "nativity" was written "Pennsylvania," not "Ireland," and for "occupation" the odd word "composer" appeared. The man brought to Bellevue that day, his name spelled incorrectly, was Stephen Foster, the nation's most popular songwriter.

A prolific artist, Foster had written hundreds of ballads in his short life, including "Oh! Susanna," "Jeanie with the Light Brown Hair," and "My Old Kentucky Home." His final years were spent in New York City, living alone. It was there, in the back room of a tavern, that he composed "Beautiful Dreamer," his most memorable song. "What killed Stephen Foster?" his biographer wrote. "Drinking too much and eating too little had reduced him to a medically tenuous state that hemorrhaging exacerbated." Days before Foster's death, his brother in Pennsylvania had received this note: "Stephen I am sorry to inform you is lying in Bellevue Hospital in this city very sick. He desires me to ask you to send some pecuniary assistance [and] if possible he would like to see you in person." By the time Morrison Foster reached Bellevue, Stephen was dead. His body, stuffed under a pile of coffins in the morgue, was claimed just in time to avoid a pauper's grave—or worse, a medical school anatomy slab.

The story doesn't end there. Fifty years later, at a musical gala honoring Foster's legacy, an elderly man approached a reporter covering the event. "He introduced himself as Dr. John Vance Lauderdale, a retired United States Army surgeon . . . and said, 'I was the intern who received Stephen Foster at Bellevue Hospital when he was admitted to the charity ward. I remember it was a bitter winter's day. . . . I learned by accident that he was a famous songwriter and I said: "This man is a genius and should receive the best of care." I turned him over to another physician and we did the best we could for him until he died.'"

"Why was the body removed to the morgue to be with the unknown dead?" the reporter asked.

"Because there was nobody to claim him at the time," Dr. Lauderdale replied, knowing how close Foster came to a trip to Potter's Field.

In the summer of 1863, the Civil War took a decisive turn. At Gettysburg, Union troops under General George E. Meade repelled the Confederate assaults of Robert E. Lee, ending the South's long-planned invasion of the North. That very day—July 4—came word of the Confederate surrender at Vicksburg, putting Union forces in control of the Mississippi River and splitting the South in two. The toll was enormous: at Gettysburg alone, more than three thousand Union troops were killed and another fifteen thousand wounded—many from New York City. Bellevue would receive 618 men in the weeks following the battle, all badly injured, a surgeon noted, "but for one or two."

The victories at Gettysburg and Vicksburg came shortly after Congress passed the National Conscription Act of 1863. With the war in its third year, the Union could no longer count on volunteers to bear the load. Casualties were mounting, and desertions were on the rise. The act required all men between twenty and thirty-five (and single men up to forty-five) to register for the first compulsory draft in the nation's history—names to be drawn at a public lottery in mid-July. New York City's quota was a staggering 24,000.

The Conscription Act fell hardest on the working classes. Among other things, it excused anyone from service who paid a $300 fee or hired an "acceptable substitute" to go in his place. (Those who paid the fee included J. Pierpont Morgan and Theodore Roosevelt, Sr., father of the future president.) For many of the city's "dollar-a-day" laborers, such exemptions made it "a rich man's war but a poor man's fight." And the timing could hardly have been worse. The Conscription Act coincided with President Lincoln's recent Emancipation Proclamation, which revived fears among white immigrant workers of a massive slave exodus from the South. Trouble seemed likely, yet there were few federal troops in New York City to maintain order. Most had gone to Gettysburg to join General Meade.

On July 11, a hostile crowd gathered in midtown Manhattan to watch the lottery. Chanting "Down with the Rich," volunteer firemen from the Black Joke Engine Company, well known for their racism, charged the building and set it ablaze. What began as a protest against the draft soon engulfed the city in murderous conflict. Long-simmering divisions boiled over: rich against poor; white against black; Catholic against Protestant; immigrant against native-born. Before it ended, five days later, more than a hundred were dead and parts of Manhattan lay in ruins.

At first, anti-draft sentiment had enjoyed wide public support. But the rioting that followed—what *The Irish-American,* New York's largest ethnic newspaper, called "a saturnalia of pillage and violence"—

had a strong ethnic tinge. Irish immigrants appeared to dominate the mobs that destroyed the townhouses of the rich, ransacked the better department stores, torched the Colored Orphan Asylum, and lynched dozens of helpless blacks in an orgy of race-based, class-fueled rage. George Templeton Strong described the rioters as a mix of "the lowest Irish day laborers . . . stalwart young vixens and withered old hags." Others reluctantly agreed. "There is no denying it!" fumed the *New York Tablet,* organ of the Catholic archdiocese. "Shame! Shame on such Irishmen; they are a disgrace to the country from which they came."

Confronting these mobs first fell to the city's outmanned, largely Irish American police force. "New York's Civil War generated its own fratricide," wrote one historian. "If many of the rioters were Irish, so were the police who challenged them in hand-to-hand combat." But it took five thousand federal troops, rushed back from Gettysburg, to finally clear the streets with bayonet charges and field howitzers fired at point-blank range.

Bellevue, meanwhile, filled up with bodies—some grievously wounded, others dispatched to the morgue. The victims included "Mary Williams, 24, a colored woman, terribly injured while being pursued by the infuriated mob," and "a colored man, name unknown, whose head was beaten to a jelly, and there is no such thing as recognizing him." There were mortally wounded policemen ("Peter McIntyre, 34, beaten with an iron pipe"), innocent bystanders ("John Mills, 8, shot through the right eye while looking out the window of his residence"), and scores of street rioters ("Patrick McSweeney, 24, barkeeper, shot in both legs," "Margaret Mullaney, 28, domestic, shot in the breast," "John Ennis, 16, plumber, injured by a club to the head"). "A gong has struck again," a surgeon wrote in his diary, noting Bellevue's emergency call. "A large [Irishman] is carried up. We visit him. A ball has gone through his body [and] he vomits blood. All we can do won't save him. We leave him to Father Larkin the priest who will get him to answer a few questions concerning his faith in the Catholic religion. This won't save him either for time or eternity, I fear."

There was irony, no doubt, in treating draft protesters where wounded Union soldiers lay. The surgeon chose his words carefully. Punish the violent lawbreakers, he wrote that evening, but don't ignore their rage. "I hope the scenes that have been enacted in this city this week will remind [us] that people, no matter how humble, are not to be trifled with. Life is the gift of every man and no one can say to his neighbor that his life is more valuable. . . . All must stand on equal footing. . . . All must be alike."

"War is the normal condition of mankind; peace is the abnormal condition," Bellevue's Frank Hamilton observed in his influential tome, *A Treatise on Military Surgery and Hygiene,* published in 1865. "This statement is not flattering to a people claiming Christianity and boasting of its civilization; but it is nevertheless true." Having seen the worst that war had to offer in his early service at Bull Run—from poor planning to outright cowardice—Hamilton devoted himself to correcting the battlefield flaws that left him helpless in the field. Well connected—his brother-in-law chaired the Senate Committee on Military Affairs—he rose to become medical inspector of the Union Army, a post with a bully pulpit built in. A food faddist, Hamilton brought changes to the atrocious army diet of salt beef, beans, and hardtack (rocklike crackers known to the men as "worm castles") by demanding fresh fruits and vegetables to ward off scurvy, dysentery, and explosive diarrhea. "The art of cookery," he insisted, "is as important as the art of defense."

Little escaped his eye. "Drawers may be necessary in the winter, but are not needed in the summer," he wrote of the proper field attire, noting that "it is sometimes advantageous to change the sock from one foot to the other, so that their seams or folds should press upon new points." But no amount of preparation, no attention to detail, could spare the country from the slaughter that followed. Combined Union and Confederate deaths in the Civil War totaled close to 750,000, with disease and infection taking twice as many lives as battlefield wounds. Much of the carnage resulted from improved weaponry at the front. New artillery pieces lobbed bigger shells longer distances with greater accuracy, and a revolutionary bullet—known as the Minié ball after its creator, French army captain Claude Minié—allowed the average soldier to regularly hit a target a fair distance away. More easily loaded, the hollow Minié spun from its barrel, increasing its power and velocity—and thus the damage it could do.*

The war became Hamilton's private laboratory, allowing him to observe and experiment on a scale that not even chaotic Bellevue could match. In terms of surgery, where his real expertise lay, Hamilton offered recommendations for every imaginable injury, from arrow wounds to gunshots of the "male organs," which, he admitted, "presented a great variety of complications." His instructions for amputation, complete with diagrams, became a bible of sorts for surgeons in the field.

Over time, in novels and memoirs, a portrait emerged of the terrified soldier—tied to a stretcher, prepared with a shot or two of whiskey, a piece of wood or metal between his teeth (thus the phrase "bite the bullet"), writhing in pain as an arm or leg is sawed off and tossed into an ever-growing pile of body parts on the floor. Union surgeons performed about thirty thousand amputations during the war, but most did, in fact, involve anesthesia. With luck, the patient avoided the two primary dangers of the operating table: blood loss and infection. Surgeons learned that the odds depended partly on body location. Amputating a hand or a foot, far from the trunk, was far less dangerous than amputating at the hip. Soldiers with gaping chest and stomach wounds rarely survived. The treatment in these cases was to make the victim comfortable—with morphine, if possible—until he died.

Anesthesia marked the first half of a surgical revolution. The second half—antisepsis—had yet to arrive. For most doctors, the concept that one could lessen the chances of infection by scrubbing his hands, wearing gloves, and sterilizing his tools seemed vaguely absurd. "We operated in old-blood-stained and often pus-stained coats . . . with undisinfected hands," a Union surgeon recalled of the typical operation of the time. American medicine in the 1860s had yet to grasp that

---

* Until recently, the accepted figure for Civil War deaths was 618,000, with 360,000 on the Union side and 258,000 on the Confederate side. A recent study, however, using the latest detailed census data, has increased that number by 20 percent, and hints that the figure may be even higher. J. David Hacker, "A Census-Based Count of the Civil War Dead," *Civil War History* (December 2011), 307–48.

people shared their world with billions of invisible organisms, and that what a surgeon didn't see around the operating table was what normally caused the most harm.

Frank Hamilton was a perfect example. Read today, his instructions are a virtual guide to death by infection. "In attempting to remove a ball by incision, the surgeon ought, if practicable, to seize upon it with the thumb and fore-finger and hold upon it firmly until the incision is made and the removal accomplished," he wrote at one point, adding: "Sometimes it is more convenient to entrust this duty to an assistant." His concluding remarks were firmer still: "Indeed, under almost all circumstances, we prefer the finger as being the most intelligent guide as causing, on the whole, as little pain as any other method of exploration." Nowhere in the 674 pages of *A Treatise on Military Surgery and Hygiene* is anyone encouraged to wash his hands.

It is unfair, of course, to judge someone by the standards of later times. "Civil War surgeons had to work without knowledge of the nature of infection and without drugs to treat it," wrote one student of the field. "To criticize them for this lack of knowledge is equivalent to criticizing Ulysses S. Grant and Robert E. Lee for not calling in air strikes." Still, few physicians used the clinical experience of the war to greater advantage than Frank Hamilton. His inventions included a serrated bone cutter, a special forceps to remove bullet fragments, and various splints to treat difficult fractures. His precise guidelines for bone settings helped many to walk without a limp, and he would even become a pioneer in the use of plastic surgery for severe facial injuries. He was, an admirer gushed, the "Surgeon Extraordinary of the Union Army."

Hamilton returned to Bellevue in 1864 a national hero. With Union forces on the offensive, he took up his old position as professor of military surgery and fractures, training medical students and interns for the final push of the war. Most were in awe of him. "I cannot recall learning anything from [other Bellevue surgeons]," a student noted. "They were irregular in attendance and entrusted almost everything to the internees. But Hamilton came regularly and punctually, usually on a large iron-grey charger and equipped with riding boots and spurs."

Among these students was twenty-three-year-old Charles Augustus Leale from Westchester County, New York, his portrait showing a slight man with long sideburns and a faint mustache. Graduating from Bellevue Hospital Medical College in 1865, Leale had been commissioned as an assistant surgeon at a military hospital in Washington, D.C., on the eve of the Confederate surrender, arriving in time to hear President Lincoln deliver a public address—it would be his last—from the White House balcony. "I was profoundly impressed with his divine appearance," Leale recalled, "as he stood in the rays of light, which penetrated the windows."

Leale saw Lincoln a few nights later when he bought a ticket to the comedy *Our American Cousin* at Ford's Theatre on the evening of April 14. Leale heard a commotion and then watched as the assassin John Wilkes Booth leaped to the stage. "I instantly arose and in response to cries for help and for a surgeon," he wrote, "I crossed the aisle and vaulted over the seats to the President's box . . . With the calmest deliberation and force of will I . . . walked forward to my duty."

These words come from a speech Leale delivered in 1909, forty-four years after the event. Leale had rarely spoken of it before then, claiming the need to honor the privacy of the fallen president. But 1909 marked the centennial of Lincoln's birth, and Leale finally agreed "to give the detailed facts as I know them." Relying on what he claimed were his personal notes from 1865, Leale placed himself at the center of the drama, put there, he insisted, by Mrs. Lincoln herself. "I grasped [her] outstretched hand in mine, while she cried piteously to me, 'Oh, Doctor! Is he dead? Will you take charge of him? Do what you can for him. Oh, my dear husband!'"

The president was slumped over, his eyes completely closed. Having seen a dagger in Booth's hand, Leale checked Lincoln's body for stab wounds, but found none. "I lifted his eyelids and saw evidence of a brain injury," Leale noted. "I quickly passed the separated fingers of both hands through his blood matted hair to examine his head, and I discovered his mortal wound." Calling upon his recent training— Leale had faithfully attended Hamilton's lectures—he "removed the obstructing clot of blood," pressed his fingers down the president's throat to open the larynx, performed mouth-to-mouth resuscitation, and vigorously pumped the chest until "a feeble action of the heart and irregular breathing followed."

Charles Augustus Leale, a few months removed from medical school, held the fate of the Republic in his hands. "Many looked on," he said, "but not once did anyone suggest a word or in any way interfere with my actions." It was Leale, in his telling, who ordered the president moved to a house across the street from Ford's Theatre, believing that the longer trip to the White House would surely kill him. It was Leale who sent for the surgeon general, then for Lincoln's personal physician, minister, and family. It was Leale who prolonged "the life of President Lincoln for nine hours" before drawing "a white sheet over the martyr's face."

The 1909 speech caused a minor sensation. Reporters, accepting Leale's version of events at face value, showed no interest in seeing the notes he claimed to have. Did they actually exist? In 2012 a researcher at the National Archives in Washington stumbled upon the twenty-one-page report that Leale had dictated in the hours following Lincoln's death. It's a remarkable piece of history—a meticulous hour-by-hour account of a hopeless medical struggle—revealing that Leale was, indeed, the first doctor to reach the stricken president. Finding Lincoln "in a profoundly comatose position," Leale did check the body for stab wounds before locating the fatal bullet hole behind the ear. From this point forward, however, the 1865 report bears little resemblance to the speech Leale delivered in 1909.

Two points stand out. First, Leale's 1865 report makes no mention of the heroics he supposedly performed—opening Lincoln's throat, giving him mouth-to-mouth resuscitation, or pumping his chest. How could Leale have omitted such vital details from his report, written hours after the assassination? And why did he choose to add them to his account in 1909? The likely answer to both questions is that Leale was determined to go down in history as having used all measures to save Lincoln's life—whether he did so or not. Since a procedure like chest compression was rarely employed in America in the 1860s, he probably did not.

In his 1865 report, moreover, Leale said that he had placed his finger deep into Lincoln's wound to look for dangerous bullet fragments.

In doing so, he was following the common practice laid out by his famous mentor. "The natural structure of the brain is so soft and fragile that when we introduce a probe it is almost impossible to determine whether we are following the track of the ball or not," Frank Hamilton wrote in his treatise on military surgery. "The finger is the safer instrument." But Leale made little mention of this in his 1909 speech, for good reason. The coming of Germ Theory and antiseptic medicine in the 1870s had ended the practice of sticking an unwashed digit into an open wound. No respectable physician in 1909 would have attempted such a potentially fatal maneuver. As such, Leale likely deleted the reference to meet modern standards of practice—and thus preserve his good name.

Leale claimed in his 1865 report that Lincoln's personal physician, Dr. Robert Stone, was satisfied with the early treatment the president had received. This probably is true. Leale appears to have faithfully carried out Frank Hamilton's instructions for dealing with the sort of wound Lincoln had suffered: stay calm, make the patient comfortable, look for clots, stem the bleeding, and feel gently for the bullet, using one's finger if need be. In the end, embellishments aside, Leale had served the president well under immensely trying conditions, doing everything he had learned to save a mortally wounded man. Leale didn't pronounce Lincoln dead on the morning of April 15, 1865, as he later claimed; that job fell to the surgeon general. But he did remain with Lincoln till the end, feeling for his pulse and gently massaging his hand. Asked why, Leale replied that common compassion demanded no less. "Sometimes recognition and reason return just before departure," he said. "I held his hand firmly to let him know, in his blindness, that he had a friend."

Word of the assassination spread quickly over the wires. In New York City, where so many had vilified the president for so long, the mood seemed especially grim. "Lincoln's death—thousands of flags at half mast—& on numbers of them long black pennants," wrote the poet Walt Whitman. "Business public and private all suspended, & the shops closed—strange mixture of horror, fury, tenderness, & a stirring wonder brewing." Lawyer George Templeton Strong, no friend of the president, was haunted by deep feelings of loss. "I am stunned as by a fearsome personal calamity . . . ," he confessed in his diary. "We shall appreciate him at last."

Bellevue's iconic surgeon Valentine Mott, now eighty, was "overwhelmed" by the news. A friend and great admirer of the president, Mott had just completed an exhausting stint as chairman of a federal commission investigating the mistreatment of "starved and tortured" Union prisoners released early from Andersonville, Belle Isle, and other Confederate POW camps. "In the whole of my surgical experience, not excepting the most painful operations on deformed limbs, I have never suffered so much in my life at the sight of anything," he admitted. "It unnerved me. I felt sick."

Mott was back in New York City recovering from the experience when the assassination occurred. "He regarded it as an omen of ill import," a friend recalled, "[and] was never himself again afterwards." A fever soon developed, sending Mott to bed. Visitors to his Gramercy Park mansion thought him "despondent" and "sick at heart," though not deathly ill. Even his former Bellevue colleague Austin Flint, a superb diagnostician, could find no physical symptoms beyond exhaustion.

On April 24, 1865, Lincoln's funeral train reached Jersey City on its long journey to Springfield, Illinois. The coffin was ferried across the Hudson River to Manhattan the next morning, then placed in a hearse led by six gray horses and driven through the streets as church bells tolled and cannons thundered. It was the largest procession New York City had ever seen, and it came within a few blocks of Mott's Gramercy Park mansion en route to the railroad depot. Mott could hear the mourners pass by, but felt too ill to join them. He died the following day—"a victim," it was said, "of the same blow that robbed the nation of its chief."

6

"HIVES OF SICKNESS AND VICE"

I s war good for medicine?" The answer for most observers over the centuries has been a clear, if sometimes grudging, yes. Trauma care, nursing, pain relief, disease control, evacuating the wounded—all have advanced dramatically through trial and error on the battlefield. "He who would become a surgeon," Hippocrates advised long ago, "should join an army and follow it."

The Civil War was no different. It came at a pivotal time for medicine, as old certainties crumbled and new ideas took hold. Anesthesia now was commonplace, as we've seen, and the "age of heroic medicine" was fading fast. Indeed, one of the lesser-known bureaucratic struggles of the Civil War involved the order by Surgeon General William A. Hammond to ban calomel and other violent purgatives from the army's medical supply chain—a move that angered many older physicians. At thirty-four, the brash, demanding Hammond also required applicants for the post of regimental surgeon to take a written examination, which most of them promptly failed. The dismal test results—Hammond privately described them as the "vague and confused" ramblings of illiterates—led him to propose a solution whose time had not yet come: a medical college for career officers.

Such efforts came at great personal cost. Until Hammond's appointment, the position of surgeon general had been something of a sinecure, filled by men of modest distinction. The pace of reform and criticism pouring from his office was unprecedented. In 1864, with a long and growing list of old-guard critics at his heels, Hammond was court-martialed and found guilty of "conduct unbecoming an officer and a gentleman" for allegedly purchasing inferior supplies for the troops—a trumped-up charge that would be discredited long after the war had ended. His army career in shambles, Hammond moved to New York City, opened a lucrative private practice, and accepted a position at Bellevue Hospital Medical College as the first professor of neurology—"diseases of the mind and nervous system"—in the United States.

As surgeon general, Hammond had been among those demanding change. But from a strictly medical standpoint, the war brought few breakthroughs of lasting note. Despite the use of anesthesia, surgical methods barely advanced, postoperative infections were rampant, and dangerous vapors, or miasmas, still explained the transmission of most diseases. One expert aptly described the Civil War as the final conflict of "the medical middle ages." Its awful fate, wrote another, was to have occurred on the cusp of a curative revolution, just "ahead of the medical care it required."

Still, Hammond's impact was substantial. He'd been recommended for the job by the U.S. Sanitary Commission, a privately funded group of reformers devoted to improving the health of the troops. As such, Hammond focused on the daily conditions in the field. He understood the dangers of bringing thousands of men together in close quarters, where facilities were crude and personal habits often revolting. He knew that many had never used a latrine, or been vaccinated against smallpox, or taught the importance of bathing and washing their clothes. For Hammond, there were more lives to be saved beyond the surgical tent than within it—through education, nutrition, and hygiene.

It seems fitting that he wound up at Bellevue following the war. The best medical handbooks for Union officers had been developed there, and the treatment of wounded soldiers had been a top priority. No civilian hospital had done more for the war effort than Bellevue, and none would put its lessons to better use.

Not all of them had been forged on the battlefield. Indeed, many of Hammond's views on sanitation had come from Bellevue surgeon Stephen Smith, who had spent most of the Civil War in New York City providing health care to the poor. The two men had become allies

in these years, facing similar problems in different domains. Where
Hammond had confronted a deeply hostile military brass, Smith had
drawn an opponent equally determined to bring him down. Dominat-
ing New York City's political landscape, it went by the name of Tammany Hall.

It would be hard to imagine a more one-sided fight: the lonely health
crusader versus New York City's ever-expanding political machine.
Named for the mythical Delaware chief said to have carved out Niagara Falls, Tammany had evolved from an elite club, whose early members included Vice President Aaron Burr and future president Martin
Van Buren, into a massive welfare agency for recent immigrants, especially the Irish. Tammany provided everything from jobs and food to
bail money and a proper burial—all without preachy condescension.
What Tammany got in return were votes, a process facilitated by its
role in helping these newcomers to become citizens. By the 1860s, it
controlled most of the elected offices and patronage positions in the
city.

The indelible face of Tammany in these years was William Magear
Tweed, the grand sachem and unquestioned leader. Elected to the
New York State Senate in 1868, and a member of the city's powerful
Board of Supervisors, Tweed pushed projects dear to the poor, such as
orphanages and public baths. He lobbied the state legislature to fund
parochial schools and he put thousands of immigrants on the city payroll, many doing Tammany's political spadework, or no work at all.
New York City—indeed, America—had never seen anyone quite like
the three-hundred-pound Tweed. A legendary brawler with a massive
appetite for food and drink, mistresses and jewelry, he embezzled funds
estimated in the hundreds of millions, lived in a Fifth Avenue mansion with "mahogany stables trimmed in silver," and became the third-
largest landowner in Manhattan. "Plunder of the city treasury . . . was
no new thing in New York," wrote James Bryce, Britain's distinguished
historian and public servant in *The American Commonwealth*, "but it
had never before reached such colossal dimensions." Tweed's bloated
persona, compliments of cartoonist Thomas Nast, would come to

symbolize the egregious corruption of urban American politics following the Civil War.

Stephen Smith could hardly have been more different. Born on a farm in upstate New York, the son of a Revolutionary War cavalry officer, he'd come to Bellevue in 1850, attracted by its clinical riches. Typhus was then at its height. Working on the wards, he discovered that many of the victims had listed the same address, a tenement on East 22nd Street not far from Bellevue itself. Smith paid a visit—and his life's calling began. "The doors and windows were broken; the cellar was partly filled with filthy sewage; every available place . . . was crowded with immigrants, men, women, and children. . . . The necessity of closing this house . . . until it was thoroughly cleansed and made decently habitable, was imperative."

Confident he had found the source of typhus in the tenement's "foul emissions," Smith tracked down the landlord—"a wealthy man, living in an aristocratic neighborhood"—who couldn't have cared less. New York City had no Board of Health to complain to, and no laws to protect tenants from neglect. "In this extremity," Smith recalled, "I visited the office of the *Evening Post* and explained the matter to Mr. William Cullen Bryant, then editor of that newspaper."

A leading poet and journalist, Bryant had big plans for New York City; his legacy would include the development of Central Park and the adjoining Metropolitan Museum of Art, and his newspaper was already sparring with Tammany over matters of fraud and corruption in civic life. Viewing Smith as a potential ally, Bryant agreed to pursue the complaint. A reporter was dispatched to interview the offending landlord, who, fearing a front-page exposé, agreed to make the needed repairs.

The incident became a catalyst for sanitary reform. Using Bellevue as his bully pulpit, Smith warned that New York faced a future of ever-widening epidemics, with thousands dying needlessly from disease. And, like Cullen Bryant, he blamed it on the pork and patronage of Tammany Hall. Real reform, both men believed, would require intervention by political forces beyond New York City.

The Civil War intervened. Social issues gave way to military concerns. At Hammond's request, Smith wrote a popular manual for Union field surgeons and inspected a number of military hospitals. Still, the tug of public health remained. Smith fumed, sometimes out loud, over the nation's misplaced priorities, at one point describing Tammany as a deadlier threat to New Yorkers than the Confederate army. "The country is horrified when a thousand victims fall in an ill-fought battle," he wrote in 1863, "but in this city 10,000 die annually of diseases which city authorities have the power to remove, and no one is shocked."

Not for long, it turned out. That fall, the cream of New York society—John Jacob Astor, Jr., August Belmont, and Peter Cooper, among them—formed a Citizens' Association to address these concerns. The timing was hardly accidental. The city had just endured the most violent summer in its history—the Draft Riots—and these men could feel the class antagonisms bubbling up from below.

What, exactly, had caused such a dramatic collapse of the social order that July, and what could be done to prevent another? Stephen Smith suggested that both questions might be answered by looking at the squalid living conditions where the violence had been worst. He recommended a survey of "the sufferings, perils, and sanitary wants" of the city, which the Citizens' Association agreed to fund. The budget was generous; dozens of young doctors—most with a Bellevue connection—were hired to do the legwork. "As a body," Smith assured the benefactors, "they represent the best medical talent of the junior portion of the profession of New York. Many occupy high social positions, and all [are] men of refinement, education, and devotion to duty."

The final report, *Sanitary Conditions of the City*, ran to 367 pages (with seventeen volumes of accompanying data). Directed by Smith, it is now considered one of the most influential public health documents in American history. The investigators—one per ward—compiled every imaginable statistic: births, deaths, and different diseases; the condition of streets and pavements; the disposal of garbage and house-slops; the location of indoor toilets and outdoor privies. There were maps and diagrams charting virtually every structure in the city: schools, churches, tenements, factories, slaughterhouses, taverns, brothels, stables, and pigpens.

More dramatic, however, were the descriptions. From the Fourth Ward inspector came this: "On a piece of ground 240 feet by 150, there are 20 tenant-houses occupied by 111 families, 5 stables, a large soap and candle factory, and a tan-yard. . . . The filth and stench of this locality are beyond any power of description."

From the Eighth Ward inspector: "The instances are many in which one or more families . . . of all ages and both sexes, are congregated in [a] single . . . apartment. Here they eat, drink, sleep, work, dress and undress without the possibility of . . . privacy. What is the consequence? The sense of shame—the greatest, surest safeguard of virtue, except the grace of God—is gradually blunted, ruined, and finally destroyed."

From the Fifteenth Ward inspector: "In a dark and damp cellar, about 18 feet square and 7 feet high, lived a family of seven persons; within the past year two have died of typhus, two of smallpox, and one has been sent to the hospital with erysipelas. . . . This occurred but a short distance from the very heart of the city."

New York was now among the most densely populated places in the world. Close to half the population lived in foul tenements or subterranean cellars that never saw the sun. As a result, its mortality rate far exceeded that of other American cities like Boston and Philadelphia, and had even passed such notorious European pestholes as London and Liverpool. Manhattan Island—blessed with two great rivers, cleansing sea breezes, and abundant vegetation—had become a frightfully dangerous place.

Worse still were the divisions *within* the city, where the mortality rate for a slum dweller was five times higher than for someone "of a better class." There always had been differences, the report noted, but not to this degree. The alarming truth was that New York had become two distinct cities: one prosperous, content, and healthy, the other marred by "filth, overcrowding, excrement, putrid exhalations, and disease."

Time was running out. The current crisis wasn't just about public health, the report insisted, but about public order as well. The Draft Riots hadn't occurred in a social vacuum; they signaled the collective rage of the perpetrators, as even a glance at their neighborhoods made clear. The "closely packed houses where the mobs originated seemed to be literally hives of sickness and vice," the report went on, quoting a witness at the scene. "[It is] difficult to believe that so much misery, disease, and wretchedness can be huddled together . . . so near our own abodes."

Armed with the survey, Smith traveled to Albany to testify before the state legislature. In scathing remarks, covered closely in the press, he blamed Tammany for the crisis and begged the legislators for help. No longer could anyone call New York a safe or healthy city, he argued, and no longer could anyone ignore the reasons why. The streets were filthy because local aldermen controlled the contracts for garbage collection, which rarely took place. Privies overflowed into drinking wells because the money allotted for inspections and repairs wound up in the pockets of Tammany hacks. Tenements resembled death traps because well-connected landlords never made repairs. "To what depth of humiliation must [we] descend," Smith pleaded, before an outraged citizenry stepped forward to say: Enough!

His testimony was, by all accounts, a withering indictment of politics run amuck. Smith had not only called out Tweed and his henchmen for corruption, he'd also accused them of jeopardizing the health and safety of their own constituents—the immigrant slum dwellers of New York. "Practically, [we] are a city without any sanitary government," he warned. "The evidence proves that at least half a million of our population are literally submerged in filth. . . . Children growing up in this pestilential atmosphere become vicious and brutal, not from any natural depravity, but because they are mentally incapable of [anything else.]"

Smith had some formidable support. Much of the business elite stood behind him, as did the prestigious New York Academy of Medicine and top Republican newspapers like the *Evening Post,* the *Times,* and the *Tribune,* always anxious to bludgeon Tammany's Democratic machine. In 1866, following intense maneuvering, the state legislature passed a landmark bill, written almost entirely by Smith, which created a Metropolitan Board of Health for New York City and the surrounding area. The key board members would be state-appointed, leaving Tweed and his followers to fume—with good reason—about the "encroachment upon our right to govern ourselves." Given the mandate to "preserve life" and "prevent the spread of disease," the board quickly replaced Tammany's forty-four part-time health wardens—a position normally handed to graft-hungry saloon owners—with a group of full-time salaried physicians.

The Metropolitan Health Act was the first of its kind in the United States. Many consider it a turning point in the history of American city life. Even Stephen Smith put aside his normal modesty to call the law "the most complete piece of health legislation ever placed on the statute books." Mortality rates in New York City had climbed so dramatically by 1870 that one child in five would not live to see his first birthday, and 25 percent of those who did reach adulthood would die before the age of thirty. Some perished in the terrifying epidemics that periodically swept the region, but many more now fell to endemic diseases related to overcrowding, poor sanitation, and miserable working conditions—in short, the plagues of modern city life.

Where to begin? Each tenement privy in New York served up to a hundred people, and there were no public bathrooms. Slaughterhouses butchered more than a million animals each year, letting the blood run into open sewers and leaving the entrails to rot in the gutters. Horse manure covered the thoroughfares, attracting swarms of flies. "Swill Milk Dairies" (so named because the cows fed on the swill, or waste products, of local breweries) sold a watery liquid almost guaranteed to sicken children. Public markets were littered with rodents and spoiled food.

As both a city health commissioner and a Bellevue surgeon, Smith saw the damage everywhere. His strategy, he recalled, was to attack some of the worst abuses in order to impress the burdened working classes and thereby neutralize Tammany Hall. It seemed to work. Using its police powers, the Board of Health closed down the vile Washington Market (which sued but lost in court) and enforced the seldom-used ordinances against driving herds of cattle through residential streets—the first step in moving all slaughterhouses, cow barns, tanneries, and glue factories out of residential neighborhoods. The board also placed hydrants throughout the city to provide safe drinking water and spent $3,500 to build a public urinal in teeming lower Manhattan, an addition described as "eminently successful and always thronged during the entire day."

Before long, Smith was claiming that New York's streets were cleaner than they'd been in years, which likely was true. But more important was the reversal of the city's alarming mortality rate, which, in the decades following 1870, began a steady decline. There were many reasons for this, as we shall see, but Smith's role was crucial. A pioneer in what he called "preventive medicine," Smith championed causes from improving childhood nutrition to developing accurate health statistics to planting shade trees in slum neighborhoods. Seeking allies, he founded the American Public Health Association, which helped turn a well-meaning social cause into a highly trained profession.

No one would do more to make Bellevue a center for medical innovation than Stephen Smith. His footprints are everywhere. The hospital ambulance, the professionalization of nursing, the use of medical photography—all would come alive, in one way or another, through his personal intervention. Generations of Bellevue interns and medical students would inherit his passion for public health.

A food faddist and something of a mystic, Smith slept with his head facing north to keep the mind sharp, while prescribing red wine for most nervous disorders. The very idea of retirement appalled him; he insisted that humans could easily reach one hundred years with the proper mental attitude and medical care. Asked for the secret of his longevity, Smith, who would live to ninety-nine, was typically brief. "Work and keep out of the easy chair," he said. Anything else? Well, yes, Smith replied with his usual foresight. "Don't eat too much meat."

7

THE BELLEVUE AMBULANCE

R ead today, a century and a half later, *Sanitary Conditions of the City* remains a medical tour de force. Combining a researcher's thirst for data with a moralist's sense of outrage, it stressed the primacy of public health in the nation's emerging urban-industrial order. Having written much of the document, as well as the legislation that followed, Stephen Smith had expected New York to become the model for other cities. And that meant finding dedicated professionals to move the agenda forward—much like the young doctors who had done the vital legwork for his survey. Among the top positions to be filled was that of sanitary superintendent, the one formerly used by Tammany to sprinkle patronage among its troops. Smith had a candidate in mind, a former Bellevue intern named Edward Dalton. It would prove an inspired choice—if not in the way that Smith, or anyone else at the time, could have imagined.

Born in Lowell, Massachusetts, in 1834, the son and grandson of physicians, Dalton graduated from Harvard, and then the College of Physicians and Surgeons, before winning a Bellevue internship, where he worked under the formidable trio of Drs. Smith, Frank Hamilton, and Valentine Mott. Small in stature, with thick spectacles and boy-ish features, he gave "the appearance of extreme delicacy," his brother recalled, and suffered constantly from illness and disease. When war came in 1861, however, Dalton did what was expected of him, joining the Union Army as a regimental surgeon.

His first tour ended quickly. Attached to a New York unit during
General McClellan's failed assault on Richmond, Dalton fell victim
to "the unwholesome exhalations of the Chickahominy swamps"—
a likely reference to malaria. But he did return to the war in time for
the savage fighting at Antietam, where his talent for medical administration caught the eye of those in command. Put in charge of several
field hospitals, Dalton wound up supervising "the removal and care
of the sick and wounded" in General Ulysses S. Grant's Army of the
Potomac during the final push toward Appomattox. The numbers were
astonishing: Dalton's largest hospital on the James River, an encampment of 1,200 tents spread over two hundred acres, treated close to seventy thousand soldiers enduring battle wounds, dysentery, pneumonia,
and other maladies. Never "in the history of the war," wrote William
Howell Reed in his magisterial account of the Union Medical Corps,
had anybody run "the complicated machinery of hospital administration . . . to such perfection."

And no part of that machinery needed more oiling than battlefield evacuation. The North had entered the Civil War without an
ambulance corps because no one believed the conflict would last long
enough to justify the expense. This oversight proved catastrophic. For
a time, the job of gathering the wounded fell to the lowest elements
of the regiment—cooks, drummer boys, and those deemed unfit for
combat—using carts, wheelbarrows, anything that moved. In 1862,
Surgeon General Hammond had begged the War Department to act,
citing "the frightful state of disorder [in] removing the [fallen] from
the field." Having seen the disaster at Bull Run, where hundreds had
died of thirst, shock, and exposure, lying untended for days, Hammond convinced General McClellan to form an ambulance corps.
Used first at Antietam, it was in full swing by Gettysburg, where close
to a thousand horse-drawn wagons, known as "gut-busters" for their
painfully rough ride, were on duty round-the-clock.

By war's end, the ambulance was widely recognized as a lifesaving
tool. The next step seemed clear enough: if thousands of wounded
men could be safely plucked from the chaotic hell of Antietam and
Gettysburg, surely this concept could be applied to civilian life as well.
But no one, least of all Stephen Smith, viewed an ambulance corps as

a top priority given the massive health problems facing New York City in 1869. Smith had picked Dalton because of his obvious administrative talents—a view reinforced by none other than General Grant, who had warmly recommended his former subordinate as "the best man in the United States" for the job. Dalton, though, was adamant. While devising plans for citywide sanitary inspections, he proposed an idea, known as "Rapid Response," that used police wagons to carry the sick and injured to Bellevue. The civilian ambulance seemed an obvious next step.

It wasn't hard to see the need. In the past, a person lying in the gutter might be comforted by caring strangers, brought to the nearest druggist for "restoratives," and then dumped into a passing conveyance for a bone-jarring ride to a hospital, or perhaps back home. These were the lucky ones: many more victims were left untreated until it was too late, much like the wounded Union soldiers at Bull Run. In pushing his case, Dalton compared the shameful neglect of these soldiers to the current situation in New York, his favorite example being an exhausted workingman who had fallen from a streetcar one night near the Battery, at the southern tip of Manhattan. "He was taken to the nearest house, and there he lay bleeding . . . while kindly passers-by tried to find a wagon to take him to Bellevue." But one man's horse had "worked all day," another's had "a stone in his shoe," and a third was "too skittish" for the trip. "It was three o'clock in the morning before [a wagon was found] and it bumped and joggled over the street, subjecting the man to exquisite pain." He died along the way.

Dalton's plan called for a small fleet of ambulances housed at a single hospital. Needing a sleek vehicle that maneuvered easily through city traffic, he approached the Abbot-Downing Company of New Hampshire, a leading stagecoach maker. Together they crafted a model of finely polished black wood, light enough for a single horse to draw, yet sturdy enough for a driver, a surgeon, and two patients lying down (or eight sitting up). The cabin stood high above the wheels for extra suspension. Each side had the word "AMBULANCE" emblazoned in gold lettering, with a gas lantern and night reflectors. A foot pedal sounded a bell to warn pedestrians. Inside were a couple of stretchers, a cabinet stocked with whiskey and bandages, a stomach pump for the poisoned and suicidal, and a straitjacket for those of "a demonstrative disposition." One writer called it "the Victorian equivalent of a portable emergency room."

Bellevue seemed the perfect testing ground. Having interned there, Dalton knew that it admitted more patients, with more injuries, than any hospital in the city. His plan linked Bellevue to local police stations by telegraph. Each message sounded a gong in the hospital's newly outfitted stables. Handed a destination slip, the ambulance team headed for the emergency, avoiding rutted alleys and cobblestone streets when they could. City traffic was the biggest obstacle. Huge steam locomotives moved freight at a snail's pace on poorly tended rails. A dozen streetcar lines jockeyed with carts, carriages, and pedestrians on thoroughfares smeared with the manure of forty thousand horses. ("Modern martyrdom," wrote the *New York Tribune,* "may be succinctly defined as riding on a New York omnibus.") By law, the Bellevue ambulance was given the right-of-way over all vehicles except the fire wagon and the U.S. mail, and that seemed to help. A reporter along for a ride noted: "As we swept around the corners and dashed over the crossings, both doctor and driver kept up a nervous sharp cry of warning to the pedestrians who darted out of the way with haste, or nervously retreated to the curb. . . . [Even] the surliest of car-drivers and the most aggressive of truckmen . . . pulled up or aside to afford passage."

The job of ambulance surgeon proved hard to fill. The twelve-hour shifts and $600 yearly salary attracted so few applicants that Bellevue took to staffing the post with new interns too intimidated to refuse. But the hospital had better luck recruiting the drivers, mostly immigrants who saw the $500 annual salary, plus room and board, as a step up from common laborer, which, indeed, it was. The driver had to know the geography of Manhattan, "with special reference to the shortest distances from one given point to another." But the key requirement was speed. The ambulance was expected to cover a mile in from five to eight minutes "in the business district," and from four to six minutes "in the less crowded part of the city." Teams competed for the fastest response times—the record held by Thomas Coughlin and his horse, Baby, on a run between Bellevue and the original Madison

Square Garden, where a circus performer had been injured. The ambulance traversed the half-mile route in under two minutes, crossing four streets and several trolley tracks, passing under two elevated railways, and taking the turns at close to full gallop.

The early Bellevue ambulance cases were not unlike those rushed to an emergency room today. A sampling from a three-month stretch in 1872 included a worker badly injured in a boiler explosion; an "intoxicated woman" who fell from a third-floor window; a "steady and hard drinker knocked down and run over by a milk wagon"; a "poorly nourished" Irish boy "caught in the wheels of a streetcar"; and "a healthy-looking German [who] attempted suicide with a butcher's knife." "Unfortunately for himself and perhaps the rest of mankind," the admitting physician scribbled, "he did not succeed."

A fair number of cases were alcoholics who had passed out on the street—policemen finding it easier to summon an ambulance than to escort the offender to the "drunk tank." Those who died along the way were sent to the morgue and placed on slabs next to a large glass window for public viewing and identification. Unclaimed bodies were stuffed into pine boxes and placed aboard the perversely named tugboat *Hope*, "a grim, black, demonic-looking craft," for the short, final voyage to Hart Island in the Bronx.

What gave the Bellevue ambulance its reputation were a series of bloody clashes in the summers of 1870 and 1871 between local Irish Protestants and Catholics. For years, New York's smaller Protestant faction had taunted its rival with a parade commemorating the Battle of the Boyne, where, in 1690, the forces of Protestant King William of Orange had crushed the army of the recently deposed Catholic King James II. As the event grew larger over the years, so, too, did the angry protests. On July 12, 1870, some two thousand well-lubricated "Orangemen" marched up Manhattan's West Side singing "Protestant Boys" and chanting "Croppies Lie Down" as they passed through heavily Irish Catholic neighborhoods. An angry, swelling crowd followed the marchers to Elm Park. "BLOODY RIOT," blared the next day's *New York Times*. "Three Killed, Six Mortally Wounded, and a Hundred Others Injured." Praising "the promptness and bravery of the police," the newspaper spotted something new—a small fleet of polished black ambulances picking up the crumpled bodies and rushing them to Bellevue. Each vehicle had a policeman sitting inside to keep the bloodied "Papists" and "Orangemen" from resuming the brawl.

A few months later, the city added five ambulances and horses to the Bellevue force. This proved fortuitous since the Elm Park riot was but a run-up to the main event. In 1871, Tammany leaders, under extreme pressure from their Catholic base, refused the Orange Order's request for a parade permit on the grounds that the city could no longer provide adequate protection for the marchers. The decision enraged New York's non-Catholics, who demanded a tough stance against "Irish hoodlums" preaching "free murder, free drunkenness, and free rioting." It bordered on extortion, they charged, to allow a raucous St. Patrick's Day Parade down the city's main thoroughfare each year while denying others the same privilege. Powerful interests, including newspaper publishers, businessmen, and anti-immigrant groups successfully lobbied the governor to overturn the ban.

On July 12, a sweltering day, the Orangemen began their march surrounded by 1,500 city policemen, most of them Irish Catholic, and four companies of largely Protestant state militia. Trouble came quickly. Angry Catholics showered the marchers with rocks, bottles, crockery, animal waste, and occasional gunfire. The militia responded with point-blank rifle volleys, while policemen waded into the crowds, clubs flying. By the time the bloodshed ended at least sixty people were dead, and hundreds more were injured. It was, in terms of civilian casualties, the bloodiest confrontation in the city's history, exceeding the worst single day of the recent Draft Riots of 1863.

Bellevue overflowed with the dead and the wounded. "The scene [there] was a sad and painful one," an observer noted, with "ambulances discharging their bloody loads at the door." No one could recall a day when more surgeries were performed and more patients were lost. "Shot while watching Parade—Died at Bellevue"; "Leg Shattered by Musket Ball—Amputated at Bellevue"; "Shot in Back by the Militia—Died at Bellevue"; "Shot by Musket in Thigh—Treated at Bellevue"; "Jaw Shot Off—Died at Bellevue"; "Pistol Shot in Chest—Treated at Bellevue"; "Musket Balls in Wrist and Abdomen—Died at Bellevue." It took several pages of single-spaced entries to document the carnage.

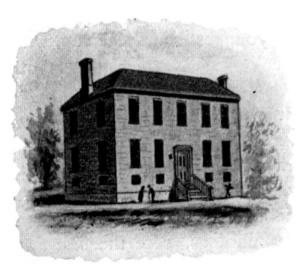

Costing £80 for building materials and fifty gallons of rum for the workmen who laid the beams and raised the roof, the New York City almshouse opened in 1736 with a single-room infirmary—"the seed from which grew the mighty oak of Bellevue."

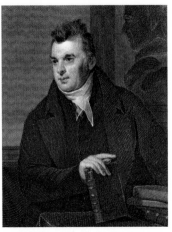

David Hosack, the leading physician for New York City's elite in the early 1800s, listed Alexander Hamilton, Aaron Burr, and steamboat inventor Robert Fulton among his patients. He also treated the sick at the almshouse and envisioned a true public hospital for the indigent.

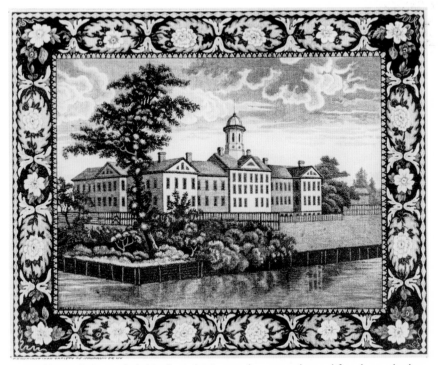

As New York's population exploded in the early nineteenth century, the need for a larger almshouse complex could no longer be ignored. Opened in 1816 on the old Bellevue estate bordering the East River, the so-called Bellevue Establishment was the largest and most expensive building project in the city's history to date, containing an almshouse, an orphanage, a lunatic asylum, a prison, and an infirmary. An infectious disease hospital would be added in 1826.

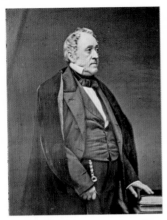

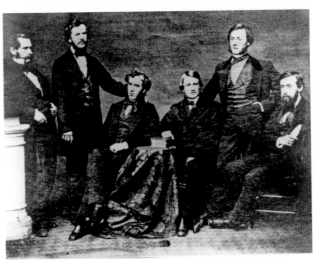

Considered the most talented American surgeon of the first half of the nineteenth century, Valentine Mott took the lead in creating NYU Medical College in 1841. His Saturday clinics at Bellevue Hospital attracted students and physicians from across the region. One prominent surgeon wrote that Mott "performed more of the great operations than any man living."

Following a series of deadly typhus epidemics that took the lives of hundreds of patients and numerous doctors at Bellevue, reforms were instituted that became a model for future hospital care. Among these was a competitive examination for beginning physicians, known as interns, who lived in the hospital and served the everyday needs of the patients. Here is the first class of Bellevue interns, circa 1856.

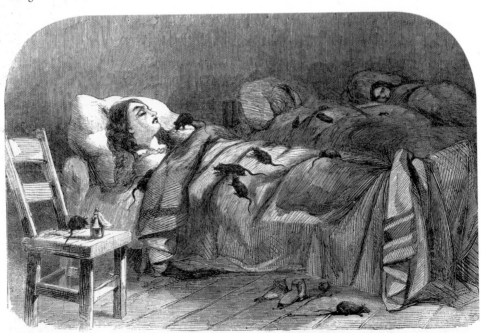

A rendering from *Harper's Weekly* showing rats crawling over Bellevue patients in 1860. The hospital received a storm of criticism after an infant apparently was gnawed to death. Though an autopsy showed that the baby had died before the rats consumed the body, sanitary problems would plague the hospital.

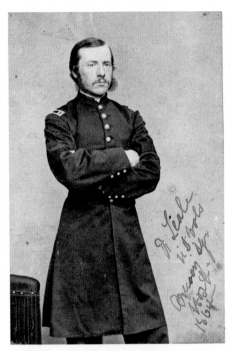

The first physician to reach the mortally wounded President Abraham Lincoln at Ford's Theatre, Charles Leale, twenty-three, a recent graduate of Bellevue Hospital Medical College, performed admirably under impossibly difficult conditions, though his role remains controversial to this day.

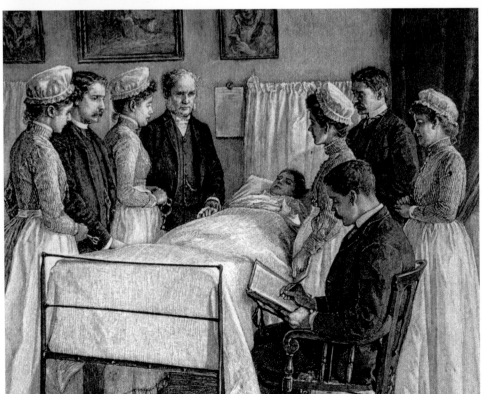

Stephen Smith (standing to the patient's right) was a founder of Bellevue Hospital Medical College and a general surgeon at the hospital for more than sixty years. His classic 1865 study, *Sanitary Conditions of the City,* warned of the disastrous consequences of ignoring the living conditions and medical needs of the poor.

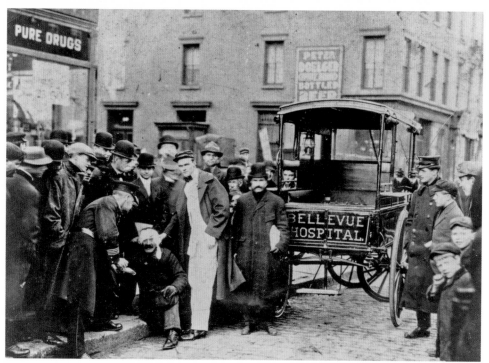

Applying the lessons he learned as a medical administrator in the Civil War, Edward Dalton organized the nation's first civilian ambulance corps at Bellevue in 1869. Here, a Bellevue ambulance surgeon provides assistance to an injured New Yorker.

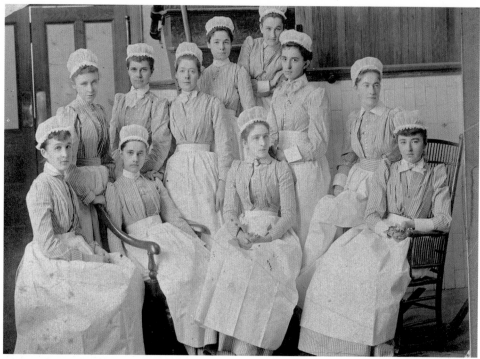

America's first professional nursing school opened at Bellevue in 1873. Preferring single, literate, religious women from cultivated families, it rejected most applicants on account of "bad breeding."

By the 1870s, Bellevue had one of the largest, most modern morgues in the world. Streams of water showered down on the faces of the corpses to keep them fresh for identification by relatives and friends. The unclaimed corpses were shipped to Potter's Field for burial.

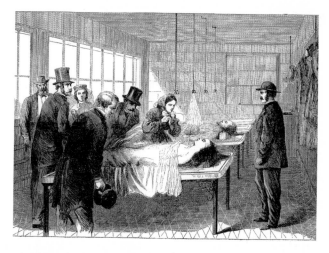

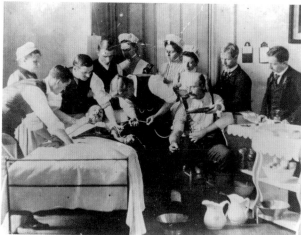

In 1876, O. G. Mason, Bellevue's official photographer, took the first photograph of a blood transfusion in progress. Carefully staged, it showed the kind of medical progress being made at the hospital.

Bellevue's Lewis A. Sayre, the nation's first professor of orthopedic surgery, invented the "tripod suspension derrick" to correct spinal deformities. His demonstration, photographed by O. G. Mason, contained overtones of eroticism at odds with Victorian norms.

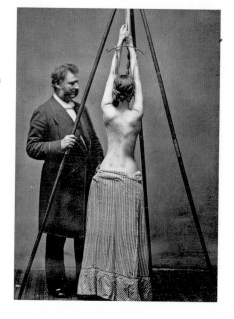

Mason's best-known photograph was of a nineteen-year-old woman with elephantiasis. With only her face shielded, and her hands clasped as if in prayer, the subject's lower body shows the full force of her disease. Some accused Mason of pandering to the P. T. Barnum "sideshow" aspects of popular culture; others viewed the photograph as an accurate rendering of a medical condition.

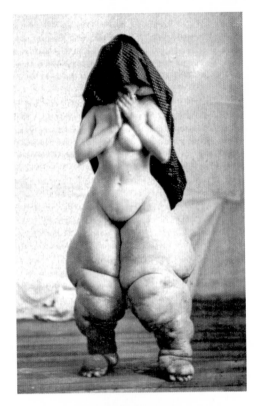

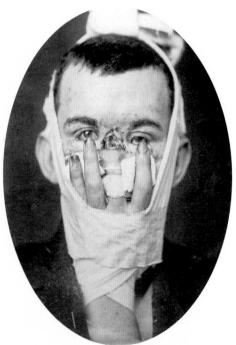

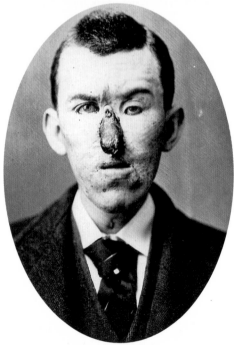

Mason photographed thousands of patients at Bellevue. His aim, he said, was to depict Bellevue as a hospital devoted to top clinical care and daring medical innovation. In this instance he followed the progress of a patient who had lost his entire nose to a dangerous infection and whose middle finger would be used to fashion a new one.

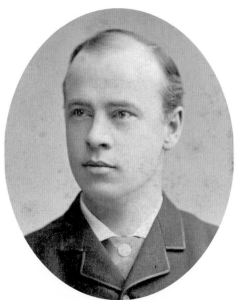

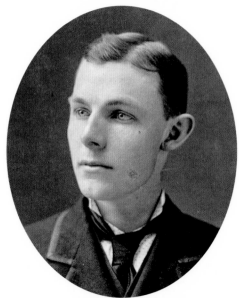

William Welch, a former Bellevue intern, introduced the nation's first modern pathology course at Bellevue Hospital Medical College. Despite intense efforts to keep him on the faculty, including a $75,000 gift from industrialist Andrew Carnegie for a new pathology building, Welch accepted a position as one of the founding members of the Johns Hopkins Medical School.

As an intern and later a surgeon at Bellevue, William Halsted worked tirelessly to bring antiseptic methods to the hospital. A brilliant innovator, his work at Bellevue was cut short by his experiments with cocaine as an anesthetic, which led to an addiction to various drugs. His close friend William Welch brought him to Johns Hopkins, where Halsted resurrected his surgical career.

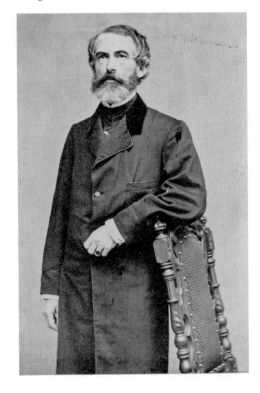

Bellevue's Frank Hamilton, one of America's finest military surgeons, was brought down to Washington to help treat President James A. Garfield following the assassination attempt in 1881 that eventually took Garfield's life. Many accused Hamilton, who did not believe in Lister's antiseptic methods, of medical malpractice in treating the president's wounds.

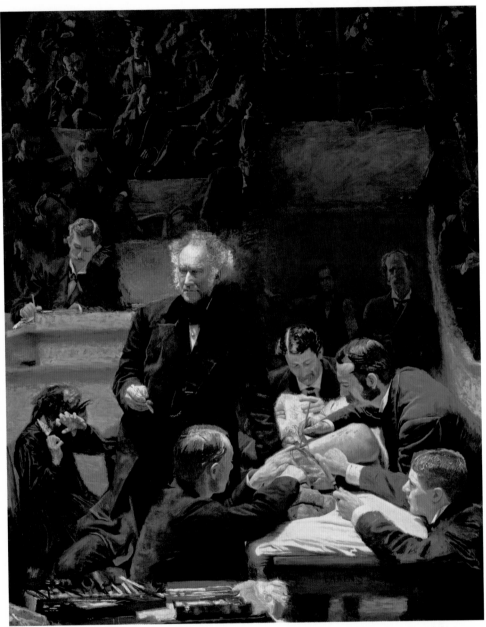

The Gross Clinic, an enormous canvas painted by Thomas Eakins for the 1876 Centennial Exhibition in Philadelphia, is one of the most important and controversial renderings of a medical subject in American history. Some see it as an unabashed tribute to Dr. Gross, who was among the greatest surgeons of his era; others see it as a subtle slap at Gross for his failure to embrace the antiseptic methods of Joseph Lister then coming into fashion.

The following day, a sea of mourners, estimated at twenty thousand, gathered at the hospital gates to accompany a shimmering line of hearses to the Greenpoint ferry and on to Calvary Cemetery, the area's largest Catholic burial ground.

The great irony of the so-called Orange Riot of 1871 was that it seemed to achieve what Dr. Stephen Smith and other reformers had been unable to: the removal of Boss Tweed. While a fair number of well-off New Yorkers had benefited immensely from Tweed's various schemes, many more had relied on him to maintain the peace. When he failed once again to do so, his usefulness came to an end. Within weeks of the Orange Riot, newspaper reports of the Tweed Ring's staggering corruption—hardly a secret—led to feverish calls for an investigation and, ultimately, to Tweed's demise. Many viewed his fall in terms of the political and economic excesses of the times, and this, no doubt, is true. But others saw it in simpler terms, as the failure of a political boss to carry out the most basic of his tasks. "That saving grace was gone," note the authors of *Gotham*, the leading history of New York City. "Tweed could not keep the Irish in line."

In 1869, Bellevue's two ambulances had responded to 74 emergencies. A decade later, its fleet of seven would answer more than 1,900 calls, the number peaking at close to 4,400 in the early 1890s. Before long, Presbyterian, St. Vincent's, Roosevelt, and New York Hospital all had ambulances on the streets. The key difference, noted the *New York Tribune,* was that "by law, private hospitals are permitted to unload free cases upon Bellevue, and the latter institution is required to receive them."

The ambulance played a dual role in this process. Crews from private hospitals were ordered to ignore street calls involving ragged-looking victims with serious injuries. And they routinely transported "problem" patients—those "likely to die"—to the one place that couldn't say no. Early on, the newspapers had reported these practices without criticism. "Patrick Carey, a horseshoer, 33, suffering from delirium tremens, was transferred to Bellevue . . . too far gone for any remedy to save him," read a typical entry in the 1880s. But as medical emergencies became more common, a different story line emerged. "THE PATIENT DIED: A Young Lad Carted from One Hospital to Another," read a *New York Times* headline in 1896. "The father, a porter in a linen house, literally gasped when he learned of the boy's death. He had not known of his removal to Bellevue."

A handful of these transfers were "nuisance" cases: Bellevue received one ambulance patient with the bizarre diagnosis of "Rheumatism and Insubordination." But most involved wounds and illnesses increasingly tied to modern city life—construction mishaps, traffic accidents, and violent crimes, with the victims invariably coming from the "lower classes." "Open your books and show me one man of wealth who has ever been transferred," a reformer fumed. The practice—known today as "patient dumping"—involved just about every ambulance corps in the city, though Bellevue's superintendent accused one in particular (almost certainly New York Hospital's) of unloading "dozens of critically ill patients each week."

This was no exaggeration. In 1900, a city health official estimated that more than a hundred of Bellevue's recorded deaths the previous year had occurred *within a day* of the patient's transfer from another hospital. There was no medical justification, the official conceded. These hospitals were "sending the poor, dying patient to Bellevue in order to lessen their [own] death rates"—pure and simple.

The original ambulance corps, based quite literally on "horsepower," didn't survive long into the twentieth century. One by one, New York's hospitals retired the horse-drawn vehicles, though not without some regret. When a huge snowstorm blanketed the city in 1915, the new gas engine ambulances proved "helpless in the drifts," while the old ones easily pulled through. "The time should never come," said one nervous official, "when the horse will be entirely discarded."

But that time did arrive. In 1924, Bellevue, the lone holdout, closed its stables for good. Only two horses remained, and they were "retired" in a poignant ceremony attended by a small crowd of doctors and nurses and retired ambulance men. "The horses, Joe and Jim, for twenty years stall mates, had tears in their eyes, according to their driver John O'Neill, who stood with bowed head as they were hitched to a wagon and driven away." Their destination was listed as "a farm

Upstate . . . where their shoes will be removed and they will be permitted to graze until they die."

The horses, it turned out, had a brighter future than Mr. O'Neill. Unable to drive an automobile, and apparently too old and nervous to learn, he received a different sort of transfer—leaving Bellevue for a lesser city job as a common laborer.

Edward Dalton's time in New York City was marred by tragedy. He lost his only child to disease in 1868, and his wife in childbirth the following year. Weakened by chest pain and a hacking cough, a likely victim of tuberculosis, he moved to California in a futile attempt to regain his health. "During all this time," it was noted, "nothing could exceed the fortitude and cheerfulness with which he bore the succession of his trials." Dalton died in 1872, far from home and remaining family, at the age of thirty-seven. "Probably no inventor has ever been more completely forgotten, or has received less credit for his work, than the New York surgeon who designed the city ambulance," an admirer wrote in 1901. "It is not likely that more than fifty persons in the country know even his name."

8

BELLEVUE VENUS

In 1867, a brief paragraph appeared in the Bellevue Annual Report stating that $281.12 had been spent on supplies for a new "Photographic Department." And it contained an explanation from the ubiquitous Stephen Smith about the importance of this infant field to the medical profession. "In all the large Military Hospitals photography is [now] regarded as an indispensable feature of the records of the sick," Smith wrote of the still-fresh Civil War experience, "and it will prove no less important in a large [civilian] Hospital."

Smith was right on both counts. Medical photography had grown immensely during the Civil War, and would continue to thrive. While much of it involved portraits of limbless veterans or scenes of corpse-covered battlefields, some photographers had boldly entered the forbidding world of the surgical tent to capture operations actually under way. The impetus came largely from Surgeon General William A. Hammond, whose order creating the Army Medical Museum in 1862 had directed field officers to collect "all specimens of morbid anatomy . . . which may be regarded as valuable . . . in the study of military medicine or surgery." A flood of material soon arrived, including photographs, instruments, bone fragments, and a small coffin containing the amputated right leg of General Daniel Sickles, lost to a Confederate cannonball at Gettysburg.

Bellevue's photographic department was another first for the hospital in the post–Civil War years. To run it, Smith wisely recommended the man who suggested the idea—a thirty-seven-year-old portrait photographer named Oscar G. Mason, with an encyclopedic knowledge of his craft. Mason's first task was to convince the skeptics that medical photography was something more than a frivolous expense for a hospital serving the poor. He did so by striking an ingenious deal with City Hall. For a small fee, Mason agreed to photograph the face of every unclaimed corpse sent to the municipal morgue at Bellevue, and to post the images on the wall just outside.

It couldn't have worked out better. As New York's population surged, so, too, did the number of anonymous corpses. Day and night, people wandered through Bellevue's dead house to inspect remains stretched out on stone tables. "A stream of cold water, from a movable jet, falls over the lifeless face, warding off decay until the last moment . . . in the hope that someone . . . will claim the body," a reporter noted, adding that "nearly all go to the Potter's Field."

Mason's "Wall of the Unknown Dead" was an instant sensation. A body might be gone within a day or two but the facial image remained there for a full year, meaning that hundreds of corpses buried in Potter's Field might be identified later, and possibly reclaimed, thanks to the magic of photography. The "unmistakable records of this gallery of death give ample proof of the humane forethought which prompted [its] establishment," Mason explained. "It is gratifying to know that public sentiment and the press continue to highly commend this feature of the department."

Though rarely given credit, Mason also played a role in creating the first criminal "mug shot," popularized by the New York City Police Department in the 1870s and modeled on Bellevue's "Wall of the Unknown Dead." Mason thought photography the perfect tool for identification. There were no embellishments, no flawed recollections, no "might be," "could be," or "perhaps." He even claimed that his photos had a "restraining influence" on violent crime, because those who were murdered could no longer be "quietly hidden from sight or easily forgotten. Their faces are always visible, waiting for recognition and testimony."

One thing was certain: Mason's Wall of the Unknown Dead allowed medical photography at Bellevue to survive. In the coming decades,

Mason photographed thousands of medical procedures and diseased patients at the hospital with the enthusiastic backing of the staff. A good example was the blood transfusion—a novel procedure in this era, and a dangerous one given the ignorance of different blood types. A number of Bellevue physicians had done these transfusions in the past, believing it made more sense to add blood to a distressed patient than to withdraw it. As a young army doctor, William Hammond had transfused several cholera victims with bull's blood, all of whom died (whether from cholera, or the transfusion, or both, is unknown). And Austin Flint, Jr., had revived a "moribund patient" with seven ounces of her husband's blood while working at a hospital in New Orleans, only to see the woman die the next day.

In 1876, Mason took the first photograph of a blood transfusion. The procedure was real, but the scene had been carefully staged. The setting is immaculate. The donor—who was carefully weighed before and after the event to determine the amount of blood taken—appears calm and healthy, while the frail recipient is receiving oxygen through the nose. Between them is a physician controlling the proper blood flow and direction. Unlike previous paintings of transfusions, nobody is unconscious or about to faint, and there are no red drippings splattered about. Everything is in perfect order.

More than likely, this photograph was intended as a promotional device. Austin Flint had recently lectured on the benefits of blood transfusion to his peers at the New York Academy of Medicine. And there was good money to be made, as Oscar Mason soon discovered, by publishing these photos in popular medical textbooks.

Mason's earliest collaboration was with Bellevue's Lewis A. Sayre, one of the founders of orthopedic surgery. In preparing his 1877 monograph, *Spinal Disease and Spinal Curvature,* Sayre employed Mason to dramatically demonstrate the treatment of skeletal deformities through photography. The result was stunning; Mason's twenty-one albumen prints completely overshadowed Sayre's meticulous text. And it wasn't hard to see why. The before-and-after images of a half-naked female patient with Pott's disease, and a photo of her on her tiptoes in Sayre's "tripod suspension derrick" with the fully clothed Sayre standing inches away, offered a whiff of eroticism deeply at odds with Victorian norms. Had this not been a "medical procedure," it might have been banned.

Other photographs showed the woman immobilized in a snug plaster of Paris cast, known as the "Sayre's jacket." How well these devices worked was a matter of debate, though they'd be used well into the twentieth century. At the very least, the enormous success of *Spinal Disease and Spinal Curvature* spurred the development of new methods for the treatment of scoliosis through bracing and body casting. And, as Sayre himself noted, the tripod suspension derrick had a side benefit as well: the patient grew a bit taller from the constant stretching.

Mason's most haunting photographs appeared in George Henry Fox's *Photographic Illustrations of Skin Diseases,* published in 1881. Almost completely forgotten today, they sparked outrage at the time for supposedly crossing the line between medical instruction and voyeuristic pandering, especially those with female subjects. The 1870s and 1880s were the height of the controversial but enormously popular "side shows" in America. Hucksters like P. T. Barnum attracted huge throngs by booking fire-eaters, sword swallowers, and "freaks" with assorted medical abnormalities, some bogus, others disturbingly real. There were the "Wild Men of Borneo" (actually two mentally disabled dwarfs from Ohio), "Jo-Jo the Dog-Faced Boy" (suffering from hypertrichosis, a profusion of body hair), "General Tom Thumb" (the world's smallest human), eight-foot giants, bearded ladies, Siamese twins, and people with humongous body tumors attached to their back, face, and scrotum. To some critics, *Photographic Illustrations of Skin Diseases* resembled a Barnum freak show masquerading as a medical text.

One of the photographs showed the hundreds of skin grafts applied to the bare chest of a thirty-seven-year-old woman badly burned by a kerosene lamp. She would die a few months later, the cause listed as "acute pleurisy," but more likely the result of blood poisoning. Mason's penultimate photo was of a nineteen-year-old woman with elephantiasis, taken against a stark white background. A black cape shields her face. Her fully naked body is normally proportioned from the waist up; her legs, ankles, and feet show the full force of her disease. She appears to be silently praying, her clasped hands pointing skyward. The text reads: "There are one or two patches of superficial ulceration, oozing a large quantity of . . . fluid. Since this oozing the legs have diminished in circumference. The general health is failing." An admirer of Mason's, perceiving a subtle blend of innocence and dignity in the photograph, dubbed it *Bellevue Venus,* and the name stuck. What happened to the patient is a mystery.

Before long, Mason had become a self-described expert on the female form. He spent his spare time as the photographer for "a very private and select coterie" of New York physicians known as the "Artistic Medical Club," whose main object, it appeared, was to find the "perfectly proportioned woman." A diligent search ensued, with various subjects interviewed and photographed, before one of the club members struck gold. "He is [her] family physician," it was reported, "and as such had exceptional privileges accorded him. He made certain measurements, comprising the young woman's height, size of waist, etc., and found them all to approach remarkably close to the ideal standard of correctness—the greatest deviation [being] the sixteenth part of an inch."

Photographing her, however, took "several months of negotiation." Mason had to promise to protect the woman's anonymity. She would pose "in various positions, her face alone concealed by a heavy veil of drapery"—much like *Bellevue Venus.* And the photographs had to remain within the Artistic Medical Club, a bargain apparently kept. There appears to be no record of anybody else even knowing about them (and they may have been destroyed). Mason's work, in this instance, was meant for fellow medical voyeurs, not for the larger profession.

At Bellevue, meanwhile, his reputation soared. His photographs had become indispensable in bringing medical procedures and oddities to an increasingly curious public. "When some eight years ago [our] department was first fully organized, through the efforts of a few of the more active and progressive members of the medical profession, some of their brethren seemed to look upon it with little favor," Mason admitted. But times had changed. Thanks to photography one could chart an operation from start to finish, or follow the different stages of disease—all done quickly, cheaply, precisely. No longer did doctors have to rely on the inexact renderings of portrait artists or the "often imperfect methods of written description." At Bellevue, even the most hardened skeptics of photography had become believers, Mason boasted, removing "any doubt as to [our department's] great importance."

Mason took so many photos in these years that Bellevue soon became the largest such repository in the world. He was particularly drawn to unique surgical procedures—the odder the better. And no part of the hospital seemed quite as fertile as the recently opened Department of Dermatology, one of the nation's first, where novel experiments in facial reconstruction were already taking place—a logical step given the needs of badly disfigured Civil War veterans and the sharp rise in violent crime and street accidents in rapidly urbanizing New York. Bellevue's leading surgeon, Frank Hamilton, had already performed twenty rhinoplasties when, in 1879, his protégé Thomas Sabine attempted a radical variation in which the patient's middle finger would be refitted as his nose. Mason eagerly photographed it all.

The twenty-two-year-old male patient had come to Bellevue suffering from a massive nasal infection, which, according to his doctors, "was finally cured, leaving him without a nose and with deformity about the eyes." After consulting with Hamilton and Lewis Sayre, Sabine began the multistage procedure by removing the nail from the patient's left middle finger and placing his left arm in a sling with the finger pressed into the exposed nasal cavity. Waiting several weeks for the surrounding tissue to bind, Sabine then amputated the finger and connected it permanently to the face with a series of silver wires. The procedure was not without complications. "Patient suffers pain from the constrained position [of the immobilized arm], relieved by hypodermics of morphine," read an early notation. "The end of the middle finger has slipped from the pocket to which it has been attached," said another. At one point, the patient required artificial respiration after the wound turned blue from oxygen loss.

Sabine and his colleagues deemed the operation a triumph. "The nose has become firmly united," a Bellevue surgeon assured the medical community. "It is about normal color. Its sensibility is quite acute. . . . The parts are looking very well indeed." This appeared to be a minority opinion, however. Years later, a former intern gave the assessment of those at Bellevue who weren't directly involved in the case. "The nose was not a great success as an ornamental feature," he recalled, "and I doubt it was very useful from a utilitarian standpoint; but, at any rate, he had a nose."

—

For all its richness and diversity, Mason's surviving portfolio is but a sliver of what occurred in the clinics and operating theaters of post–Civil War Bellevue. No photograph could possibly illuminate the diagnostic genius of an Austin Flint, who used the newly discovered binaural (two-eared) stethoscope to describe the first heart murmur and listen for the symptomatic wheezes and crackles of lung disease. And no photograph could illustrate Flint's remarkably prescient instincts in recommending moderate exercise for cardiac patients—"indolence" led to "degeneration" of the heart muscle, he warned—and urging them to substitute fruits and vegetables for "fatty substances," especially meat.

The same went for Bellevue's Job Smith and Abraham Jacobi, the acknowledged "Fathers of American Pediatrics," whose insights were better suited to the printed word than to the telling photograph. Or Francis Delafield, whose stunning experiments in microscopy were performed at his workbench, invisible to the naked eye. Or William Hammond, whose ingenious lectures on the importance of drugs and electrotherapy in treating disorders like insomnia, vertigo, and paralysis were heard and read by thousands of medical students and physicians. Even Lewis Sayre, one of Mason's favorites, discouraged photographs of himself performing his most controversial procedure—circumcision—though he did allow occasional "before" and "after" shots of the children who had undergone it.

Sayre's interest in circumcision had come about quite accidentally. In the early 1870s, a colleague had asked him to examine a five-year-old boy "unable to walk without assistance or stand erect," whose knees were bent at a 45-degree angle to his trunk. "This little fellow," the colleague wrote him, "has a pair of legs that you would walk miles to see."

Sayre was intrigued. Already a leader in orthopedics, he was among a handful of surgeons to perform a gruesome operation called a tenotomy, in which the hamstring tendons are severed to expand movement in the legs. Sayre had no idea what had caused the problem until the boy's nurse warned him: "Oh, doctor, be very careful—don't touch his pee-pee—it's very sore." What Sayre discovered was a penis so tightly wound in its foreskin as to literally cripple the child. A few days later, in the surgical amphitheater at Bellevue, Sayre first tried a scissors and "the thumbs and finger nails of each hand" to perform an emergency circumcision. Within weeks, the lad was walking "with his limbs quite straight."

It was, Sayre recalled, a eureka moment. If circumcision worked so well in this case, what else might it do? Sayre would spend much of his professional life seeking the answer. His experiments on Bellevue children and others regarding the dangers of the "constricted penis" led him to boast, often ludicrously, of having cured patients with club foot, epilepsy, bladder disease, extreme sexual urges, and serious mental conditions. Lecturing to a group of doctors in 1876, Sayre spoke of turning two wild boys—one "an idiot," the other a "vicious lunatic"—into veritable angels through the simple act of circumcision. "This is almost a miracle," he said. "It is beyond the power of man to comprehend it unless you see these cases from the start." But further trials upon children at the local asylum proved disappointing. While Sayre claimed some "improvement" in his subjects, none was deemed well enough to be discharged.

Sayre would never quite find the "magic bullet" he so relentlessly pursued. What he did do, however, was to almost single-handedly bring circumcision into public view. "When a man of Sayre's experience, reputation, and professional standing insisted that [serious conditions] could be cured by a comparatively simple operation on the foreskin," an observer noted, "the medical world was prepared to take him seriously." In the coming years, more and more doctors would come to view circumcision as essential to the nation's public health. Using the 1880 U.S. Census, for example, John Shaw Billings, a founder of the Johns Hopkins Medical School, singled out immigrant Jews for their greater longevity, smaller number of "defective classes" (idiots and epileptics), and lower rates of cancer, syphilis, and other diseases—most of which he simplistically attributed to circumcision. (Several studies of that era suggested that Jews were better off because circumcised people masturbated less frequently.) Thanks largely to Sayre's persistence, an obscure religious ritual became, by 1900, a routine medical procedure for millions of American boys.

—

O. G. Mason amassed a remarkable résumé in his lifetime. The list includes one of the first lunar photographs, the first image of a lightning flash in a thunderstorm, and the first known photo album "for the safe storage and sharing of portraits." When Bellevue purchased one of the first X-ray machines in 1896, Mason naturally became the house radiographer. (He retired in ill health in 1909, blaming the X-rays.) But Mason's greatest service was his public depiction of Bellevue as a place of clinical riches and original research—a place where bold, creative, if sometimes bizarre and Frankenstein-like, experimentation prevailed. Hospitals earn their stripes, the illustrious Dr. Oliver Wendell Holmes had told the graduates of Bellevue Medical College in 1872, when "men of well-sifted reputations" arrive to turn them into "true centers of medical education." Bellevue had approached that status, he declared, by attracting extraordinary talent and then disseminating the work.

Thanks, in some measure, to the vision of O. G. Mason and the medical photography he so deftly pioneered.

9

NIGHTINGALES

M edical progress comes in many forms. Sometimes a shift in public perception can be as valuable as a lifesaving scientific advance. During the Civil War, Americans were forced by circumstance to reassess one of the most reviled symbols of antebellum medical care. As the casualties mounted with each new military campaign, tens of thousands of soldiers found themselves in a place they'd never been before—a hospital. A farmer from Iowa now shared a ward with a shopkeeper from New York; a blacksmith from Ohio recuperated next to a carpenter from Maine. For sick and wounded veterans, the commonly held perception of the hospital as a dumping ground for the poor no longer matched their personal experiences. Many claimed to have been well treated, and what they remembered most fondly, according to their diaries and letters home, was yet another practical innovation of the war: the female nursing care made possible, in part, by the good works of Florence Nightingale in a faraway conflict a decade before.

In English history, notes the website of the British National Archives, the Crimean War of the 1850s "is principally remembered for three reasons: the charge of the Light Brigade, maladministration of the British army, and Florence Nightingale." In almost all wars in that era, more soldiers had died from sickness than from enemy fire. But the British experience in Crimea had been alarmingly one-sided: 4,774 men lost to battlefield wounds, 16,323 to illness and disease. The public took notice—and the government almost fell—as newspaper correspondents in the field, using the newly discovered telegraph, relayed their gruesome stories in current time. The London *Times,* in particular, exposed the frightful state of the transports that ferried the wounded across the Black Sea to military hospitals in Turkey, where conditions were even worse. "Cause of death" in these places read like a medical encyclopedia: cholera, dysentery, gangrene, malaria, scurvy, typhus—even frostbite. When a witness at the main hospital asked an orderly why a wounded soldier lay unattended, his uncovered wounds crawling with lice, the orderly replied: "It's not worthwhile to clean him: he's not long for this world."

Under enormous pressure, England's war minister, Sidney Herbert, authorized Nightingale to lead a team of female nurses to Crimea. "Her interventions, considered at the time to be revolutionary, seem in hindsight to be acts of common sense," an admirer noted. Nursing had long been scorned because the job attracted women Nightingale herself described as "too old, too weak, too drunken, too dirty, too stupid, or too bad to do anything else." Those who accompanied her to Crimea, by contrast, were well-trained devotees (including fifteen Catholic nuns) with a fetish for cleanliness and order. Once there, they scrubbed down the wards, emptied the waste buckets, bathed the patients, cleared their bodies of lice, laundered the bedding, and threw open the windows for fresh air. Nightingale never saw much good in bleeding or purging a wounded man, or in providing opiates to dull his pain. What she did see was a "clear relationship between the diseases killing [her] patients and the filth in which they lay. . . ."

Nightingale viewed the hospital as the best place for nature to run its course. Nourishment, hygiene, and patient comfort were the keys. "Recovery from sickness in the vast majority of cases depends [more] upon pure air and pure water, with suitable diet, than upon any medical treatment, however skillful," she insisted. A meticulous record-keeper, Nightingale proved her point with a series of "mortality diagrams" showing the dramatic improvements in Crimea once she and her fellow nurses took charge of the day-to-day care. Deaths went down dramatically; epidemics eased; patients recovered. Disease—or much of it—disappeared.

Word of her work soon crossed the Atlantic, winning converts like

Surgeon General William Hammond. Among his initiatives would be the construction of one-story Civil War "Pavilion hospitals" providing more light, better ventilation, and extra space between the beds. The most impressive of these, the enormous Satterlee Military Hospital in West Philadelphia, contained a maze of low-slung buildings with large windows and wood plank construction to let the fresh air in and the bad air out. At its height, following the Battle of Gettysburg, Satterlee held more than 3,500 patients, making it one of the largest hospitals in the world.

The sheer number of casualties also led Hammond and Army Secretary Simon Cameron to recruit female volunteers as military nurses, a bold step at the time. There were no training schools like the one Nightingale had created in London because nursing wasn't yet a recognized profession in the United States. American doctors generally viewed women as too delicate and flighty for the serious demands of medical work. How would they react to the odor of a pus-filled wound or the sight of gushing blood? And what sort of woman would voluntarily tend to the most intimate needs of a male stranger, beyond a lonely spinster or a self-absorbed busybody with nothing better to do? As one doctor sneered, "Can you fancy half a dozen or a dozen old hags, for that is what they are, surrounding a bewildered hospital surgeon, each one clamoring for her little wants?"

The greatest fear, however, was that trained female nurses might challenge the doctor's authority—or worse, try to become doctors themselves. The American Medical Association spoke directly to this problem when it described nursing as "an art and a science" in the hands of properly trained women, while also listing the deficiencies that prevented them from ever becoming good physicians: "uncertainty of rational judgment, capriciousness of sentiment, fickleness of purpose, and indecision of action."

Treading lightly, army officials recruited the most competent (and least objectionable) nurses they could find: single women from religious orders, the best known being the Catholic Sisters of Charity. Having spent years working in orphanages, poorhouses, and hospitals like St. Vincent's in New York City, the Sisters didn't require on-the-job training. Indeed, the wounded soldiers at Satterlee took to calling them

"Angel" and "Mother" for their remarkable skill and devotion. Even better, the Sisters presented no risks to the male medical staff. They were deferential to a fault; they saw nursing as a duty, not a profession; they had no desire to become doctors; and they were extremely good at what they did—so good that both sides, Union and Confederate, actively sought them out. The problem, quite simply, was that there weren't enough Sisters to go around. As a result, much of the nursing in the early months of the war fell to runaway slaves, convalescing troops, even prisoners of war.

To plug this gap, Secretary Cameron chose Dorothea Dix, the noted social reformer, to create the Women's Nursing Corps. On paper, at least, the qualifications were severe. Fixed in her ways and determined to avoid trouble, Dix vigorously applied the Victorian standards of the day. The proper nurse must be single, literate, and over thirty, she ordered, "plain almost to repulsion in dress and devoid of personal attractions." That meant "no bows, no curls or jewelry, no hoop skirts"—nothing, in short, to excite the baser instincts of the wounded troops. Socializing was strictly forbidden. The nurse "must be in her room at taps, must not go to any place of amusement" or—worse yet— "allow a [man] in her room." For reasons of prejudice—or perhaps jealousy at the powerful bond created between wounded soldiers and the Sisters of Charity—Dix instructed her charges "not to speak to those Catholic nurses." She also rejected Catholic applicants "if a Protestant could be substituted."

Thousands of Northern women volunteered for nursing duty during the Civil War. Some attracted wide attention: Clara Barton for her bravery on the front lines at Manassas and Antietam, where a bullet grazed the sleeve of her dress and killed the wounded soldier she was attending; Harriet Tubman, whose extraordinary nursing skills included the use of herbal remedies; and Louisa May Alcott, whose letters home, published as *Hospital Sketches*, showed off her literary gifts in the years before *Little Women* became a national sensation. In New York City, the ninety-one applicants chosen for duty in the Nursing Corps were sent to Bellevue or New York Hospital for a thirty-day training course in "making beds, cooking food properly for the sick, washing and dressing wounds, and ventilating and caring for a ward." (A survey of their motives showed "philanthropy, patriotism, and Christian duty" heading the list.) Those who stuck it out—a fair number dropped away—spent the war in field hospitals, on military transports, or at places like Satterlee. Their experiences would lay the groundwork for professional nursing in the United States.

"I had never been in a hospital before," Elizabeth Hobson recalled of her first visit to Bellevue in 1872. "The sight of the patients and the loathsome smells sickened me so that I nearly fainted." Having first inspected the laundry, which operated without soap, and then the kitchen, where a "huge negro" prepared greasy soup while "pauper women" huddled together peeling potatoes, Hobson reached her limit in the ladies' surgical ward. The beds were "unspeakable," she noted, and the single helper—"an Irishwoman of a low class"—slept in a washtub filled with trash. It seemed a hopeless place—"an Augean stable"—and it buckled her knees.

Hobson hadn't gone alone. She was part of the "Local Visiting Committee to Bellevue Hospital," a group of several dozen women of "wealth and high social position" determined to improve "the mental, moral, and physical [condition] of the patients." What bound them together, besides "representing the very best class of our citizens," was their volunteer work during the Civil War. Led by Louisa Lee Schuyler, a descendant of Alexander Hamilton, they hoped to keep that spirit alive by focusing on local issues such as "nursing the sick, protecting the children and caring for the aged whom they may find in the institutions of the City."

The timing certainly was right. Stephen Smith's *Sanitary Conditions of the City* had just alerted wealthy New Yorkers to the dangers of leaving festering social problems unaddressed, while Edward Dalton's ambulance corps had shown that wartime medical advances could be put to civilian use. Meanwhile, the recent fall of Boss Tweed had spawned a cluster of reform efforts, including the curious inspection of Bellevue Hospital by Miss Schuyler and her well-heeled friends. "We are aware, owing to the many years of corruption and dishonesty in the administration of affairs in New York . . . that economy is one of [our] first duties," the Visiting Committee noted. "We strive to . . . confine our demands to the real necessities."

The most critical need they identified was nursing care, which ranged from primitive to none at all. Bellevue had long relied on inmates from the Tombs prison—vagrants and prostitutes known as "Ten Days Women" for the length of their sentences. When Bellevue separated from the almshouse in the 1840s, funds were provided to hire a handful of female "nurses" and male "orderlies," but the pay was so low, the working conditions so wretched, that the new system seemed hardly different from the old. "The nurses, or rather those employed as such, were nearly without exception to the last degree incompetent," wrote Dr. Robert Carlisle in his nineteenth-century *Account of Bellevue Hospital*. "They were ignorant, indifferent, dishonest."

Determined to open the nation's first professional nursing school, the Visiting Committee went directly to the source. A liaison was dispatched to London to study the methods of Florence Nightingale, whose iconic "Letter of Advice to Bellevue" offered both a blueprint for the project and an endorsement of its goals. Applicants must be "moral" and "cultivated," she wrote, and, above all, know their place. They were "*there, and solely there, to carry out the orders of the medical and surgical staff,* including, of course, the whole practice of cleanliness, fresh air, diet, etc." As to the day-to-day operation of the school, Nightingale was equally blunt. A trained *woman* superintendent must be the sole manager and disciplinarian, with full authority over the students. "Otherwise," she warned, "nursing is impossible."

Opened in 1873, the Bellevue Training School for Nurses closely mirrored Nightingale's views. The superintendent would select the entering class and supervise its training. Only single, literate, religious women need apply, a flyer stated, with a preference for the "daughters and widows of clergymen, professional men, and farmers throughout New England and the Northern states." Most of the candidates were rejected on account of "bad breeding." The first class had just six members, the second twenty.

Progressives like Austin Flint and Stephen Smith strongly supported the school. But others thought it a fool's errand, almost certain to fail. "I do not believe in the success of a training school for nurses," a Bellevue surgeon declared. "Our patients are such a difficult class to deal with, and the service is so hard, that the conscientious, intelligent women you are looking for will lose heart and hope long before the two years are over."

But the Visiting Committee pressed ahead, raising $24,000 to provide living quarters for the students and salaries for the staff—the biggest donor being Mrs. William Henry Osborn, whose husband ran the Illinois Central Railroad. Following strict "Nightingale procedure," the training stressed "deportment, patience, industry and obedience." A Bellevue intern described the students as "slavishly afraid" of their supervisors. "They had military discipline," he said. "They didn't go out [with men] except surreptitiously." And they worked twelve-hour shifts, seven days a week, for little more than room and board. Should a patient pose a medical question, the proper answer—the *only* answer—was: "I don't know—ask your doctor."

Still, resentments grew as the Training School assumed a larger presence in the wards. A confrontation was inevitable, and it erupted in 1874 over the Visiting Committee's demand that student nurses be posted on the Bellevue maternity floors. The rationale was the rising death rate among mothers who had just given birth. Everyone knew the cause to be puerperal fever. The larger issue was what, if anything, could be done to prevent it.

Puerperal (or childbed) fever, a bacterial infection of the female reproductive tract, had plagued Bellevue for years. In 1851, eighteen of the 207 women who delivered babies there had contracted the fever, and twelve had died. "Every effort has been made to arrest its progress by isolating the patients, purifying the wards, and changing the attendants," a doctor noted—but nothing had worked. The fever seemed to float on the miasma clouds that permeated every nook and cranny of the hospital.

In Europe, meanwhile, a breakthrough seemed at hand. In 1847, a young physician named Ignaz Semmelweis noticed a pattern to puerperal fever at his hospital in Vienna. The maternity ward run by the midwives had far fewer cases than the maternity ward run by the obstetricians. Semmelweis had no concept of Germ Theory; that would come later with the discoveries of Louis Pasteur, Robert Koch, and Joseph Lister. What Semmelweis did observe, however, was that the obstetricians, unlike the midwives, regularly conducted cadaver dissections in the hospital's dead house, and few of them bothered to wash their hands before entering the maternity wards to deliver babies. This must be the cause of puerperal fever, he thought. Doctors were transferring deadly "particles" from the morgue to the birthing rooms.

In fact, these "particles" came from numerous sources—not simply cadavers—but Semmelweis was on to something. He urged his colleagues to soak their hands in a chlorine solution before each delivery, a procedure that did, indeed, reduce contamination among those who tried it. The problem was that Semmelweis proposed no scientific mechanism to explain his claims to those he indelicately accused of killing their own patients. "His genius [had] led him to a discovery for which the world was not yet prepared," wrote one biographer. "He violated the most basic of the principles that underlie the hunting-rules of those who would track down Nature's secrets: an idea must never be presented before its time."

Deaths from puerperal fever had climbed steadily at Bellevue in the post–Civil War years, from seventeen in 1865 to thirty-three by 1872. The patient logs describe a slow, agonizing demise, about two weeks in duration. "Case XXXII . . . aged 25, single, delivered a boy . . . following a labor of 27 and a half hours." Her symptoms began that evening with a rapid pulse and a temperature of 105. Day by day, her condition worsened: "sweating profusely . . . excited and nervous and often wanders . . . vomited a dark green liquid . . . tongue dry and covered with a brown coat . . . face flushed and burning hot." Her nourishment included "brandy and milk . . . a pint of beer and as much beef-tea" as she could hold down. The treatment relied on quinine, morphine, and "tincture of veratrum viride," a toxic plant extract used to slow a rapid heartbeat. The last notation read: "Respiration 26, pulse imperceptible at the wrist, temperature 107. Died 4:15 p.m."

Theories abounded as to its spread, the most popular still blaming dangerous "miasma clouds." "All admit that the saturation of the air with the exhalations of surgical and puerperal patients is eminently toxic," wrote Bellevue's Fordyce Barker, past president of the New York Academy of Medicine and personal physician to Ulysses S. Grant. Others added commentaries of their own—none more peculiar than the observation of Bellevue's chief obstetrician, William T. Lusk, that his birthing wards were filled with guilt-ridden "unwed mothers" who *wanted* to die. "Few people realize the appalling mental condition of some of these poor outcasts," he declared. "Without money, or friends, or sympathy . . . it is difficult to keep under control the suicidal propensities of the more desperate."

There was a better explanation, of course. With a new medical college at Bellevue, as well as a larger morgue for dissection, the chance of bacterial transmission had dramatically increased. Dozens of students and instructors now moved freely between the dead house and the maternity wards, ignorant of the dangers involved. (Fordyce Barker's widely read Bellevue lectures on puerperal fever, published in 1874 and running to 512 pages, make no mention of Semmelweis.) Further, these wards sat directly above the general operating rooms, where fatal infections—due, in part, to the role of anesthesia in permitting more invasive procedures—were also on the rise. While puerperal fever had invaded hospitals everywhere, Bellevue seemed ideally suited to its spread.

In 1874, Schuyler and her Visiting Committee issued a scathing report calling for Bellevue to be torn down and replaced by a series of low-slung, Pavilion-style structures. Citing the work of Florence Nightingale and William Hammond, they charged that Bellevue's "defective ventilation [and] construction" had created a death trap, "its walls saturated with the poisonous emanations of disease." No patient was safe from these "fatal influences," Schuyler claimed. Pyaemia, erysipelas, gangrene, puerperal fever—all thrived within this teeming, decrepit, filth-ridden disgrace.

The logic may have been faulty but the problem was disturbingly real. An in-house survey of fifty-five amputations performed at Bellevue in 1869 showed more than half the patients (twenty-seven) dying within a month of their surgeries. The survey didn't note the cause of death in all cases, but when it did, blood poisoning was mentioned almost every time. ("Died on the 14th day from pyaemia," read a typi-

cal entry.) And a follow-up of fifty-eight amputations at Bellevue in
1872–73—"not including fingers and toes"—counted "30 recoveries"
and "28 deaths," with pyaemia (11), exhaustion (8), and shock (4) top-
ping the list. Small wonder that a black-lettered sign in one of the
wards read: "PREPARE TO MEET YOUR GOD."

Bellevue was hardly unique. All urban hospitals in these years
recorded horrifying fatality rates from infections following surgery.
"Everything swam in pus," recalled an intern at Boston City Hospital.
"We [had] so much . . . gangrene that all operations were suspended
for several weeks because to cut a man meant to kill him." The difference was one of scale. Bellevue was massive: more patients meant more
surgical procedures, and more surgical procedures meant more deaths
from infection.

While razing the hospital struck most who worked there as extreme,
it did have the support of two high-profile Bellevue faculty members:
Frank Hamilton and William Hammond. Hamilton had long warned
of deadly miasma clouds, which he blamed for virtually all of surgery's
current ills. "The best place to treat a sick or wounded man is always,
other things being equal, where he can get the most and the purest
air," he wrote in his popular *Treatise on Military Surgery*. Hammond,
the driving force behind Satterlee and other Pavilion-style hospitals,
had moved to Bellevue following his controversial dismissal as surgeon
general, and quickly found trouble again. A snippet from one of the
Bellevue faculty meetings explained why: "Dr. Hammond [has] been
disloyal to the college . . . in remarking to persons not members of the
faculty that the Hospital was infested and should be destroyed." The
well-regarded Hamilton easily survived the crisis; the more disagreeable Hammond did not.

In the end, a compromise was reached. Bellevue would remain
standing, but student nurses would take over the patient care in the
birthing wards, despite angry protests from the physicians in charge.
But even this did no good. By 1874, the mortality rate among new
mothers at Bellevue was one in three—and climbing rapidly. Desperate for answers, Elizabeth Hobson consulted several physicians familiar with the disease, who told her that the controversial theories of
Ignaz Semmelweis—a name she, and most Americans, hadn't heard

before—appeared to be gaining ground. Many European hospitals were now requiring his chlorine solution; some had banned physicians who performed autopsies from delivering babies, and a few had even constructed separate maternity buildings, with excellent results.

In a dramatic confrontation, the Visiting Committee demanded that Bellevue close its birthing wards and send the patients somewhere else. "Gentlemen, we have learned the cause of the mortality," its spokeswoman told the Bellevue Medical Board. "We give you forty-eight hours to remove those women. If they are here at the end of that time, the whole story will be published in the *Evening Post*." While no doubt furious at an ultimatum from society-types based on "specula-tion" from Europe, the board quickly caved in. The maternity wards were closed and the patients moved to Charity Hospital on Blackwell's Island, along with nurses from the Bellevue Training School.

Progress came slowly. Flare-ups of puerperal fever would continue until 1877, when Hobson and her supporters funded a new birthing facility in an old firehouse near the Bellevue grounds. Run jointly by the Bellevue Obstetrical Service and the Training School, it observed a strict new set of rules. Hands were to be washed thoroughly in a chlo-rine solution and no staffer was permitted "to be present at autopsies [and then] to assist at surgical operations or the dressing of wounds." Puerperal fever virtually disappeared.

The victory helped bring professional nursing out of the shadows. In the late 1870s, the Training School had attracted fifty applicants a year. That number would reach 200 in 1880; 1,370 in 1890; and close to 1,800 by the new century. The most striking change, for both crit-ics and supporters at Bellevue, was the sense of order that had spread within the crumbling shells of the buildings, reminiscent of Night-ingale in Crimea. "I can still see the wards there," an intern recalled. "The floor was gleaming, every bed in perfect alignment, the sheets tucked in so tight the patients couldn't possibly dislodge them." In terms of basic care, he thought, the nurses "left little to be desired."

Looking back on the years of struggle to bring professional nursing to Bellevue, Elizabeth Hobson took understandable pride in the prog-ress that had occurred. "The early prejudices, the opposition we had to contend with, have long since vanished," she wrote in 1916. "Now a surgeon would not undertake an operation of any importance without the attendance of a trained nurse." A sure sign of this advancement was the expanded nursing curriculum, which added classes in anatomy, physiology, and the basic sciences. Even the once hostile Bellevue Medical Board had come to view the Training School as "an incalculable benefit to [our] hospital."

But problems remained. Most graduates of the school looked beyond Bellevue and other public hospitals to careers in the private sector, where the pay was better, the hours shorter, the workload less intense. And while the prejudice against nursing per se had surely eased, the public perception of nurses as "all-purpose female service workers," rather than carefully trained professionals, still lingers. Nightingale's emphasis on deference and discipline had actually retarded progress, some believed, by endorsing the power gap between doctors and nurses to the point where it became a fixed and natural part of hospital life. "When my mother became a registered nurse [in 1903]," wrote Lewis Thomas, a former NYU Medical School dean, "there was no question in anyone's mind about what nurses did as professionals. They did what the doctor ordered," from hanging up his hat and coat to following his precise instructions, though they knew the patients far better than he did. Eighty years later, Thomas could only marvel that so many of his male colleagues still viewed their nurses as glorified "ward administrators and technicians," despite the immense improvements in nursing education.

Ignaz Semmelweis never got to see the fruits of his labor. Fired from his hospital position in Vienna, he moved from job to job, a hero to some, an outcast to others. He died in 1865, following his commitment to a mental institution, but the work he pioneered would be studied, and refined, in laboratories across Europe. Known collectively as Germ Theory, it would soon divide America's medical community as few things had before—nowhere more so than at Bellevue Hospital.

10

GERM THEORY

By 1870, Bellevue was the uncontested giant of American hospitals. With 1,230 beds, its sheer size attracted elite physicians for whom the lure of "interesting" patients outweighed the fear of deadly "miasmas" and physical blight. So great was the clamor for a visiting position that the Medical Board agreed to split the hospital into four divisions—one for each of the city's major medical schools (Physicians & Surgeons, Bellevue, New York University), and one for "unaffiliated" doctors. Each division would be independent, with the power to appoint senior staff (physicians and surgeons) and house staff (interns and residents): the former chosen by pull and reputation, the latter by pull and examination.

Competition at the low end was especially intense. With America's medical schools producing thousands of graduates each year, those seeking an internship, the key to a successful practice in the larger cities, often found themselves shut out. An internship required a hospital willing to provide one, and there simply weren't enough hospitals to meet the demand. Though "merit" supposedly drove the selection process, the criteria could be flexible, to say the least. When applying for an internship at the Massachusetts General Hospital, young William James spoke of the shameless "toadying" that included "courtesy calls" to the homes of trustees. "I have little fears, with my talent for flattery and fawning, of a failure," James rightly boasted.

City hospital positions were the most coveted and cutthroat. Dr. Her-

ogs—a future giant in the field of public health—described Bellevue internship as the "highest honor" a medical school graduate could achieve. Biggs had dutifully enrolled in a "prep course" that tutored applicants for their entrance exam. He hardly seemed to need it—"[You] have passed with the rank of No. 1," he was told—but dozens of his peers signed up in the hope of gaining an edge. "I am undecided whose course I should take," a Bellevue applicant wrote home in 1878. "If I take Professor Smith's class it will cost me fifteen dollars, and if I take Prof. Loomis, it will cost twenty-five. I almost believe it would pay to take Loomis, for . . . I would at least have his goodwill [and] he is one of the examiners."

In this case, the extra ten dollars seemed very well spent. "Prof. Loomis' private class is excellent," the applicant noted, though that was hardly the reason he signed up. What drove him was the chance to buy favor with the right professor, which, he admitted, "is a trick that is frequently done." Lacking the talent of a Hermann Biggs, the young man did the next best thing. "I think I can count on Prof. Loomis," he wrote, and he probably was right. His exam went smoothly, and his internship came through.

Few hospitals could match the young talent that Bellevue attracted. In the late 1870s, its list of interns included two men destined to revolutionize their fields. One was William Welch; the other William Halsted. Both men hoped one day to make Bellevue their permanent home, though neither man did. Their stories, complicated and intertwined, speak volumes about the workings of the hospital in that era and the deep medical divide that eventually drove them away.

William Welch, the son of a Connecticut country doctor, had been a top student at Yale and P&S before arriving at Bellevue in 1875. "It is certainly the most completely appointed hospital in New York and [perhaps] in the world," he gushed in a letter home. "We have the best visiting physicians and surgeons in the city; we have the advantages of daily clinics and pathological examinations in the Dead House." In short, a medical bonanza—cradle to grave.

Welch found a mentor of sorts in Dr. Francis Delafield, a remote presence who ran the morgue and performed the autopsies. One learned from Delafield through silent observation; a wizard with a microscope, he spent long hours stooped over his workbench studying the pathology of disease. Delafield's case reports on tumors of the lung and the kidney are still considered among the classics of microscopic pathology. The problem, Welch realized, was that he'd gone about as far as he could at Bellevue or any other American hospital; a dead end loomed ahead. In Europe, there were dozens of Delafields working on subjects barely explored in the United States. Welch saw no choice but to follow his internship with two years of study abroad. "Even assuming that I do not obtain any position in a medical college," he wrote his father, "the prestige and knowledge which I should acquire . . . would decidedly increase my chances of success in a large city. The young doctors who are doing well in New York are in a large proportion those who have studied [in Europe]."

William Halsted, the son of a leading New York City merchant, had graduated from Yale two years after Welch, their paths rarely crossing. Halsted rowed, played baseball, and captained the first eleven-man football team in school history. Bored with his studies—there is no record of his ever borrowing a book from the Yale library—he bought a copy of *Gray's Anatomy* after attending a few lectures at the medical school with a friend. Somehow, a light clicked on. Deciding to forgo the family business for a career in medicine, Halsted chose the College of Physicians and Surgeons, where his father, conveniently, was a trustee.

Though every bit a proprietary—or profit-making—institution, P&S had a lineage and reputation that few medical schools could match. And it sat only a few blocks from the Halsted mansion on lower Fifth Avenue, adding convenience as well. The lectures at P&S were dull and redundant, Halsted recalled, but the clinics in medicine and surgery—often held at Bellevue—made the drudgery worthwhile. Like Welch, Halsted performed splendidly, writing the best examination essay in his graduating class. And like Welch, he moved on to Bellevue.

Halsted began his internship just as Welch departed for Europe. "In 1876, the year I [first] walked the wards of Bellevue Hospital, New

York," Halsted recalled, "the dawn of modern surgery had hardly begun." He was referring to the era between the discovery of anesthesia and the triumph of antiseptic methods—a time when the horrors of postoperative infection still haunted the operating room. Determined to be a surgeon, Halsted worked closely with Bellevue's best, including Stephen Smith and Frank Hamilton. Halsted admired both men, calling them the finest teachers he had known. Where Smith and Hamilton differed, however, was in their opinion of a British surgeon named Joseph Lister. Smith admired him; Hamilton did not. The stakes for American medicine could hardly have been higher.

In 1876, the United States celebrated its hundredth birthday with a dazzling display of technology and consumerism known as the Centennial Exhibition. Held in Philadelphia from May through November, it attracted ten million visitors—equal to 20 percent of the country's population. President Ulysses S. Grant opened the festivities, flanked by fellow Union generals Philip Sheridan, Winfield Scott Hancock, and William Tecumseh Sherman in full military dress. For many Americans, the Exhibition proved a respite from troubled times. To the west of Philadelphia, coal mine owners were locked in a violent struggle with immigrant miners, led by the Molly Maguires. From the Great Plains came word that General George A. Custer and his entire cavalry regiment had been wiped out by Sioux warriors at the Little Big Horn. In the South, vigilante violence against newly freed blacks threatened to unravel a decade's worth of federal policy known as Reconstruction. On top of this, the nation faced a constitutional crisis in which both major presidential candidates—Republican Rutherford B. Hayes and Democrat Samuel Tilden—claimed victory in the 1876 election, raising concerns about who would govern the Republic.

A more optimistic scene awaited visitors to the Centennial Exhibition. For 50 cents, one could climb through the unassembled right arm and torch of the Statue of Liberty, awaiting its final trip to New York harbor. In Machinery Hall, one could watch Alexander Graham Bell show off his telephone, and then tap away on a Remington "typographic machine," which switched seamlessly from uppercase to lowercase letters with the stroke of a key. A nearby food court show-cased a new condiment known as "ketchup" from the Heinz family of Pittsburgh, and a caramel-flavored soft drink called "root beer" from the Philadelphia pharmacist Charles Elmer Hires. While the Exhibition was an international event with numerous foreign pavilions, there seemed little doubt about who owned the future. "The products of the industry of the United States [have] surpassed our own," lamented the *Times* of London. "They revealed the application of more brains than we have at our command."

There was one notable exception to the claim of American superiority. The 1876 Exhibition also hosted the International Medical Congress, five hundred strong, whose speakers included the English surgeon Joseph Lister. Lister had come to America with a radical idea. He believed that the recent discoveries of Louis Pasteur had forever changed the practice of medicine. Pasteur had shown that putrefaction—the decomposition of organic matter—depended on "minute organisms," or "germs," suspended in the air and the water, invisible to the naked eye. These microbes, said Lister, were responsible for the postoperative infections that turned the average operating room into a slaughterhouse. Like Ignaz Semmelweis, Lister blamed the problem of infection not on deadly "hospital air," but rather on the careless habits of the surgical staff. Unlike Semmelweis, Lister supplied both a theory of causation and strong clinical evidence to make his point.

Pasteur had employed intense heat and intricate filters to prevent bacterial contamination—neither of which could be used during surgery. Lister thought a chemical compound might work, so he experimented with carbolic acid, a common treatment for neutralizing the stench of sewer gases. At the Glasgow Infirmary, he dipped everything in carbolic acid—hands, fingernails, instruments, table surfaces, towels, and dressings—while using an atomizer to spray the air. The infection rate dropped so dramatically that Lister published his findings in *The Lancet*, England's leading medical journal. "Comparing the aggregate results," he wrote, "we have—

Before the antiseptic period (1864–1866), 16 deaths in 35 [amputations]; or 1 death for every 2 ⅕ cases;

During the antiseptic period (1867–1869), 6 deaths in 40
[amputations] or 1 death for every 6 ⅔ cases."

Antiseptic surgery had dramatically reduced the risk of blood poisoning and hospital gangrene, Lister noted. "Its effects upon the wards
lately under my care [in Glasgow] were in the highest degree beneficial,
converting them . . . into models of healthfulness."

The American response was predictable. Medical theories from
Europe had long faced stiff resistance, and the battle over antiseptic
surgery would be no different. Lister, forty-nine years old at the time
of the Centennial Exhibition, had been invited to speak by Samuel
Gross, seventy-one, president of the American Medical Association.
Immensely self-assured—his relentlessly immodest autobiography
ran to 855 pages—Gross was so revered for his surgical skills that the
International Medical Congress, which Gross also headed, had com-
missioned a mural of him at work by a local artist named Thomas
Eakins.

Today *The Gross Clinic* is considered a masterpiece, one of the finest
American paintings of the nineteenth century. The enormous canvas,
eight feet high and six and a half feet wide, depicts Dr. Gross pausing in
reflection beside an operating table, a bloody scalpel in his right hand,
as one of his numerous assistants leans over to probe the partly clothed
patient's open wound. In the foreground lies an open box of menacing
surgical instruments; to the left sits a grief-stricken woman, likely the
patient's mother, her arm slung feebly over her eyes; in the background
are row upon row of spectators, the clearest of whom (often identified
as Eakins himself) is intently scribbling notes.

The mural was supposed to hang in the Centennial Exhibition's
main gallery. But critics were so stunned by its realism, calling it "a
picture strong men find difficult to look at," that a decision was made
to move it to an army hospital far from the Exhibition grounds. Some
questioned Eakins's motive. Was the mural intended as a tribute to the
medical craftsmanship of Dr. Gross, or was it something more sub-
versive? What is obvious—to modern eyes, at least—is the absence of
basic antiseptic methods. Gross and his assistants are wearing business
suits. There is no water for washing the instruments and no carbolic

acid in sight. The patient is wearing the soiled clothing he arrived in, his dirty socks prominently displayed. Blood is everywhere—on scalpels, dressings, and bare hands. Was Eakins making a statement about the willful ignorance of Dr. Gross—a man who scoffed at Pasteur's theories and needlessly exposed his patients to disease?

Furthermore, why would Gross ask Lister, of all people, to address the International Medical Conference? The most likely answer—aside from an actual interest in the subject matter—is that Gross hoped to debunk Germ Theory and antiseptic surgery on a grand stage. Gross had invited a number of skeptical surgeons, including Bellevue's Frank Hamilton, to question Lister on his methods. One by one, they rose to challenge the need for antisepsis and to present their own remedies for combating surgical infection, a list that ranged from "cold water" sprinkled on the open wound to "rest—quietude of the limb."

Then it was Hamilton's turn. "A large portion of American surgeons seem not to have adopted [Lister's] practice," he began, "whether from a lack of confidence or for other reasons, I cannot say." Hamilton didn't belittle the Englishman; he simply ignored him—much as he ignored Germ Theory as a silly notion that would mercifully disappear. For his part, Hamilton endorsed something called the "open air treatment" in which "no dressings whatever are employed," leaving the wound free to excrete pus until it healed on its own. "At Bellevue Hospital," he said, citing no real evidence, "this method has been employed recently, in quite a number of major amputations, with remarkable success."

Lister had come to America to spread his gospel. Philadelphia was the first leg of an extensive cross-country tour. A genuinely humble man, he took pains to praise the medical advances made in the United States, singling out anesthesia as the greatest gift "ever conferred upon suffering humanity." At times, his remarks bordered on pandering, as when he described American surgeons as "renowned throughout the world for their inventive genius, boldness, and skill in execution." Lister spoke for three hours that afternoon, linking germs to infection and demonstrating his techniques. To those who worried about the time and effort involved, he assured them it was well worth the trouble. "It is the close attention to these minute details that renders this system so absolutely certain and safe," he said. And to those who questioned the science behind it, he linked himself directly to Pasteur. "The germ theory of putrefaction is the foundation of the whole system of antiseptic surgery," Lister declared, "and if this theory is a fact, it is a fact of facts that the antiseptic system means the exclusion of putrefactive organisms."

Few minds were changed. Some in the audience grumbled about Lister's complicated instructions, while others fretted that carbolic acid might irritate their hands. Mostly, though, there was bewilderment that anyone should listen to an Englishman spouting the theories of a Frenchman about the dangers of particles too small for anyone to see.

Lister's Philadelphia presentation did not go entirely unnoticed, however. In the audience that day was an apothecary's apprentice from New Brunswick, New Jersey, named Robert Wood Johnson. Inspired by the science of the presentation, the young man imagined a future in which Lister's ideas would be the norm for operating rooms, doctors' offices, and medicine cabinets across the land. Joining with his brother and a few friends, he would begin a company producing sterile bandages for a market that barely existed: Johnson & Johnson.

Welch and Halsted were two of the thousands of young American physicians who visited Europe in these years in search of better clinical and laboratory training. One historian described this migration as the largest "movement of professional men over so great a distance . . . in the annals of human experience." Previously, such visits were limited to cities like Paris, London, and Edinburgh. But times had changed. Those seeking the latest techniques in bacteriology, pathology, and surgery now flooded the labs and clinics of Leipzig, Vienna, and Berlin. Welch began his two-year odyssey through Central Europe in 1876. It was expensive—he, unlike Halsted, wasn't wealthy—and it meant learning German. Welch adapted rather well, commenting with his usual fussiness about everything from the food (heavy and monotonous) to the local medical students he met (arrogant and condescending) to the alien street life ("You can see the original Shylocks in the shape of Polish Jews who are swarming here"). What most impressed him, however, was the German passion for evidence-based science. "Don't be alarmed," Welch wrote his sister. "I do not expect to [settle here] but I do think that the condition of medical education [in America] is simply horrible."

Welch was particularly taken by Germany's embrace of Lister. "You must go to [Leipzig] if only for a couple of days," he urged a friend. "Such results as they have there are simply astounding to me—42 successive cases of amputation of the thigh [without] one death. If you are not a convert to Lister, you [are] stubborn to fact."

Welch returned to New York in 1878 determined to spread the word. Ignoring these breakthroughs was more than an affront to science, he believed; it was a brazen attempt by parts of the medical community to prevent new and better ideas from taking hold. Welch turned first to his medical school professors at P&S. Offered a lowly, unpaid lectureship in pathology, he replied that a successful course required an actual laboratory, which the college didn't have and was unwilling to build. Welch then approached his friends at Bellevue, with modestly better results: a small stipend was promised, along with three bare rooms for a laboratory and $25 worth of supplies. Begging and borrowing, Welch collected his own specimens by combing the local marshes for frogs. That fall, with half a dozen Bellevue students and an equal number of "antique microscopes," he offered the first pathology course at an American medical school.

It proved an instant success. As word spread that the European-trained Welch was offering a pathology course with a laboratory component, medical students from across the city clamored to get in. A few months later, a new offer arrived from P&S. Lab space had been found; an alumni group would provide the supplies; and a modest salary was attached. Given the school's powerful reputation, it seemed a perfect fit for Welch, a recent alumnus. "We've got to get you back," he was told. "We must have pathology here."

Welch was sorely tempted. The offer meant that two major medical schools now recognized pathology as a discipline worth pursuing. It was a heady moment for the son of a country doctor, not yet thirty years old, who had returned from Europe with few prospects for academic success. But Welch turned down the offer. "I felt I would be a traitor after all that they had done for me at Bellevue if I abandoned them, so I declined very reluctantly," he recalled.

While immensely popular with medical students and the house staff,

Welch earned mixed reviews from Bellevue's senior physicians, some viewing him as "a laboratory man," unable to do "anything practical." One episode is particularly revealing. Upon learning that Germany's Robert Koch had isolated the tubercle bacillus, Welch explained its momentous implications at his next lecture, drawing bursts of applause. Word of this reached Alfred Loomis, a Bellevue faculty don and president of the elite New York Academy of Medicine. A few days later, Loomis openly mocked the discovery in the hospital's packed amphitheater. "People say there are bacteria in the air, but I cannot <u>see</u> them," he said, peering dramatically into space. Welch wisely let it pass. He wasn't about to pick a fight he couldn't win. "That's too bad," he told the student who reported the remark to him. "Loomis is such a nice man."

As Welch gained a modest foothold at Bellevue, William Halsted began his own journey to Central Europe. Returning to New York City in 1880, he took on several jobs before settling primarily at Bellevue, where he and Welch, formerly acquaintances, became fast friends. Like other young surgeons, Halsted faced a senior staff bitterly divided over Germ Theory and antisepsis. At one end of the spectrum stood Frank Hamilton and his allies, conceding nothing to these "foreign ideas." In the middle were those like James Rushmore Wood, a founder of Bellevue Medical College, who had begun his surgical career before anesthesia existed and could amputate a leg in nine seconds. Wood wasn't opposed to Lister per se. He conspicuously washed his hands before operating because he believed in personal cleanliness, not because he supported—much less understood—what Germ Theory implied. As a result, Wood made no attempt to sanitize his instruments, or the operating table, or the patient's wound—and few in the audience seemed to mind.

At the other end of the spectrum were surgeons like Stephen Smith, who had met Lister during his American tour in 1876 and was among his early converts. Smith had come to Germ Theory the hard way—by watching dozens of his patients survive the operation only to die shortly thereafter of infection. "We may summarize the conditions regarded as essential to success as follows," he wrote of his new surgical routine: "A clean operator; clean assistants; a clean patient; clean instruments; clean dressings."

Frank Hamilton viewed Smith's methods as "demented," and some shunned Smith entirely. Walking through the hospital, he could hear the mocking cries of "There's a bacillus, catch him!" The conflict led Halsted to worry whether he could continue to practice at Bellevue—a place, he fretted, "where the numerous anti-Lister surgeons dominated and predominated." This was an exaggeration. The lecture notes of Bellevue medical students in these years show a fair number of faculty endorsing Germ Theory and antisepsis. "Pasteur has demonstrated that 212 degrees heat destroys germ life," read a typical student entry. "To [prevent] poison in the blood use carbolic acid about wound and in room freely—metastatic abscesses should be opened early and washed out."

What troubled Halsted were the methods of the old guard—surgeons who held instruments in their teeth, passed unwashed artery clamps from patient to patient, and closed wounds with catgut discolored by filth. Refusing to work in the same operating space used by these men, Halsted got permission to build a private surgical tent on the hospital lawn, personally raising the $10,000 it would cost. "The floor was of maple laid almost as finely as a bowling alley," Halsted recalled. There were "large and numerous portholes [for] ample light. Water, hot and cold, and gas were piped to the tent and patients were rolled [in] on a platform." It was, some believed, the most sanitary operating room in the country.

In 1880, controversy surrounding Joseph Lister and his methods was largely unknown to Americans beyond the medical profession, but this was about to change. Less than a year after Halsted's return from Europe, a political tragedy of epic proportions struck the United States, bringing esoteric terms like Germ Theory and antisepsis into the national dialogue in an unimaginable way.

11

A TALE OF TWO PRESIDENTS

On the morning of July 2, 1881, an assassin named Charles Guiteau approached President James A. Garfield in Washington's main railroad depot and fired two shots at point-blank range from a snubnosed revolver. Convinced that he had been responsible for Garfield's victory, and demanding an ambassadorship in return, the deranged Guiteau exacted his revenge. One bullet grazed the president's arm; the other entered his back, missing the spinal cord but breaking two ribs before settling behind the pancreas. Those who first attended him thought the wound to be fatal, as did Garfield himself. "Doctor, I am a dead man," he told a physician at the scene. Only forty-nine, he'd just taken office in March.

The assassin's bullet, we know today, did not cause Garfield's death. It had lodged in fatty tissue, skirting vital organs and major arteries. Had the responding physicians been followers of Joseph Lister, or had they done nothing more than make Garfield comfortable, he almost certainly would have survived. Instead they searched clumsily for the bullet, inserting unwashed fingers and filthy probes into the open wound. Rushed back to the White House, the new president appeared to rally; in truth, the fatal damage likely had been done.

The lead physician was Doctor Willard Bliss, a family friend. (His hopeful parents actually named him Doctor.) Though Bliss spoke boldly of his ability to handle the case, Secretary of State James G. Blaine, Garfield's political confidant, was less certain. Blaine had been standing alongside the president when the shooting occurred. Taking charge, he summoned two of the nation's top surgeons to the White House—David Hayes Agnew, sixty-three, a professor at the University of Pennsylvania Medical School, and Bellevue's Frank H. Hamilton, now sixty-eight. "The President, while doing well, is still in a very critical condition," Blaine telegraphed Hamilton on July 3. "It would do much to relieve Mrs. Garfield's anxiety to have you here to consult with the attending Physician. Will you come by first train?" Hamilton left for Washington that evening.

He and Agnew examined Garfield the following day—July 4—without pausing to wash their hands or clean their instruments. The problem, Hamilton told reporters, was that "the ball seems to have entered the liver and remains in the abdominal cavity beyond the reach of detection." Actually, Hamilton had no idea where the bullet lay, and wouldn't find out until the autopsy was performed. Worse yet, he threw caution to the wind. "The President is getting better," he assured the nation. "The chances are all in his favor."

Hamilton furthered this fantasy by returning to Bellevue. With Garfield's condition now "stable," a full recovery was predicted. "Dr. Hamilton's Views: No Danger of Pyaemia or Other Complications—The President's Life Safe," the *New York Times* declared. But when Garfield didn't recover—he got progressively worse—Hamilton was summoned back to Washington. At a tearful private meeting on July 23, he recalled, Mrs. Garfield begged him to remain by her husband's side, and he dutifully agreed. "From this moment until the death of the President," he wrote, "my time and thoughts were given wholly to the sufferer in the White House."

No stone was left unturned. In attempting to cool down Garfield's sweltering bedroom, a group of engineers designed what one historian has called "the country's first air conditioner"—a huge fan "that forced air through cheesecloth screens soaked in ice water." With the X-ray machine yet to be invented, Garfield's advisors invited Alexander Graham Bell to try to find the bullet believed to be responsible for Garfield's grave condition with a primitive metal detector called the "induction balance." It didn't work. What had caused Garfield's reversal? Some blamed the presidential mansion, then in awful disrepair. The pipes leaked, the floors were rotted, and rodents had the run of the place. Surrounded by swampland, it often stank of sewage. In one of the more bizarre episodes of the assassination drama, Garfield's doctors, suspecting dangerous "miasmas" to be the cause of his troubles, brought in a sanitary engineer to inspect the plumbing, cesspools, and local marshes for dangerous odors. His report, never made public, confirmed the worst: the White House was a deadly mess. "The President," said one alarmed physician, "is now in much greater danger from the pestilential vapors of the Potomac flats than from Guiteau's bullet." What influence, if any, this had on the future course of events is not known. But three weeks later, Garfield was moved by train to a house on the New Jersey Shore, where "the cool breezes of the sea coast" allowed "air of the right kind to [filter] into the invalid's chamber."

There is no evidence, however, that his treatment changed course. In an era before antibiotics, there was little to be done once a massive bacterial infection set in beyond draining the pus and easing the pain, which meant morphine, alcohol, and nourishment through the rectum, since Garfield could hold down little of the food he ingested. Still, the cheerful updates kept appearing. "I regard his case as making good progress toward an almost assured recovery," Hamilton announced on August 1. Two days later, he publicly applauded Garfield's medical team—himself included—for its heroic efforts on the president's behalf. "I have had a great deal of experience with gunshot wounds in the course of my life, having seen many thousands of them," he stated, "and I think I may safely say that I have never seen a case more judiciously managed."

Not everyone agreed. As the weeks passed without a sighting of the bedridden Garfield, rumors spread that he might indeed be suffering from pyaemia, or blood poisoning. If true—if something this serious had so long escaped detection—"it does not give a happy impression of the acuteness of the doctors around the President," remarked the *New York World*. But Dr. Hamilton's resolve remained rock solid through the crisis, and his sterling reputation helped ease the doubts. Many physicians—including several Bellevue colleagues—lined up loyally in support. "The case," said Alfred Loomis, "could not possibly be progressing more favorably." As late as September, with Garfield now hovering near death, most newspapers still expressed confidence in Hamilton, calling him "the prince of surgeons" and "a model gentleman." A typical headline read: "The President's Best Day: His Condition Growing More and More Hopeful."*

Garfield died on September 19 at the oceanfront home in Elberon, New Jersey. Ravaged by multiple infections, "his ribs stuck out, his arms and legs resembled matchsticks and his face appeared skeletal." He had lost close to one hundred pounds in ten weeks. The autopsy listed the cause of death as a "secondary hemorrhage" near the path of the bullet but noted, without further comment, two enormous abscesses (or collections of pus), one "in the vicinity of the gall bladder," the other "between the loin muscles and the right kidney."

The findings were controversial. And their publication seemed to accomplish what Joseph Lister's Centennial Exhibition address had failed to do five years before: ignite a full-scale debate over the value of antiseptic surgery. For some, the abscesses clearly indicated pyaemia, which raised serious doubts about the care that President Garfield had received. Writing in the prestigious *Boston Medical and Surgical Journal*, Dr. John Collins Warren Jr., a rising star in the profession, took direct aim at Hamilton's methods. "We might criticize the introduction of the finger of several surgeons into the wound," he wrote, adding: "These examinations were not in accord with prevailing present theories."

Even those who had stood solidly behind Garfield's doctors during the crisis seemed shaken by the death. Perhaps other approaches

---

* Whether Hamilton's optimism was based on his medical judgment, wishful thinking, a desire to calm public opinion, or a combination of these factors is unknown. Garfield's medical team kept a daily medical log. The notations include July 27: "The President slept sweetly last night. . . . His general condition is improving." July 30: "The discharge of his pus is satisfactory in quantity and quality." August 17: "The President's condition is even better than it was this morning. . . . Two teaspoons full of beef extract have been twice administered by mouth and not rejected. The wound continues to do well." As late as September, the log spoke of Garfield's "unusually good night" and "reassuring general condition." The final notation on September 19 reads: "He awoke complaining of a severe pain above the region of his right heart. He almost immediately became unconscious and ceased to breathe at 10:35." Complete Medical Record of President Garfield's Case, Washington, D.C., 1881.

could have been tried; perhaps more could have been done to reverse the downward spiral. "The collision of opinion on [Lister's methods] is exemplified by the varying practices of surgeons working in the same hospital everywhere," wrote the *New York Herald Tribune*, "and the fair-minded observer is indeed puzzled to know on which side he should take his stand."

Others, however, mocked Hamilton as a fossil in his own institution. "If Garfield had been a 'tough,' and received his wound in a Bowery dive," a doctor sniffed, "he would have been brought to Bellevue Hospital in an ambulance, operated on without fuss or feathers, and would have gotten well." Furious, Hamilton replied that dressings dipped in carbolic acid *had* been applied to Garfield's wound. What he couldn't comprehend was that antisepsis required precise daily effort—it couldn't be done casually, hit or miss. There was no compensating for the single thrust of a germ-ridden finger. The slightest deviation could be fatal. At his murder trial that fall, Garfield's soon-to-be-hanged assassin refused to accept blame for the president's death, shouting: "Nothing could be more absurd. . . . Garfield died from malpractice." Sadly there was truth to what he said.

Whatever goodwill Garfield's doctors had earned from their vigil at the failing president's bedside vanished instantly when word leaked out regarding the size of the bill each man sent Congress. "For professional services as consulting surgeon and physician," Hamilton's read, "rendered to the late President of the United States, James A. Garfield, Deceased, from July 3, 1881, to September 19, 1881, inclusive, Twenty Five Thousand Dollars, $25,000." Hamilton justified the sum (worth close to $600,000 in 2016 dollars) by claiming to have led each consultation and surgical procedure "until the hour of Mr. Garfield's death," and remaining, "as was my duty, to take part in the autopsy." But his tone-deaf explanation only made things worse. "Sir, the bill you have submitted . . . is exorbitant in the extreme," an anonymous "Friend of the late President" wrote him, and he wasn't alone. The public response proved so hostile that a special congressional committee was formed to investigate "the Expenses of the Last Illness and Burial of President Garfield," with an eye toward lowering the bill. The majority recommended the sum of $15,000, noting that a surgeon of Hamilton's standing often earned that much overseeing a serious case, while the minority, furious over both the bill *and* Garfield's medical treatment, opposed the majority's recommendation as "excessive." In the end, Congress cut the fee to $5,000, including expenses. Hamilton returned to Bellevue a bitter, humbled man.

When he died five years later from tuberculosis, his friends recalled him as a skilled surgeon, a generous mentor, and a decent soul. "To younger practitioners and medical students, he was most considerate and kind," said one, and to the poorest charity patients he was as courteous as to the wealthy. Hamilton's main eulogy was delivered by his "favorite pupil," Charles Augustus Leale. "As a tribute of love, I take pleasure in placing on record the history of my early preceptor and dear friend," said the physician who had rushed to Lincoln's aid at Ford's Theatre in 1865. Leale's "history" didn't include their fateful bond—two surgeons linked by their roles, two decades apart, in treating a stricken president. Frank Hamilton "stood erect to the last," Leale concluded, accomplishing "so much for the good of his profession and also of his fellow-man." There was not a mention of James A. Garfield, Joseph Lister, or the future of antiseptic medicine.

As Welch and Halsted pushed the Listerian agenda at Bellevue, their bond grew stronger. Both were young and single, graduates of Yale and P&S—though their differences were substantial. Halsted was tall, lean, and athletic. A meticulous dresser, he wore tailored suits from London and expensive Italian shoes. (For a time, he actually sent his linen shirts to be washed and pressed in Paris because he couldn't find a local laundry that met his absurdly exacting standards.) Welch, by contrast, was short, paunchy, and disheveled. He avoided physical exercise and had no interest in sports. His greatest love, aside from medicine, appeared to be eating. His longtime friend, the critic H. L. Mencken, described a lunch the two had shared when the two-hundred-plus-pound Welch was almost eighty years old. "The main dish was country ham and greens, and [he] had a large portion," Mencken observed, "washing it down with several mugs of beer. There followed lemon meringue pie. He ate an arc of at least 75 degrees of it, and eased it into his system with a cup of coffee. Then he lighted a six-inch panatela and smoked it to the butt. And then he ambled off to a medical meeting and to prepare for dinner."

Like Halsted, who had insisted on his own surgical space, Welch never felt truly comfortable at Bellevue. His teaching philosophy, though popular with students, was clearly out of step. "I shall make the leading features of [my] course the demonstration of fresh pathological specimens and the making of post mortem examinations," Welch declared. "In doing this I must sacrifice to a considerable extent systematic didactic instruction." What this meant, in simple terms, was the substitution of the microscope for the textbook, the laboratory for the lecture hall. And it included subject matter viewed by some as the "passing nonsense" of foreign minds. In the words of the ubiquitous Dr. Loomis: "The [germ] theory, which so recently has occupied medical men, especially in Germany, is rapidly being disproved, and consequently is rapidly being abandoned."

There was more to it than the clash of teaching philosophies, however. Unlike the wealthier Halsted, Welch constantly had to scramble to make ends meet in New York. He took on so much outside work to supplement his income—performing autopsies, tutoring students, examining private patients—that there was little time left for what most interested him: laboratory research. Privately, Welch longed for the chance to pursue his academic passions without the drudgery of earning a living.

In 1884, an offer arrived from a new university in Baltimore named for its main benefactor: Johns Hopkins. At his death in 1873, Hopkins, a bachelor with no heirs, had left the largest philanthropic gift in American history to that point, $7 million, for the construction of a university and a hospital, with a medical school to follow. "What are we aiming for?" asked Daniel Coit Gilman, the university's first president, at his inauguration. "The encouragement of research . . . and of individual scholars, who by their excellence will advance the sciences they pursue, and the society where they dwell."

Welch deeply admired the Hopkins medical school model, built on German thinking, with a four-year curriculum, a major laboratory component, and a college degree required for admission. At Bellevue, a medical school had been created to serve the interests of the hospital; at Hopkins, a hospital was being built to serve the interests of the medical school. "Mr. Gilman is looking out for men to fill positions in his university," Welch had written his father in 1876. "It seems folly to me to aspire to attaining [one] when there are so many distinguished men in the country who have already acquired great reputation."

Eight years later, Welch was high on Gilman's list. The report on him summed up exactly what Hopkins wanted: "a gentleman in every sense . . . a good lecturer . . . an excellent laboratory teacher [with] a keen desire for an opportunity to make original investigations." In short, "the best man in this country."

An offer quickly followed. Welch would receive a handsome starting salary—$4,000 a year, with raises to follow. Even better, he could count on "such laboratory facilities and assistants as may be requisite" through a personal endowment, something unheard of at an American medical school. President Gilman attached a personal plea to the offer: *"You must come."*

Welch was more than flattered; he was intrigued. Staying at Bellevue had its advantages: good friends, fine museums and restaurants, and a hospital filled with brilliant, if sometimes combative, peers. "I have [tasted] the pleasures and comforts of New York," Welch noted, "and they are not easy to relinquish." The problem lay elsewhere. "I do not feel as if [I'm] accomplishing what I want to do," he confessed to his father. "My energies are split in too many different directions and are likely to be [as] long as I remain here." At Hopkins, Welch could focus on his laboratory work, free from the demands of seeing private patients, running student tutorials, and (he sheepishly admitted) "the drudgery of teaching."

Given the unique pull of Hopkins, a serious counteroffer was required. The point man would be Frederic Dennis, a Bellevue surgeon who had known Welch since prep school and prized their companionship in ways that Welch himself did not. "Willie Welch came to see me," Dennis would gush in his teenage diary. "Willie Welch and I went to the woods and read a book. . . . Went swimming in Mill Pond with Willie Welch. . . . Willie is visiting me. . . . I went with him to New York and we walked up Broadway." When Welch left for Yale, the fawning Dennis had flooded him with mail. "I should have answered your letter sooner if I had not been afflicted with the mumps," Welch would eventually reply. Or, "I've delayed answering so long [because] I was sick with boils." Or, "You are no doubt surprised that I have not written before this. The reason is that I have been troubled with a sore eye." Upon exhausting all known medical excuses—a swollen foot, headaches, mental fatigue—Welch requested a break. "For if we write oftener," he wearily explained, "I shall be obliged to expatiate upon nothing, which besides being tedious for me to do must be very uninteresting for you to hear."

Dennis came from serious money. His family—like Halsted's—belonged to New York City's commercial elite. Growing up, Dennis had showered gifts upon Welch, who accepted them without complaint. The Dennis family had even paid for Welch to accompany Fred to the clinics of Europe following their Bellevue internships, and Welch had traveled to medical conferences in the Dennis railroad car, which he described as "furnished with kitchen, dining room, staterooms, balcony and every sort of luxury." Whatever his ambivalence about Fred Dennis, Welch kept the relationship alive—partly out of need, partly out of respect. Dennis was a terrific surgeon with wide-ranging interests. He would be among the first Americans to employ Pasteur's treatment for rabies and to grasp the importance of antibiotics in battling bacterial disease. And nobody at Bellevue had better social connections than Dennis, whose celebrated patients included Andrew Carnegie, one of the richest men in the world.

In 1884, Carnegie had yet to discover philanthropy—a failing he would acknowledge five years later by vowing, in a famous series of essays titled "The Gospel of Wealth," to give away much of his fortune and urging fellow plutocrats to do the same. But Dennis approached him anyway, explaining the importance of the medical research being done in Europe and the need to bring it to the United States. The pitch was successful: Carnegie responded with a sum large enough to build the nation's first fully equipped pathology laboratory adjoining the Bellevue Hospital grounds. "Gentlemen," the steel king wrote his bankers, "Please pay drafts of Frederic S. Dennis upon you to the extent of fifty thousand dollars and charge same to my [account]." A week later, the Bellevue Medical Board appropriated $45,000 to buy the land on which the building would be constructed.

Carnegie's gift was very big news. The *New York Times* described it as a triumph for American medical research. "In Germany," it said, "[such] facilities are amply provided by the Government. In this country they can only be furnished by private beneficence. . . . The purpose of Mr. Carnegie's gift is to supply in the city of New York advantages for which now the student goes abroad. . . . The building will belong to the Bellevue Hospital Medical College, but will be open . . . to members of the medical profession throughout the country."

The *Times* had missed the main purpose of Carnegie's largesse: keeping Welch at Bellevue. The rub, however, was that Hopkins had offered Welch something even more precious—a *guaranteed endowment* covering his laboratory expenses and an annual salary for him and his assistants. Bellevue refused to go that far. Dennis believed, no doubt correctly, that Welch's earning potential in New York City was enormous. Students would flock to his tutorials; private patients would line up at his door. "I know in ten years his income [here] will be twenty thousand dollars and more as contrasted with a salary of ten thousand [in Baltimore] and . . . a life in isolation [as] a scientific recluse," Dennis wrote Welch's brother, begging him to intervene. "His ideas imbibed in Germany are impractical. . . . He [will] cut himself aloof from everything in the way of sacred associations and of true friendships . . . for an ideal, which cannot ever be realized."

In fact, the German research model had dramatically raised Welch's profile in the United States. The recent discovery by Robert Koch that the causative agent of tuberculosis was a bacterium *visible* through a microscope had served both to demolish the Miasma Theory and propel the fields of pathology and bacteriology into the spotlight. Even the more reluctant Bellevue dons took notice. In perhaps the most remarkable turnabout, Alfred Loomis, who had publicly mocked Koch and Germ Theory only months before, now begged Welch to stay. "I shall resign my position in Bellevue Hospital within a few years and you shall be my successor," he wrote privately. "We mean to make Bellevue the finest Medical College in this country and we wish you to help us."

It wasn't enough. Welch had made up his mind: Hopkins it would be. How could this happen? Why would an ambitious researcher turn down the prestige and potential of the Bellevue-Carnegie offer in favor of an infant institution in a notoriously run-down city? The answer was simple: Welch's New York friends had either misunderstood or chosen to ignore what truly mattered to him—the chance to do his research free of distractions and to help build a medical school different from any other in the United States.

Dennis was furious. His role as intermediary having failed, he accused Welch of deceit and disloyalty in a note that Welch dutifully threw away. ("Your letter is destroyed, as you requested.") But Welch saw no reason to apologize. Indeed, he thought *himself* the injured party. "I am conscious that I have acted throughout in good faith and that I have done nothing which needs defense," he responded. "I was ready up to the last moment to stand by the conditions which I made and which I cannot consider were fulfilled." The decision, while not an easy one, was now final. "It seems clear," Welch added, "that the opportunity which everyone should seek in this world of doing the best which is in him is for me in Baltimore."*

Before Welch left for Baltimore, his remaining friends threw him a farewell party. The toasts were mostly good-natured, the guest of honor recalled, with a strong dose of amazement at what had just transpired. Who else among them would have chosen such a path? "Well, good-bye," Welch later described the mood that evening as tongues loosened and the wine flowed. "You may become a connoisseur of terrapin and Madeira, but as a pathologist, good-bye."

They could not have been more mistaken.

* The friendship was severed. Welch would write Dennis a condolence note in 1890 upon the death of his father, and a second note of congratulation upon his election to the Royal College of Surgeons in 1899. There is no record that Dennis responded. On Welch's seventieth birthday in 1920, however, Dennis sent along his best wishes. Welch was thrilled. "I wish, Fred, that you would come down and stay awhile with me," he replied. Six years later Dennis did visit Welch during a business trip to Baltimore. "It quite took my breath away to find you waiting for me," Welch wrote of the encounter. The two maintained a cordial relationship thereafter. Frederic Dennis Folders, William Welch Papers, Chesney Medical Archives, Johns Hopkins University.

—

Halsted, meanwhile, continued to thrive. He would never be busier or happier than during his "Bellevue days" of the early 1880s, described as "the most vigorous period of his life." Elected to the exclusive New York Surgical Society, he seemed destined, at the age of thirty, to revolutionize his field. The meticulous ledgers at Bellevue show him performing dozens of operations, from amputations to hernias, from setting fractures to draining infected joints. In one case, Halsted did extensive plastic surgery on the face of a woman who had fallen into the flames of a kerosene lamp; in another, he grafted the muscle of "a healthy dog" onto the forearm of an industrial accident victim. (The result is unclear.) Germ killers were precisely employed. Halsted's case notes are dotted with descriptions such as "arm thoroughly cleansed and disinfected," "dressing of carbolized gauze aseptic," and "parts washed with Thiersch's solution [a strong antiseptic] and powdered with iodoform."

As one who followed the latest medical news from Europe, Halsted was especially intrigued by a paper delivered in Germany about the potential of cocaine as a numbing agent in cataract removals. The problem, in a nutshell, was that general anesthesia sometimes induced vomiting and the shakes, making it risky in cases requiring a perfectly still patient. Halsted instantly grasped the importance of the German research. A safe, easily delivered local anesthetic would benefit everyone, dentists included, whose work caused excruciating pain. In December 1884, the *New York Medical Record* published an article about the breakthrough, noting: "A body of gentlemen in this city composed of willing medical students and intelligent surgeons have been experimenting . . . to determine the hypodermic effects of cocaine."

Halsted was among the leaders. He not only recruited these "willing medical students" and "intelligent surgeons," he also took the drug himself, believing he had a duty to do so before experimenting on others. In 1886, he scribbled some thoughts on the subject in a piece "Practical Comments on the Use and Abuse of Cocaine; Suggested by Its Invariably Successful Employment in More Than a Thousand Minor Surgical Operations." The writing bordered on incoherent—

Halsted had become severely addicted to cocaine by this point—but the operations he listed ranged from the removal of minor skin lesions to the circumcision and even amputation of the penis.

Cocaine did, indeed, work wonders as a nerve blocker when injected locally under the skin. But those who used it liberally experienced something more: a rush of energy and exhilaration that temporarily banished depression and fatigue. As word spread, cocaine quickly became a recreational craze in Europe and the United States, available in wine and soft drinks, cough drops and cigars. People of means could now look to a host of new drug firms like Squibb, Searle, and especially Parke-Davis to satisfy their personal and professional needs. Little was known at this point about addiction. Indeed, Bellevue's William A. Hammond cheerfully described cocaine as no more habit-forming than tea or coffee, and some doctors pushed it as a miracle drug for everything from melancholy to malaria. Its users soon included the likes of Sherlock Holmes creator Arthur Conan Doyle, the cancer-ridden former president Ulysses S. Grant, and (it was strongly hinted) Pope Leo XIII.

By 1885, Halsted was fully hooked, as were most in his inner circle. His behavior became so erratic that he failed to show up for scheduled operations and even fled Bellevue when hearing his name paged in emergencies. Word of Halsted's trouble soon reached William Welch in Baltimore. Determined to save his friend, Welch took a short leave from Hopkins and hired a schooner to sail the two men to the Windward Islands in the Caribbean. The trip went badly. While accounts vary, it appears that Welch encouraged Halsted to bring some cocaine, hoping to decrease the dosage over time. When the supply ran out, however, Halsted broke into the ship captain's medicine locker in search of drugs—most likely morphine. His desperation, wrote one biographer, had turned him "from a model of patrician rectitude to a thief."

At Welch's urging, Halsted left New York City to seek treatment at Rhode Island's Butler Hospital for the Insane, one of the few facilities then specializing in drug and alcohol abuse. The regimen—fresh air, long walks, good food, and daily sessions with an "alienist," as psychiatrists were then called—lasted seven months. When it ended,

Welch took Halsted to Baltimore and installed him in his laboratory as a "special graduate student" in pathology. There would be no return to Bellevue. That chapter was closed.

Halsted went on to a distinguished career at Hopkins. Some consider him the most influential American surgeon of his generation, on par with previous luminaries like Valentine Mott. With Welch opening doors, Halsted soon became an associate professor of surgery and then surgeon-in-chief at the Johns Hopkins Hospital, leading the way in areas ranging from gallstone removal to suturing techniques to breast cancer. His radical mastectomy is perhaps his best-known and most controversial legacy.

Halsted also remained a strong voice for Germ Theory and antiseptic surgery. And his demanding methods led to another breakthrough in an unintended way. Shortly after arriving at Hopkins, Halsted found himself attracted to his scrub nurse, Caroline Hampton, who complained about the constant rashes on her hands and forearms caused by the harsh chemicals Halsted employed as disinfectants. To resolve this, Halsted met with representatives of the Goodyear Rubber Company to design a set of sterile surgical gloves that would become standard fare in operating rooms across the country. He also married Caroline Hampton.

What Halsted couldn't resolve, however, was his dependence on drugs. His daily routine in Baltimore would include three grains of cocaine, often supplemented by morphine, and he'd sometimes disappear for a week or two, enduring what one historian has called "a life of controlled addiction." William Welch rarely mentioned the subject, and never related the full scope of the problem. "As long as he lived he would occasionally have a relapse and go back to the drug," Welch supposedly told a confidant after Halsted had died. "He would always go out of town for this and when he returned he could come to me, very contrite and apologetic, to confess." It was the price that Johns Hopkins silently paid to have the brilliant Halsted around.

At Bellevue, meanwhile, the well-financed Carnegie Laboratory had become a world leader in bacteriology and public health. Led by Frederic Dennis and Hermann Biggs, its research penetrated deep into disciplines like surgery, where change was needed most. Indeed, Dennis developed the antiseptic routine to guide each operation at Bellevue: "The surgeon scrubs his forearms and hands for five minutes with a sterile brush and hot water and tinctures of green soap. Fingernails are cleaned with a sterile orange stick, then hands are rubbed with lime and soda for three minutes and then rinsed in sterile water. They are then immersed in a 1-3,000 bichloride solution of mercury for two or three minutes, and finally rinsed in a saline solution."

Surprisingly, one of the best examples of the antiseptic revolution would remain hidden from public view. Bellevue physicians already had treated two stricken presidents—Lincoln in 1865 and Garfield in 1881. (Moreover, Bellevue's Fordyce Barker had warned former president Grant to have his throat checked for a possible malignancy, which turned out to be fatal.) And it happened again, in 1893, under circumstances so delicate that the incident went untold for the next twenty-four years, when one of the attending surgeons broke his silence in a spectacular confession in *The Saturday Evening Post*.

The president was Grover Cleveland, a hard-drinking, cigar-smoking bear of a man who stood five feet eleven inches tall and weighed somewhere north of 250 pounds. Noticing a rough patch near the roof of his mouth, Cleveland had alerted his personal physician, Bellevue's Joseph Bryant, who sent a piece of the "ulcerative lesion" to pathologists at the Army Medical Museum. When the result came back malignant—confirmed by none other than William Welch—an immediate operation was prescribed. But Cleveland resisted—not out of fear or denial, but because he worried, with good reason, that the news would alarm a nation already enduring one of the worst economic depressions in its history. Absolute secrecy was required for the procedure, which ruled out a hospital or even the White House, where the coming and going of surgeons would surely be noticed.

Dr. Bryant took charge. A former student of Stephen Smith's, he had spent decades teaching surgery at Bellevue Hospital Medical College. His professional life had closely mirrored the battle over antisepsis, with Bryant reluctantly accepting the ways of Joseph Lister. Upon learning of Cleveland's biopsy, Bryant put together a six-man surgical team that included two Bellevue colleagues—Dr. John Erdmann, a trusted assistant, and Dr. Edward Janeway, a brilliant diagnostician. Erdmann would help perform the operation, while Janeway would monitor the vital signs. President Cleveland suggested that the operation take place aboard the luxury yacht *Oneida,* owned by his friend Commodore Elias Benedict, a New York banker. And he insisted there be no telltale changes to his face—meaning no external incisions and no disappearing mustache.

On the morning of July 1, 1893, the *Oneida* sailed up the East River toward Long Island Sound. "So careful were we to elude observation," wrote one of the physicians, "that Dr. Bryant and all of us who might have been recognized by some of the staff at Bellevue Hospital deserted the deck for the cabin below." That afternoon, the president had a "gelatinous mass," along with five teeth, removed in an operation lasting about an hour and a half. The six medical men wore starched white coats and boiled their instruments. They rinsed Cleveland's mouth with Thiersch's solution, favored by finicky surgeons like William Halsted. As one team member put it: "Fresh, pure air, disinfected quarters, and skilled doctors all had to be provided lest blood poisoning set in."

The operation was successful. Tissue samples examined many years later showed a slow-growing form of squamous cell carcinoma common to heavy smokers. Cleveland would die of a heart attack in 1908, his life extended, in no small part, by the bitter legacy of James A. Garfield.

12

THE MAD-HOUSE

Reputations can be remarkably immune to change. In 1878, *Harper's New Monthly* published a lengthy piece about New York City's major hospitals. At one end of its spectrum was private, tidy, well-managed New York Hospital, the perennial favorite of social reformers, and recently upgraded to an ornate brick-and-stone building on 15th Street compliments of its generous trustees. The great bulk of its 163 patients were respectable working-class folk, most paying a modest fee to enjoy "the exquisite cleanliness" of its spacious wards. The modern kitchen, the polished maple elevator, the sun-drenched solarium—all reminded the writer of what future hospitals might happily provide for the unfortunates who had no choice but to use one.

At the other end stood Bellevue, a bare-bones receptacle "for the poorest of the poor, the dregs of society, the semi-criminal, starving, unwelcome class, who suffer and die unrecognized." There were no luxuries to be found in this "ponderous dull gray mass of granite," and that was a good thing, the article explained, because New York already attracted too many foreign paupers, compounding the "hopeless misery" that had once distinguished American cities from the urban cesspools of Europe.

The writer did throw a bone Bellevue's way. Students and professors from New York City's leading medical schools could be spotted in every ward and corridor. Following one class through its bedside rounds, the writer marveled at the endless variety of human suffering on display, the professor "explaining the cases and operations [with] so much perspicuity and simplicity that the thickest-headed student would have unimaginable difficulty in not understanding." Of Bellevue's limited virtues, the sheer range of afflictions seemed to stand out most.

The writer wasn't seeking gray areas, just black and white. There was no mention that Bellevue housed many of the nation's finest medical researchers; that its attending physicians and residents were among the best in the city; that professional nursing had raised the quality of care in the wards; or that, unlike New York Hospital, it didn't get to pick the patients it cared to treat. When an ambulance arrived with the victim of a robbery, or a trolley accident, or a boiler explosion; when a paddy wagon dropped off an alcoholic suffering from delirium tremens; when the police court sent over an unruly suspect for mental observation—all were taken in.

On one point, at least, the article got it right. Physically, Bellevue was a wreck—a crumbling former almshouse so overcrowded that patients could be seen sleeping on the floor. And so underfunded that a survey of the nation's hospitals in 1883 found the "cost-per-patient-per day" at Bellevue to be 49 cents—the lowest figure by far in New York City and well behind other metropolitan hospitals like Boston City ($1.24) and Cook County ($1.01).

Worse, the 49-cent figure included supplies routinely pilfered from Bellevue, where staff thievery was a way of life. Like many hospitals of this era, patient recovery depended on generous alcohol use. "Spirits" at Bellevue accounted for about 20 percent of its annual budget, twice the figure for "medicines." By one estimate, however, barely 5 percent of the beer, brandy, whiskey, and wine actually reached the mouths of the intended. "It is a mighty dry place," wrote the rarely sarcastic *New York Times,* noting "the wonderful evaporating power of the atmosphere around Bellevue Hospital."

Not surprisingly, *Harper's New Monthly* paid scant attention to the subject that would come to dominate Bellevue's standing in the popular mind: its treatment of the insane. There was little reason to bring it up; the connection was still rather vague. Where *Harper's New Monthly* had told a lively if familiar tale of poverty and physical neglect, a more sensational piece of journalism, fusing Bellevue to the hidden world of bedlam, was about to change the hospital's image forever.

From its earliest times, the city almshouse had kept a small number of "idiots" and "lunatics" isolated in the basement, often in chains. As their numbers grew, however, this segregation disappeared. "The invalid, the aged, the infirm, the vagrant, and half lunatic are [now] confined together, and are allowed the most unrestrained intercourse," a grand jury reported in the 1840s, calling the situation an affront to "every Christian."

The solution, as we have seen, involved a small rocky island in the East River. When the Blackwell family had first put the 107-acre property up for sale in 1784, there were no takers. It wasn't until decades later, as the almshouse complex and the jails reached overflowing, that public officials took notice of the island's unique potential— uninhabited, surrounded by water, with "a rapid and violent current" to discourage escapes. In 1828, the Common Council purchased Blackwell's Island—now called Roosevelt Island—for a handsome $32,000. The following decades would see the construction of a new almshouse, an orphanage, a prison, and a fever hospital. But the island's grandest structure was a lunatic asylum containing two four-story wings connected by a five-story rotunda of blue-gray stone known as the Octagon.

Bellevue in these years would continue to house a pavilion for the insane. But its role was limited to examining those brought in for observation and then deciding whether to release them or send them on to Blackwell's Island. These examinations were done quickly; mental patients now remained at Bellevue for a month or less, their fate decided by a young, untrained house staff (interns and residents) acting on little beyond their intuition.

Among the early visitors to Blackwell's was Charles Dickens, on a grand tour of America's public institutions. While impressed by the Octagon's size, he could hardly wait to leave. "The moping idiot, cowering down with long, disheveled hair; the gibbering maniac, with his hideous laugh and pointed finger; the vacant eyes, the fierce wild face, the gloomy picking of the hands and lips, and munching of the nails; they were all without disguise, in their naked ugliness and horror." Dickens declined to visit the wards where "the violent were kept under restraint," claiming he'd seen quite enough. "I never felt such deep disgust and measureless contempt," he wrote, "as when I crossed the threshold of this madhouse."

There'd be few other visitors in the coming years. The press showed little interest, running occasional stories about the harmless delusions of the patients, like the one who claimed to be the king of Scotland or the sister of the pope. And every so often, a reporter would profile the asylum's longest-tenured inmate, a woman who insisted she was the widow of President James Buchanan and the mother of his children, all of whom were cats. "I had the honor of stroking the back of the president's oldest son," read one such account, "who purred as though his sire had no political difficulties to disturb his repose."

Each year, the asylum superintendent would issue a report complaining of the crowded conditions and his inadequate budget, yet filled with descriptions of happy patients "planting vegetables" and "learning to play instruments." The reports sent a jarring mixed message—and almost certainly went unread. In the early 1880s, a superintendent candidly admitted that one of his main accomplishments lay in keeping the asylum out of the news.

But not for long.

When Joseph Pulitzer bought the *New York World* from the robber baron financier Jay Gould in 1883, the paper was in trouble. Deeply in debt, with barely fifteen thousand readers, it ran well behind competitors like the *Times, Tribune,* and *Sun.* Having made his publishing mark in the heavily immigrant city of St. Louis, Pulitzer had a good feel for what could work in New York. The *World* quickly found its niche as the voice of the laboring classes, with lurid stories, vivid graphics, and simple words. It created the city's first sports section and ran splashy headlines—"FRENCH SCIENTIST AND EXPLORER DISCOVERS A RACE OF SAVAGES WITH WELL-DEVELOPED TAILS" being a prime example. A master at mobilizing public opinion for causes that benefited both his newspaper and the city, Pulitzer put the *World* on solid footing with a campaign to finance a pedestal for the Statue of Liberty, which had just arrived from France. "We must raise the money," he thundered. "The *World* is the people's paper, and now it appeals to the people to come forward. . . . Let us not wait for the millionaires to give us the money." The campaign caught fire in New York's immigrant communities, anxious to honor their adopted land. More than 125,000 donors responded, each receiving a mention in the *World* no matter how small the gift. The Statue of Liberty got its pedestal and the *World* shot up to first place in reader circulation.

Pulitzer fancied himself a "muckraker." Having exposed all sorts of corruption in St. Louis, he expected to find more of the same in New York City, especially scandals involving the abuse and fleecing of the poorer classes. The *World* relied heavily on undercover work—some called it the "new journalism"—in which the newspaper planted a reporter inside a factory, a politician's office, or a public institution to get the "real" story. An entire generation of writers would come to prominence through these sensational exposés—none more daring than Elizabeth Jane Cochran, known to the public as Nellie Bly (pseudonyms for women writers being quite common at the time).

Arriving in 1887 from Pittsburgh, where she'd covered debutante balls and flower shows for the local newspaper, Bly literally begged her way into a job at the *World*. A handful of women, led by the iconic Ida Tarbell, were now doing spirited journalism, and the *World* was looking to expand the undercover reporting that had become its trademark. Bly, for her part, proved fearless and inventive. Before long, she was posing as an unwed mother to penetrate a baby-buying ring and getting herself arrested to check out the city jail. In 1889, inspired by the Jules Verne novel *Around the World in Eighty Days,* Bly would circle the globe with the aid of Pulitzer's wealthy friends, beating Verne's "record" by more than a week. But her first major story for the *World* was probably her most important, appearing in two lengthy installments and then as a book titled *Ten Days in a Mad-House.*

Contrary to most accounts, it wasn't Bly's idea. At her job interview, she spoke of exposing the dangers of immigrant travel to America, but the editor wanted something bolder. His plan, Bly recalled, was to "have [me] committed to one of the asylums for the insane in New York, with a view to writing a plain and unvarnished narrative of the treatment of the patients."

Though "plain" and "unvarnished" weren't exactly hallmarks of the *World*'s reporting at the time, she jumped at the chance. More important, Pulitzer wanted the story done. The *World* had recently run some editorials about the rumored mistreatment of patients on Blackwell's Island. What it needed was confirmation from a source planted inside.

Bly was given an assumed name she could easily answer to—Nellie Brown. Her editor cleared the caper with a friend in the district attorney's office so she wouldn't be prosecuted for entering a city institution under false pretenses. After spending several hours in front of a mirror "practicing to be a lunatic," Bly checked into a boardinghouse for young women and behaved so oddly that she was carted off to police court, where the judge ordered her taken to Bellevue's Insane Pavilion for observation. Psychiatry in the 1880s had yet to become a specialty; the young doctors in charge received no training. Their job was to separate the moderately disturbed from those requiring "further attention" on Blackwell's Island—a subjective process, to be sure. Bly spent two days at the Insane Pavilion pretending to hear voices and act "deranged." She obviously performed well. The staff declared her "undoubtedly insane." And that earned her a ferry ride to the Octagon.

Each step along the way had its pitfalls. The police court of the 1880s was fertile ground for curious reporters, and "Nellie Brown," an attractive, well-dressed woman with no apparent sense of who she was or what she was doing in New York City, seemed ripe for attention. "If there is anyone who can ferret out a mystery it is a reporter," Bly recalled. Claiming to be cold and frightened, she chose a wide-brimmed hat with a black veil for her disguise. "Who Is This Insane Girl?" the *New York Sun* asked its readers, hoping to crack the case. Even the stodgy *Times* took notice. "A Mysterious Waif: Bellevue Shelters a Girl of Whom Nothing Is Known," it declared, adding, "She gives evidence of both in her speech and manner of good breeding."

Bly portrayed Bellevue as "the third station on my way to the island"—the boardinghouse and police court being stations one and two. She vividly described the crowded wards, the freezing temperatures, the filthy bedding and moth-eaten clothing. But a careful reading of her exposé showed Bellevue to be more of a clueless institution than a brutal one. The main problem, as Bly saw it, was the failure of its four "Lunacy Examiners" to make an informed diagnosis. "I began to have a smaller regard for the ability of doctors than I ever had before," she reported. "I felt sure now that no doctor could tell whether people were insane or not, so long as the case was not violent."

There was one skeptic, however. Unbeknownst to Bly, she had crossed paths in the Insane Pavilion with longtime Bellevue superintendent William B. O'Rourke, who had seen his share of mental illness over the years and was dubious of the fuss surrounding "this girl of whom nothing is known." Speaking to reporters, O'Rourke branded Bly's condition "humbug." He was right, of course, but his remark struck the public as callous and self-serving.

The real focus of Bly's exposé was the Octagon on Blackwell's Island—the hidden expanse of sadism and neglect. Under the banner headlines "BEHIND ASYLUM BARS" and "INSIDE THE MAD-HOUSE," her articles appeared in back-to-back installments of the *World*'s new Sunday section, another Pulitzer innovation. Bly spared no details in the telling. "My teeth chattered and my limbs were goose-fleshed and blue with cold," she wrote at one point. "I got, one after the other, three buckets of water over my head—ice cold water, too—into my eyes, my ears, my nose, and my mouth. I think I experienced the sensation of a drowning person as they dragged me gasping, shivering, and quaking from the tub. For once I did look insane."

Bly became an overnight celebrity, rewarded with a byline from the *World* and a handsome check from her publisher. Describing her as "very bright" and "very plucky," Pulitzer called her work the very essence of the journalism he had in mind. "She thoroughly understands the profession she has chosen," he beamed. "She has a bright future before her."

She did, indeed. The *World* soon demanded an investigation of conditions at the Octagon, and two weeks later a grand jury visited Blackwell's Island with Bly herself in tow. What they found was a place scrubbed clean of the horrors she so graphically described. The wards were spotless, the attendants were friendly, and the inmates Bly had portrayed in her articles as "appearing sane" had simply vanished—the authorities insisting that no such patients had been treated there. "I had hardly expected the grand jury to sustain me, after they saw everything different from what it had been while I was there," Bly reported. "Yet they did."

When the city voted a record-breaking budget increase for the Department of Public Charities and Corrections, which included Bellevue Hospital and the Octagon, Bly naturally took the credit. "I have one consolation," she wrote of her brief tribulations. "On the strength of my story the committee of appropriations [provided] $1,000,000 more than was ever before given, for the benefit of the insane."

This wasn't exactly true. Just before Bly's exposé appeared, the Board of Estimate had received a budget from the Department of Charities requesting $1.5 million in additional funds for various improvements. And the Board, a few weeks later, had responded more favorably than anyone could have imagined—with Bly's exposé playing a crucial role. In the end, the city would approve an $850,000 increase for the entire department, not simply for the insane. The Octagon received a $60,000 increase, with Bellevue getting somewhat less. Hype aside, Nellie Bly had modestly served her cause.

For Bellevue, however, great damage had been done. "ALL THE DOCTORS FOOLED," screamed the headlines. Bly's dramatic narrative had made no real attempt to separate one stop from another in her ten-day descent into hell. Bellevue and Blackwell's Island were fused together—two snake pits, equally culpable, equally dark. The stories played perfectly upon Bellevue's reputation as the Grim Reaper of American hospitals, ignoring its primacy in public health, medical research, nursing care, clinical instruction, and so much more. From this point forward, the name "Bellevue" would be linked, above all, to a particular strand of illness: insanity.

New York's fascination with the exposé soon became an obsession. Bellevue's medical wards may have been for the poorer classes, but the Insane Pavilion had a wider reach. Anyone acting oddly could be sent there involuntarily for observation, making it a human-interest bonanza. A sampling of newspaper headlines in a single year—1897—showed the results:

"Imagines Himself a Mosquito—Now an Inmate at Bellevue"
"Crazed by Smoking: Victim of Cigarettes and Worry Goes Insane, Taken to Bellevue"
"Wealthy Woman Is Insane: Mania for Shopping Lands Her in Bellevue"
"Chased Mother with a Knife: She Escaped . . . He Was Sent to Bellevue"
"Rich Man's Son in Insane Ward: Secretly Taken to Bellevue"
"She Raves of a Beast: Sent to Bellevue"

In this new age of muckraking and circulation wars, some stories had a rougher edge. There were reports of dangerous maniacs roaming Bellevue's halls ("Hospital Patient Slain: Woman in a Straight-Jacket Strangles Another"), staffers snapping under pressure ("Nurse for Insane Goes Crazy Herself"), and botched diagnoses ("Sane Man Held as Crazy at Bellevue"). But the most damaging pieces alleged the sadistic treatment of patients, and no publication took more pride in uncovering it than Pulitzer's *New York World*.

In 1900, the paper decided to secretly revisit the Octagon—Nellie Bly *Redux*. The plan was virtually identical to the one she had employed thirteen years before. A young reporter, Thomas Minnock, would feign insanity, go to police court, fool the doctors at Bellevue, and wind up on Blackwell's Island. But Minnock never made it that far; the story he found—big enough to dwarf even the Nellie Bly caper—unfolded at Bellevue, where he claimed to have witnessed the murder of an elderly French mental patient at the hands of three sadistic male nurses.

In Minnock's telling, the three men, enraged by the patient's refusal to eat, had pummeled him before placing a knotted sheet around his neck. Under the banner headline "SHOCKING BRUTALITY OF MALE NURSES IN INSANE PAVILION AT BELLEVUE," he wrote: "I was horrified. No big, strong, healthy man could have lived under that awful strangling. The patient was weak and feeble."

Murder charges followed. The trial judge had to change courtrooms to accommodate the overflow crowds. In his opening remarks, the prosecutor called the crime "the most terrible treatment that was ever given to an insane man," adding: "No writer of fiction could have put them in a book. They would appear so improbable and monstrous that his manuscript would have been rejected as soon as offered to a publisher." The press dubbed it "The Case of the Garroted Frenchman."

The trial grew wilder by the day. The prosecution's only witnesses beyond Thomas Minnock were two Bellevue mental patients who claimed to have seen the assault. While acknowledging that New York state had never before allowed an "admittedly insane" person to testify under oath in a criminal proceeding, the judge swore them in anyway, ruling that "in a lunatic asylum, the patients are often the only witnesses to outrages upon themselves and others."

Under cross-examination, both witnesses were pressed about their mental conditions. "Why did you go to Bellevue?" the defense lawyer asked the first man. "Why, because I was crazy," came the reply. "What cause did your wife have to put you in an asylum?" the lawyer asked the second man. "That's a personal matter," the witness replied, "and I decline to answer." The judge dutifully entered both diagnoses into the record: paranoia and dementia.

Still, the evidence seemed compelling. The coroner's report spoke of an apparent strangling, and the key witness in the case, reporter Thomas Minnock, could hardly be accused of insanity. Well-spoken and college-educated, a rarity in this era, he had the press solidly on his side.

Minnock's story had opened a window into a little-known aspect of hospital care: the role of the male nurse. The Victorian world of late-nineteenth-century America placed a premium on sexual modesty. Even a progressive thinker like Bellevue's Abraham Jacobi, the father of American pediatrics, believed that some hospital procedures offended both a female nurse's "sense of chastity" and a male patient's "sense of decency." Furthermore, certain parts of Bellevue, including the Insane Pavilion, were said to require a strong male presence to maintain physical order. The best solution, it appeared, was to open a training school for male nurses.

Bellevue did just that in 1887 with a gift from Darius Ogden Mills, a prominent philanthropist, but the school faced problems from the start. Recruitment lagged; the stigma of men working in a female profession took an obvious toll. Applications to the Mills School were never very high, and those who came rarely stayed for long. Some simply quit; others were expelled for a long list of personal failings: "too nervous," "too childish," "too slow," "dishonest," "neglect of duty," "insubordinate," "disobedient," "intoxication," "cocaine," "an uncontrollable temper." One student was "unable to stand the odor of ether," another was described as looking "too much like a colored man." Those who graduated, however, found quick employment in the male wards at Bellevue and other institutions.

The three nurses on trial were Mills graduates. They claimed that the Frenchman's death had been unavoidable—"a wild melee by a crazy man." The patient had become violent, they said, sprinting down the hall and crashing into tables before striking his head on the floor. One nurse had put his knee on the patient's chest to restrain him. The other two had picked him up and put him in bed, where he died in his sleep.

Fearing for the school's future, Darius Ogden Mills hired one of New York's top attorneys, Francis Lewis Wellman, to defend the nurses in court. A master of cross-examination, Wellman got Minnock to admit that he had lied freely about his past, written stories for other newspapers that turned out to be untrue, and placed himself at events he had never, in fact, attended. Minnock left the witness stand in tears. The nurses were acquitted.

The verdict, however, did little to build confidence in the Mills School. The Bellevue superintendent publicly complained that too many of the students were "rough, unkind, dishonest, addicted to the use of alcohol, or neglectful." He personally thought them more trouble than they were worth. Then, in 1909, came the final indignity: a male patient at Bellevue accused a Mills trainee of "unnatural advances and acts," leading to the young man's "resignation." The incident triggered a chaotic student meeting at which charges of "effeminate practices" flew back and forth. And that led the trustees to hold closed-door hearings of their own.

Minutes taken but never released showed a variety of student "confessions"—one admitting to an affair with a man he "loved very much." A trustee privately described his colleagues as "ready to puke." "The details of the investigation are of such a nature that I do not think you would care to hear them," he wrote New York's mayor William Jay Gaynor, adding: "The evil appears to have been pretty well eradicated."

Twenty-seven of the sixty-five students at Mills either resigned or were dismissed. The official who ran the day-to-day operations was discharged "on grounds of economy." And there was talk of closing down the school. "Nursing is essentially a woman's work," a trustee argued. "[It] is very closely allied to the domestic life and the more nearly we approach the domestic and home atmosphere in our hospital wards, the better the results for us all." The director of the Insane Pavilion went a step further. "The average man does not select the profession of nurse," he declared, "unless there is something wrong with him."

Darius Ogden Mills lived just long enough to learn of the accusations. He had recently agreed to donate four building lots near Bellevue for a new men's dormitory. At his death, his family members voted with the other trustees to graduate the remaining students and accept no more. As a substitute, Bellevue agreed to recruit and train a group of male "attendants" for tasks that men might do more effectively than women. The trustees were quite specific about what they had in mind: "the care of alcoholics, the insane," and men with "rectal" diseases.

Fortunately for Bellevue, the details of the Mills episode were never released. But the previous decades had been extremely unkind to its image—the Bly exposé and the Minnock spectacle serving as bookends to a relentless flogging in the press. Fairly or not, America's largest hospital entered the twentieth century under a pile of bad news, shaken by charges of brutality, incompetence, and neglect.

13

THE NEW METROPOLIS

We cannot have too much of New York City," a local politician boasted near the turn of the twentieth century, and it was easy to see why. Hard times had passed. The brutal depression of 1893 had run its course. New York was on the move, with a robust economy, record-breaking immigration, and the merger of Brooklyn, Manhattan, Queens, the Bronx, and Staten Island into a single behemoth of 303 square miles and 3,437,000 people. Massive construction defined its frenetic pace—a subway system; enormous bridges connecting the boroughs; elegant hotels, museums, athletic venues, railroad stations, and boulevards. New York now ranked second to London in population among Western cities, having overtaken Berlin, Paris, and Vienna. Once mocked by the caustic Washington Irving as a vast wasteland called "Gotham," it entered the new century at a pace unrivaled in the world.

The city's look was molded in no small part by the architectural firm of Charles McKim, William Mead, and Stanford White. A survey of its work would include Gilded Age masterpieces like Pennsylvania Station, the old Madison Square Garden, the Columbia University campus, the ultraexclusive Harvard and Century Clubs, the north and south wings of the Metropolitan Museum of Art, and the iconic Washington Square Arch. In 1902, however, the city paid McKim, Mead & White a $75,000 retainer for a master plan that caught many by surprise: a new hospital complex on the Bellevue grounds. The firm had no track record in that field, after all, and Bellevue seemed an odd choice for an elaborate makeover. The plan called for the demolition and replacement of the current buildings at a huge price. "COST OF NEW BELLEVUE WILL BE $11,000,000," the *Times* declared. "World's Greatest Hospital Will Shelter 3,000 Patients—To Cover Three City Blocks."

The initial design was stunning. By 1900, Manhattan's better hospitals had moved north to larger plots in less congested neighborhoods. Bellevue, though, had stayed put. The master plan envisioned a phalanx of brick-and-granite structures surrounding an Administration Building with an elegant glass dome atop a marble rotunda—not unlike the one in Penn Station. All construction north of the rotunda (the uptown side) would be for "surgical use," and south of it (the downtown side) for "medical use." The wards facing east (the river) would house patients "undergoing continued treatment," while those looking west (First Avenue) would contain the units for short-termers, including alcoholics and the mentally ill.

The plan included a gymnasium, tennis courts, and a swimming pool to keep the doctors in "good health." There would be Corinthian columns, marble floors, and winding staircases with wrought iron railings in the public areas; imposing fireplaces and oak-paneled libraries in the living quarters for house officers. Each ward had a full-length balcony for patients (often with tuberculosis) to catch the fresh river breezes. Medical waste would be channeled through a series of pneumatic tubes to a proposed crematory. The new morgue contained a 240-body cold storage unit, with more space for "the public inspection of the unidentified dead."

The internal memos of McKim, Mead & White show a firm determined to win the final bid—and socially positioned to get it. "Dear Charlie," Stanford White wrote his partner in 1904. "Do you think it advisable to pull any wires with Tammany on the hospital? I am sure . . . we could get hosts of help if you thought it best to make a fight." McKim told him not to worry: all was going well. "Dear Stanford," he replied. "As we are on the best terms with the trustees of the hospital, it would be most unfortunate to risk any disturbance." Should "the situation alter," McKim added, there'd be "time enough to call to our aid the men you speak of."

—

Why the sudden interest in upgrading a public hospital that had been neglected for decades? It was no accident that calls for change had resounded during the sensational trial of the three male nurses in 1901. "Grand Jury Denounces Bellevue Management," read a typical headline feeding the flames. As a result, Mayor Seth Low, an anti-Tammany progressive, had replaced the patronage-driven Board of Charities and Corrections with the newly created Department of Bellevue and Allied Hospitals, run by seven unpaid trustees from the city's medical and civic ranks. It was, observers noted, about as decent a body as New York could muster. And among its top priorities were the expansion and makeover of the city's flagship hospital.

The need was obvious. Beginning in the 1890s, New York had witnessed a surge of new immigrants—most coming from parts of Europe with few connections to the United States, and many in need of acute medical care. In the past, improvements at Bellevue had followed a distinct pattern: heavy immigration accompanied by an epidemic of some sort, cholera and typhus being prime examples. And it happened once more around 1900, the offender this time being tuberculosis. Also known as phthisis and consumption, TB wasn't new to the city. In fact, it had been the leading infectious killer in New York for generations, though its numbers had fallen since the discovery of the tubercle bacillus by Germany's Robert Koch in 1884 and the strict sanitary measures put in place by public health officials. But tuberculosis now appeared to be making a comeback—many blaming the new immigrants and calling it by names like "tailor's disease" after newly arrived Jews working in the city's slum-ridden sweatshops.

As usual, Bellevue bore the brunt of it. The problem, said Dr. John Brannon, chairman of the hospital's Board of Trustees, was that most immigrants suffering from tuberculosis had been admitted for another reason—an accident, a pregnancy, an alcoholic stupor. Since Bellevue had no quarantine facilities beyond two jam-packed chest wards, one male, one female, the victims were mixed in with regular patients—coughing, spitting, spreading their germs. Small wonder that twenty of Bellevue's sixty-five interns had come down with the disease in a single year. "When we consider the number of nurses and physicians who have contracted tuberculosis during their services at our hospital," a Bellevue doctor complained, "I think we have a conclusive responsibility to eliminate such dangers of infection as far as possible."

Brannon had a personal stake in this. Having been "cured" of tuberculosis as a young man, he greatly admired the work of Bellevue's Hermann Biggs, the city's premier bacteriologist, who had convinced a skeptical medical establishment, or much of it, that TB could be more easily controlled by making it a mandatorily reportable disease. The campaign, opposed by some as an invasion of privacy, led Robert Koch to send Biggs this note of congratulation: "I wish to cite the example of the free American people who of their own free will accepted the limitation of their own liberties for the sake of public health."

Given the hundreds of TB patients scattered across Bellevue, Brannon expected the new plan to include a separate building for their quarantine and treatment. Meanwhile, by sheer coincidence, a wealthy young doctor named James Alexander Miller had joined Columbia's First Division at Bellevue, giving him a peek at "how the other half lived"—and it wasn't pretty. "There was no attempt to give instruction in the sanitary disposal of the sputum," he wrote of the primitive TB wards. Germs were shooting everywhere, and the "treatment" consisted of a cough mixture laced with morphine and whiskey.

Urged on by Biggs and Brannon, Miller created the Bellevue Chest Service in 1903. His approach in this post–Germ Theory but pre-antibiotic era was rather like Florence Nightingale's: good food, plenty of rest, lots of fresh air. Miller quarantined his patients, bundled them up in heavy blankets, and propped them on open roofs and balconies for hours at a time. Milk and eggs replaced morphine and whiskey, compliments of a new women's group called the Auxiliary to Bellevue. In perhaps his most celebrated move, Miller partnered with the auxiliary to buy the *Southfield,* a retired Staten Island ferryboat. Docked in the East River, it became a fresh air "summer camp" for poor children with "incipient or moderate" tuberculosis.

Supporters of the McKim, Mead & White master plan used examples like the *Southfield* to show Bellevue's deep connection to the city. This wasn't another run-of-the-mill public hospital, they argued; it was a research center, a teaching facility, a beacon of compassionate care. For all its troubles, Bellevue had always served New Yorkers in times of need—its history intertwined with the wars, riots, epidemics, and assorted calamities that had marked the city's raucous past. Only years earlier, its staff had treated hundreds of victims of the Great Heat Wave of 1896, a ten-day August inferno of record temperatures and eerily still air. "Doctors stripped [one] man and placed him in a large tub filled with as much as half a ton of cracked ice," a reporter noted. "A thermometer placed in the man's mouth registered the maximum: 110 degrees. Attendants grabbed large chunks of ice and rubbed the patient's skin. After ten minutes the man's temperature dropped three degrees. A few more minutes, and his temperature was back down to a normal 98.6." Newspapers marveled at the effort.

Then, in the very midst of the master plan discussion, came an unspeakable disaster. An excursion boat, the *General Slocum,* caught fire in the East River on its way to a church picnic, killing more than a thousand of the 1,358 passengers on board. Bellevue's entire ambulance corps rushed to the water's edge carrying staffers and supplies. Survivors filled the wards, and bodies lay stacked in the morgue. For years afterward, stories circulated about the horror and courage of that awful Sunday afternoon. "He dived overboard seventeen times to make rescues and brought a total of 145 bodies to the Bellevue dock aboard his vessel," read the obituary of a ferryboat captain four decades later, citing the hospital's steady hand when tragedy struck.

Still, criticism of the master plan was intense. Some saw the site itself as outmoded. Why not move it farther uptown to follow Manhattan's northward migration? Others grumbled at the expense, which, by current estimates, would equal one third the cost of the entire subway line then under construction from City Hall to the Bronx. Couldn't improvements be made on a smaller scale? Did a hospital for the poor really need the look of a lavish train station or a fancy college campus?

Under growing pressure the trustees backed off. Their memos to McKim, Mead & White became more critical: Be "less pretentious." Try "a simpler design." At last, a firm order came down: "It is the sense of the Trustees that all unnecessary or expensive features be dispensed with."

A slimmed-down version soon appeared. The gymnasium vanished, along with the tennis courts and swimming pool. The pneumatic tubes were scuttled, and the living quarters scaled back. The ornate touches—save the Corinthian columns, wrought iron railings, and patient balconies—largely disappeared. Cement replaced tile in the bathrooms; the granite finishes gave way to brick. Gone, too, was the most visible symbol of excess. "OMIT DOME and put regular flat roof in [its] place—SAVINGS, $420,000," read the "REDUCTIONS" memo prepared by the trustees. It was the safest way, they understood, of keeping the Bellevue project alive.

The new plan called for two thousand beds, a third fewer than before. And to spread out the costs, the old buildings would be torn down and replaced over years, not months. In 1910, Bellevue opened the four-hundred-bed medical pavilion, followed two years later by a new pathology building and morgue. Then came the five-hundred-bed surgical pavilion, with its massive operating theater. Not everyone was pleased. The "blandness" of the structures surprised those expecting greater vision from the likes of Stanford White. A planner hired by the city to evaluate the project could barely hide his contempt. The pavilions were oddly spaced, he thought, creating a maze of corridors. The ceilings were too high, the windows too small, the wards too long and narrow. "It is my opinion," he said, sticking the knife still deeper, "that [comfort] has been sacrificed too much to architectural line, although the architecture of the buildings, in spite of the sacrifice, is somewhat disappointing."

The price tag, meanwhile, was approaching $20 million, almost twice the original budget, with half the buildings yet to break ground. "It seems a great deal more money than ought to be expended on any one hospital," griped the *New York Times*.

Aesthetics aside, a modern behemoth was taking shape. And it wouldn't take long to fill the extra beds. Near the end of the nineteenth century, immigration to the United States took a dramatic turn. Until that point, the vast majority of foreigners had come from the British Isles, Germany, and Scandinavia. Between 1890 and 1920, however, a series of major crises, from anti-Semitic pogroms to radical changes in landholding and agriculture, brought a flood of immigrants from Southern and Eastern Europe. The number of foreign-born Italians in the United States rose from 250,000 to 3,339,000 in these decades, while the number of foreign-born Russians (overwhelmingly Jewish) soared from 258,000 to 3,871,000. Many listed New York City as their final destination.

The reaction was not unlike the one that greeted the Irish a half century before. A government study, "The Foreign Immigrant in New York City," questioned whether any municipality could assimilate so many newcomers holding such alien beliefs. The study's author wasn't shy—few were in those days—about the "special traits" of various ethnic groups. Italian children, she wrote, were "fair students, better than the Irish, but not as good as the Hebrews and Germans at book work." Fortunately, they weren't a problem in class, despite their limited attention spans, because Italian parents showed "a somewhat terrifying eagerness to add discipline on their own part in the shape of corporal punishment to that already administered by the school."

Many viewed these immigrants as purveyors of disease. Where the Irish had been accused of bringing cholera and typhus to New York in the 1830s and 1840s, now Jews were suspected of spreading tuberculosis, despite its low incidence in their neighborhoods, while Italians would be blamed for causing the city's first polio outbreak in 1916. There was no shortage of explanations—biological determinism often heading the list. Steerage passengers from Southern Europe "show a depressing frequency of low foreheads, open mouths, weak chins, poor features, skew faces, small or knobby crania, and backless heads," wrote the prominent sociologist E. A. Ross. "Such people lack the power to take rational care of themselves; hence their death rate in New York is twice the general death rate and thrice that of the Germans."

Bellevue naturally mirrored the city's rapidly changing population. In 1890, foreign-born Irish had comprised 31 percent of the hospital's admissions, with foreign-born Germans at 11 percent, Italians at 3 percent, and Russians too few to count. (Bellevue didn't list the ancestry of its American-born patients.) By 1913, the ground had shifted. Foreign-born Irish and German admissions to Bellevue had dropped from 42 percent to 20 percent, while foreign-born Italian and East European admissions had jumped from 4 percent to 12 percent—and were climbing fast.

Close to one third of these foreign-born patients in 1913 were "noncitizens." What rankled Bellevue officials was the fact that so many of them had come to their hospital within "a day or less" of reaching Manhattan—meaning their "illness" had been overlooked by the steamship operators who brought them over from Europe and the public health doctors who examined them at Ellis Island. For the already overburdened Bellevue staff, treating hundreds of "mandatorily excludible" cases—"idiots, imbeciles, epileptics, alcoholics, those with tuberculosis and dangerous contagious diseases"—would become a routine, if disagreeable, part of the job. And there was no use complaining about it because federal authorities weren't interested in enforcing the law. In 1913, the Immigration Service rounded up a grand total of seven Bellevue patients for deportation.

The irony, of course, was that Bellevue had never been popular with the groups now pouring through its doors. Previous generations of Jews and Italians had scrupulously avoided the place, viewing it as a death trap and a refuge for the "low Irish." For years, rumors had abounded in the city's immigrant neighborhoods about the "black bottle" used at Bellevue to "bump off" patients who "weren't worth saving." "The opinion is prevalent . . . that Bellevue is a school of experiment for the instruction of young surgeons, and that only cases of peculiar novelty are of interest there," a city health officer explained. "In cases of lingering sickness . . . they are supposed to hasten the end by administering a fatal dose from the mysterious black bottle." Or, as immigrant legend had it, "they give you a drink, and that's the end of you."

New York's small Jewish community had long favored Mount Sinai in emergencies, while Italians preferred Roman Catholic Columbus Hospital, where their native tongue was spoken. But times had changed. Private (or "voluntary") hospitals could no longer handle the sheer volume of foreigners now seeking admission—nor, in some cases, did they want to. At Mount Sinai, officials were quite open about favoring "the better conditioned of people" over the unwashed masses, just off the boats. "In the philanthropic institutions of our aristocratic

German Jews you see beautiful offices, desks all decorated, but strict and angry faces," a recent immigrant complained. "Every poor man is questioned like a criminal, is looked down upon; every unfortunate suffers self-degradation and shivers like a leaf, just as if we were standing before a Russian official."

Given a choice, many new arrivals preferred Bellevue's rough egalitarianism to Mount Sinai's stern condescension. Bellevue asked no questions. It was less judgmental, and a lot closer to the teeming immigrant slums of the Lower East Side—Mount Sinai having moved uptown to better serve its well-heeled patients. The 1890s had seen a sprinkling of Jewish and Italian names in the Bellevue ledgers, an occasional "Isaac Levy, Russia, tailor" or "Guiseppe Amato, Italy, longshoreman" among the scores of Callahans and Kellys. In 1907, a small synagogue opened at Bellevue for "Hebrew worshippers" and a translator was hired to accommodate Yiddish-speaking patients. By 1915, the sprinkling had become a steady stream. A look at Bellevue's pediatric files that year shows a clear majority of Jewish and Italian names: Julia Cohen, Morris Fink, Solomon Iskowitz, Sam Katz, Joseph Schwartz, Ada Nutelli, Agnes Pellegrino, Dominic Rossi—the list goes on. By 1920, more Jewish and Italian immigrants would be entering Bellevue than any other hospital in the city.

Bellevue's growth in these years was stunning. Admissions rose from 6,546 in 1879 to 45,470 by 1920. And Bellevue wasn't alone. Hospitals throughout the city were expanding, though the reasons owed little to the immigrant explosion or the medical needs of the poor. What had changed—and quite radically—was the public's negative perception of the hospital itself. Once viewed as a dumping ground for the lower classes, it had begun to attract "respectable" folk long accustomed to being treated at home. The era of the "private" patient had arrived.

The concept wasn't new. As far back as the 1860s, St. Vincent's had made a few rooms available for those wanting something more than a ward bed. But it wasn't until the turn of the century that voluntary hospitals started to build separate quarters for private patients in a serious way. New York Hospital opened a ten-story structure in 1900 with "brass bedsteads, couches, and open fireplaces," followed quickly by Mount Sinai, its private rooms overlooking Central Park, its charity wards facing the side streets. A survey of New York City hospitals in 1924 showed close to 30 percent of all patients occupying private or semiprivate rooms. The trend has "had a beneficial influence," the authors noted, because "the hospital [has] ceased to be regarded as exclusively the refuge of the sick poor."

What, exactly, had made a hospital more appealing to patients in 1910 than it had been in 1880? The most obvious answer is the remarkable impact of science and technology. Surgical operations had become safer, thanks to Pasteur, Semmelweis, and Lister. Trained nurses could sterilize wounds and monitor a patient's vital signs. Blood and tissue samples could be sent to well-equipped laboratories for examination. The newly discovered X-ray was coming into use. "Today," a writer observed in *Popular Science Monthly*, "the patient approaches [the hospital] with . . . the hope of life rather than the fear of death."

But well-heeled patients weren't about to mingle with the charity cases or forgo the luxuries of home. And they no longer had to. A stay at New York Hospital or Mount Sinai might now include a room with fresh-cut flowers and plush Persian rugs. So, too, gourmet meals and full-time nursing care. Even the bathrobes and bedsheets of private patients were color-coded to separate them from the laundry of the hoi polloi. For the privileged few, the hospital had come to resemble a medical resort, described by the *Times* as "a hotel for rich invalids."

There was space for the middle classes as well. Those unable to afford the staggering $40 to $75 a week for princely quarters could find a "semi-private room" or a "pay ward" at a fraction of the price. It wasn't luxurious, but it did segregate them from the putrid smells and poorer elements they hoped to avoid. The end result was an institution increasingly split by social class, with paying patients getting preferred space and a lion's share of the resources. One medical journal, sensing that a corner had been turned, implored its readers to step back and search their souls. "In the spirit of fairness and in the name of charity . . . we ask, 'Is it right?'"

It would be hard to overstate the importance of science, sanitation, and material comfort in creating the modern American hospital. But there was another factor as well. Those who had avoided hospitals in the past normally used a trusted family physician—someone familiar with their needs. Would they now enter a place filled with doctors they didn't know?

Hospital privileges had long been restricted to those who taught at a medical school and did some clinical research. The rule hadn't mattered much in the era when hospitals were filled with the lower classes. But the new competition for private patients depended heavily on referrals from family doctors whose wants—and resentments—could no longer be ignored. As one of them fumed: "Why is it that when our patients enter a hospital we must surrender them to self-styled and Lord-knows how appointed professors . . . who assume ownership and charge of them . . . in absolute disregard of our rights in the matter?" Opening the hospital door to family doctors no doubt diminished the power of the elite medical practitioner; but keeping them out severely restricted the number of paying patients—a far greater concern.

The expansion of these privileges spoke to a profession in flux. Physicians had rarely charged for services rendered in a hospital because the typical patient lacked the ability to pay. Surely that would change. And what of the relationship between the family doctor and the hospital staff? Was a nurse or an intern expected to carry out his wishes? Who would order the various tests? Or determine when the patient was well enough to be discharged?

For a public hospital like Bellevue, such questions were moot. There would be no wooing of private patients and no temptation to segregate by class. But the changing landscape of patient care would seriously complicate its role. Though New York's voluntary hospitals would continue to accept charity cases, the pace already had begun to slow. Meanwhile, private referrals were pouring in. Among the many examples was Mount Sinai, where the number of paying patients would more than triple—from 9 percent to 30 percent—in the years between 1889 and 1909, while charity care languished.

Public hospitals had no choice but to pick up the slack.

Working at Bellevue in the late nineteenth century had marked a man as a fine doctor and an even finer Christian. The surroundings may have been decrepit, the conditions sometimes threatening, but the medical care was as good as one could hope for, given the challenges of the job. Where else, the *New York Times* had boasted, could "a pauper without a rag to his back . . . command the services of [giants] like Dr. Austin Flint, Sr., Stephen Smith, and Dr. A. L. Loomis?" And how better for a pauper to repay his debt than by supplying the "clinical material" required for teaching and research?

For decades, Bellevue had recruited its doctors through a byzantine arrangement with the city's top medical schools. Changes had occurred—the merger of Bellevue and NYU in 1898; the addition of newly opened Cornell—but the concept of "separate fiefdoms" remained firmly in place. Columbia (P&S) ran the First Medical and Surgical Division at Bellevue; Cornell the Second Division; NYU/Bellevue the Third Division; and "non-affiliated doctors" seeking postgraduate training the Fourth (a much smaller operation). On paper, at least, it seemed to work. Students were trained; research flourished; patients got free care; and the city fulfilled its obligation to the poor.*

Bellevue had even survived the pen of Abraham Flexner, whose heralded Carnegie Foundation report, *Medical Education in the United States and Canada,* published in 1910, had portrayed the typical medical school as a wretched diploma mill run by incompetent doctors looking to make a fast buck. While not a physician himself, Flexner had immersed himself in the German model of medical education, which stressed the combination of clinical training and laboratory work. He particularly admired Johns Hopkins, where entering students held col-

---

* In 1898, the separate NYU and Bellevue Medical Colleges merged into a single institution known as the University and Bellevue Hospital Medical College. The stated reason was a fire on the Bellevue grounds that damaged parts of the Bellevue Medical College building, though both institutions had been struggling financially for years. The merger allowed the colleges to pool their resources and to trim overlapping faculty. The acrimony it produced—who would stay and who would leave—was substantial. Indeed, a number of departing faculty members negotiated with Cornell University, which then offered a two-year "preparatory curriculum" in medicine in Ithaca, New York, to create a four-year medical college in New York City, which opened in 1898 with substantial funding from Cornell alumni. Given its solid financial standing and Ivy League credentials, Cornell Medical College had no trouble getting off the ground. In short order, its faculty and students were fully integrated into Bellevue Hospital for clinical instruction. In 1935, Bellevue/NYU formally changed its name to NYU Medical College.

lege degrees, the medical school was attached to a hospital, and the operating expenses were covered by an endowment, not simply tuition and fees—the very arrangement that had led William Welch to depart Bellevue for Baltimore two decades before.

Flexner had visited almost every medical school in both countries. "FACTORIES FOR THE MAKING OF IGNORANT DOCTORS," read the *New York Times* headline of the scathing report. The good news, said the newspaper, was that New York City "is practically free from the things [Flexner] condemns." Cornell, P&S, and NYU/Bellevue "are favorably commented upon in the report." This was mostly true. Of the eleven medical schools in New York State, Flexner had given the highest grades to Cornell and Columbia, with NYU/Bellevue a distant third. Cornell and Columbia required at least two years of college for entering students; NYU accepted high school graduates (soon to be upgraded). Cornell and Columbia admitted fewer applicants and had fair-sized endowments; NYU relied on tuition and fees to cover its costs. What the three schools held in common, however, was their link to the largest public hospital in America.

The main problem at Bellevue, in Flexner's view, was the lack of coordination among the separate divisions. There was no mechanism in place to hold them accountable for clinical training and patient care. "The schools skate on thin ice," he wrote, calling their "lack of unity" a threat to the hospital they served.

The Flexner Report is considered a watershed document—one that changed the course of medical education in North America. And its release coincided with the efforts of other reformers in the Progressive Era to hold the various professions, including law and medicine, to a higher standard, while protecting society's most vulnerable groups. New York City would be a major testing ground for reforms involving child labor, worker safety, and stricter health codes. In 1914, it undertook a massive study of its public hospitals, looking, above all, to increase their efficiency—another goal of the Progressive Movement. Running to more than seven hundred pages, the study dissected every imaginable aspect of Bellevue's operation, from the maternity wards to the morgue, from the high turnover among menial workers (described as "downs and outs" and "periodic drunks") to the pay grades for drivers of "horse ambulances" and "motor trucks." There even were statistics showing the amount of food routinely wasted in the dining rooms for doctors ("On one day, 25 pounds of porterhouse steak were returned with the plates") and for nurses ("89 pounds of steak and chicken were returned, [along] with 55 pounds of Irish stew and veal").

The heart of the report, however, addressed patient care. And most troubling, it appeared, was the poor coverage on the wards. The attending physicians from the medical schools were spending too little time at Bellevue—not out of laziness, but because they relied on private patients to earn a decent living. The end result, said the report, was a ripple effect whereby the burden of care had shifted even further to interns and residents "inexperienced in the diagnosing of disease." A survey of the hospital's records showed a disturbing pattern of premature patient discharges—some out of ignorance, others because the intern handling the case thought it "uninteresting." In fact, the report had hit upon a problem that would only grow larger over time: the reliance upon a badly overworked and clearly under-supervised hospital house staff.

The report had an immediate impact: salaries at Bellevue went up across the board. Menial workers (or "hospital helpers") saw their meager wages double, from $60 to $120 a year, with free room and board, while the minimum pay for nurses rose to $360. Regarding the medical schools, the city agreed to supplement the salaries of each division chief, a full-time job, which raised the pay to $5,000 a year—a handsome sum in that era, but well below the earnings of an elite faculty member with a private practice on the side. This gap would become painfully clear when four consecutive Columbia physicians turned down the chance to lead the First Division before a fifth agreed to take it on. "Financially, the position would demand considerable sacrifice," one candidate admitted. New York Hospital not only encouraged its attending physicians to admit their private patients, it also allowed them to charge for their in-hospital services. "This is not allowed at Bellevue," he said, and "it would mean a [financial] loss greater than I could, in justice to my family, afford."

Between 1915 and 1922, the three medical schools serving Bellevue accepted their first women. It was a progressive move, though hardly a daring one. Johns Hopkins Medical School had been coed since its founding in 1893; Harvard, by contrast, would remain all-male until 1945. But women seeking an internship after graduation were largely out of luck. Though the hospitals in New York City selected their house staffs by competitive examination, the process excluded women, blacks, and, in most cases, Jews.

Bellevue was the first to break this taboo. With a doctor shortage looming as the nation prepared for World War I, the idea of using female residents to replace the young men joining the armed forces seemed a natural step. Though Bellevue would house these women on the farthest reaches of the property, where "rats of heroic East River dimension came up through the floor at night and playfully scampered across their faces," the opportunity rarely went begging. "My choices were extremely limited," recalled Dr. Connie Guion, a 1916 graduate of Cornell Medical School. "I could apply to the New York Infirmary for Women and Children, which was run entirely by women, or I could go to Bellevue, which had just begun to take women as interns." Wanting "the full experience," Guion chose Bellevue, noting: "I don't think there was a disease in Osler's *Textbook of Medicine* that I didn't see."

By the 1920s, twelve of Bellevue's ninety-nine interns would be women. They came with medical degrees from Columbia, Cornell, or NYU, recommended in careful prose, free of superlatives, to avoid offending the hospital's old guard. Words like "acceptable," "creditable," and "well-disciplined" dotted the paper. "Her services," a typical letter ended, "will have no cause for regret."

African Americans faced a tougher climb. Close to 85 percent of the nation's 1,500 black physicians in these years were graduates of "Negro medical colleges," Howard (in Washington, D.C.) and Meharry (in Nashville) heading the list. Some Northern medical schools were known for accepting a small number of black men, including Michigan, Northwestern, and Western Reserve. The University of Pennsylvania took in three each year starting in the 1880s—with two of them expected to "fail out" before graduation. And Johns Hopkins, which had led the way in opening doors for women (in return for a $300,000 gift from a feminist donor) would remain an all-white preserve until the 1970s, not surprising given its location in a racially segregated city.

Roscoe Conkling Giles exemplified the plight of ambitious black doctors in this era. A child prodigy, the son of a Brooklyn minister, Giles had won a full scholarship to attend Cornell University in 1907. Graduating with honors, he became the first African American accepted at Cornell Medical School—and the first to earn a degree. Denied housing and threatened by a gun-wielding student, he graduated on schedule in 1915 and took the competitive examination for a prized Bellevue internship, which had never been offered to a Negro.

Giles failed the exam. Furious, he accused the hospital of discriminating against him on account of his color, which almost certainly was true. Bellevue officials barely blinked. "In plain English, he was outclassed," said one, adding that Giles should accept the verdict in a "sportsmanlike manner and not go about claiming that he had a race grievance."

Indeed, it would take the political weight of City Hall to get the first African American intern placed at Bellevue. His name was U. Conrad Vincent, and he'd applied after graduating from the University of Pennsylvania Medical School in 1917 because no hospital in Philadelphia would accept him. Applications in those days required a photograph, and that alone doomed Vincent's chances. But his cause gained an unlikely ally when Mayor John F. Hylan, anxious to court the city's rapidly growing black vote in future elections, lobbied Bellevue officials to reexamine Vincent's credentials and test scores, which they did.

Vincent was accepted, but the progress ended there. Bellevue would award only four other internships to African Americans in the years between 1920 and 1950, though most hospitals, in truth, offered none. Even a medical degree from Columbia, Cornell, or NYU did little good. In 1926, for example, Bellevue rejected two NYU graduates who stood near the top of their class: May Chinn and Aubrey Maynard. Dr. Chinn, an accomplished pianist, was black *and* female, while the Guyanese-born Dr. Maynard was, in Chinn's words, a "very, very dark" Negro man who would never be allowed to examine a white female patient. Both took their internships at Harlem Hospital, in a neighborhood undergoing dramatic racial change.

All four went on to remarkably successful careers. Roscoe Conkling Giles became the first African American to win certification from the prestigious American Board of Surgery and the first to have the word "colored" removed from his title in the AMA's Official Directory. His success in the white medical world was a source of pride—and some unease—among other black physicians. "Dr. Giles is one of us," a leading black medical journal declared. "We are proud of him. We are sure that this honor will not be used to lift him away from his constituency but to help to elevate them."

Drs. Vincent, Chinn, and Maynard would remain part of the Harlem community—Vincent opening a TB sanitarium that trained a generation of black physicians, Chinn promoting early cancer detection in women, and Maynard specializing in thoracic surgery at Harlem Hospital, where, in 1956, he operated on a visiting young minister who'd been stabbed by a deranged woman while signing books in a local department store. "Days later, when I was well enough to talk with Dr. Aubrey Maynard," the victim recalled, ". . . I learned that . . . the [letter opener] had been touching my aorta, and that my whole chest had to be opened to extract it."

Maynard had saved the life of Dr. Martin Luther King, Jr.

For Jews, ironically, the problem was reversed. They'd been readily accepted into medical schools and hospital internships throughout the nineteenth century, when their numbers were small and their origins were German. But the mass immigration from Eastern Europe had set off alarm bells at the nation's leading universities, which were clustered in the regions where these immigrants had settled. Following World War I, Harvard, Yale, Columbia, and Cornell would lead the way in establishing undergraduate quota systems to limit the percentage of Jews, with their medical schools following suit. As Columbia's dean of students Herbert Hawkes put it: "We have honestly attempted to eliminate the lowest grade of applicant and it turns out that a good many of the low grade men are New York Jews."

Hawkes wasn't alone. College administrators of this era routinely described Jews as "radical," "pushy," "asocial," "unstable," and "commercially inclined." Their quota systems were designed to ensure "civility" and "balance" in the student body. And they required no great overhaul, just a tweaking of the application. Where the form had once asked for name, place of birth, a college transcript, and a faculty recommendation or two, it now added categories such as "religion," "maiden name of mother," "place of birth of parents," and a photograph (which helped weed out African Americans as well).

The quota system proved devilishly effective. At Yale Medical School, the dean had the applications marked with an "H" for Hebrew and "C" for Catholic. His instructions were remarkably precise: "Never admit more than five Jews, take only two Italian Catholics, and take no blacks at all." According to one detailed study, the percentage of Jewish admissions to Columbia Medical School dropped from 47 percent in 1920 to 19 percent in 1924 to 6 percent by 1940. The same held for Cornell Medical School, which normally took about 80 students each year from a pool of 1,200 applicants—700 of whom were Jewish. With the new system in place, Cornell cut the number of Jewish acceptances to between eight and twelve. As word spread, many Jewish students, knowing the outcome, simply stopped applying to these places. Arthur Kornberg, a graduate of the overwhelmingly Jewish City College of New York and a future Nobel Laureate, recalled his bitterness at the vulgar anti-Semitism he faced. The hardest part, said Kornberg, was learning that an endowed scholarship for a CCNY graduate to attend Columbia Medical School "went begging for nine years because there were no candidates. To this day it rankles me."

The harshest quotas were found in the New York City area, where Jewish applicants abounded. On average, a study in the early 1930s concluded, 63 percent of gentile applicants gained admission to a city medical school, as opposed to only 15 percent of Jews. And things would have been even worse had it not been for Dean John Wyckoff of NYU Medical School, who insisted that academic achievement was the best predictor of success in medical school—and beyond. When Wyckoff presented his findings at a conference in 1927, the dean at Columbia sniffed that "many traits" merited attention, such as "the personal side of the man, his ability to get on with other men in his class, and various other things."

A look at Columbia's "preferred" lists for medical internships showed exactly what he meant. One candidate, "standing in the middle third of his class," had "an attractive personality and is a nice chap to deal with." A second was "tall, good-looking," and—better yet—"a graduate of

Princeton." A third, alas, was "a homely chap," but "very intelligent." A typical list would contain two or three females ("fine family background . . . the most desirable type of woman") and perhaps one or two Jews ("an exceedingly bright, mature, pleasant, and well-rounded boy").

Dr. Joe Dancis, a Columbia undergraduate in these years, recalled a conversation he had with a medical school professor there who apparently took a liking to him. Suspecting that Dancis, who was Jewish, might ask him for a recommendation, the professor called him into his office "for a chat, during which he defended the fact that they had a cap on Jews at Columbia . . . and went on at great lengths to explain that this was an attempt to have a more diverse student body." Dancis went to medical school at St. Louis University before interning at Bellevue and joining the NYU faculty, where he chaired the Department of Pediatrics for three decades. "I didn't ask any questions," he said. "I accepted it as a way of life."

Since NYU Medical School had no formal quota system, its average class was more than 50 percent Jewish, providing a refuge for future research giants like Albert Sabin and Jonas Salk—and fodder for critics who sneeringly dubbed it "NY-Jew." Moreover, because NYU chose so many of its own graduates for internships in the Third Medical and Surgical Division, Bellevue (along with Mount Sinai) became the best option for Jews seeking house staff positions in a time of clubby prejudice and tightly closed doors.

There never was a time when Bellevue appeared even remotely trouble-free. Its list of challenges in the new century—half-completed buildings, fickle city budgets, surging immigrant numbers, conflicting medical school agendas, the private patient revolution—seemed no larger, or bleaker, than before. Bellevue was Bellevue, a municipal eyesore most New Yorkers couldn't imagine living without. Even those who would never think of setting foot inside understood its need to exist. A writer for the *New York Times* captured Bellevue's essence in Dickensian prose: "It gathers the dead and dying from the rivers and streets and is kept busy night and day with the misery of the living."

In the late summer of 1918, as World War I turned in America's favor, a pandemic of biblical proportions swept the globe. Some scholars have traced its origins to Spain; others to an American army camp in Kansas; still others to the battlefield trenches in France. Before it ended, the so-called Great Influenza would kill more people, in a shorter time, than any other outbreak in history, with fifty to eighty million lives lost worldwide. One American in four would contract it before the pandemic subsided, and close to 700,000 would die. No statistic can properly convey this horrific damage, but one comes close: in 1918, the life expectancy of the average American dropped by twelve full years.

Previous influenza epidemics had taken their greatest toll among those with fragile immune systems, especially the very young and very old. This flu was different; the highest death rates would occur among adults in their twenties and early thirties. Numerous theories have appeared to explain this anomaly, the favorite being the "cytokine storm" in which a vigorous immune system responds so forcefully to the invading microbes as to literally drown the lungs in gooey phlegm, dead cells, and assorted debris. William Welch was stunned by the carnage he saw in the quarantine wards at Fort Devens, Massachusetts, in 1918. "This must be some new kind of infection. Or plague," he told a young army physician, who never forgot the look of panic that crossed the great man's face.

Bellevue received its first influenza cases in mid-August—three sailors from the Brooklyn Navy Yard, all dead within the week. "High temperature, short of breath, and bluish," noted the resident in charge. By September, the disease had felled hundreds, then thousands, of New Yorkers. As it spread, the Health Department banned spitting in public as well as "promiscuous coughing and sneezing." To prevent crowding on the subways, stores and factories staggered their working hours, and theaters cut their ticket sales in half. The public schools remained open, but only because the health commissioner thought the classrooms to be safer for children than the slums where so many of them lived. Before long, public libraries had stopped lending books, gauze face masks had become regular attire, and people had stopped shaking hands.

In October, Bellevue saw more admissions than it had at any time in its history. Resident Connie Guion was soon treating five hundred victims by herself. There was little to be done for them beyond some aspirin and whiskey to dull the pain. "It got to the place where I would only see the patients twice—once when they came in and again when I signed their death certificate," she recalled. With so many bodies in the morgue, the city hired extra gravediggers to handle the overflow.

Guion's most vivid memory was of a teenage Italian boy who had lost ten members of his family to the epidemic. The father, now dead, had run a neighborhood cigar store. The boy asked her, "Doc, what do you think I should do? Should I use up all my money burying [them] or do you think I should let them go to Potter's Field?" Guion told him to save the cigar store and let the city assume the burial costs. The store survived—a small sign, she thought, of the enduring human spirit.

Patients weren't the only casualties. So many nurses and doctors took sick that city officials wondered whether to limit new admissions to public hospitals until the crisis eased—a suspension of Bellevue's most sacred rule. They decided against it; no one would be turned away, though some patients wound up sharing a bed or sleeping on the floor.

The city's voluntary hospitals played a lesser role. Their policy was to accept as many influenza patients as their charity wards could normally hold. When a bed opened, a new admission would occur. There would be no doubling up, no cots in the hallways, and no invasion of the rooms set aside for private patients.

Meanwhile, work proceeded on a flu vaccine, led by Hermann Biggs and his disciple, William Hallock Park. Both men had trained at Bellevue, and both held appointments at NYU Medical School, where the field of virology was rapidly taking hold.

To develop an effective vaccine, one must isolate the responsible pathogen—an impossible task in 1918 given the mysteries of the endlessly mutating influenza virus. Park did his best in an atmosphere of growing alarm as his own staffers fell, one by one, to the disease. Believing, correctly, that the high death rate had less to do with the initial bout of influenza than with the bacterial pneumonia that followed, Park injected one group of volunteers with weakened strains of pneumococcus to produce an antibody reaction, while simply observing the other group. The results were discouraging. Those who received the vaccine had twice as many lung infections as those who didn't.

Park was beaten. "Our final conclusion," he admitted, "is . . . that the micro-organism causing this epidemic has not yet been identified." A decade later, in 1929, the biographer of Hermann Biggs described the vaccine debacle as "a chastening experience for [those] who had come to feel that modern science had placed in their hands weapons of almost unlimited power for defense against epidemic disease."

The Great Influenza disappeared as suddenly as it had come. Belle-vue had been staggered, at times overwhelmed by the crisis, but its credo remained intact. When it came to treating the sick, whatever the circumstances, there was always room for one more.

14

CAUSE OF DEATH

The 1920 U.S. Census revealed a country barely imagined a generation before. The population now exceeded 100 million, more than double the figure in 1880, and larger than that of any European nation except the infant Soviet Union. Even more telling were the demographic changes: America, the land of farms and open frontiers, had officially become "urban." More people were living in cities than in rural communities—a shift accelerated by mass immigration from Europe and the exodus of Southern blacks to the industrial North and Midwest. Manufacturing jobs were there for the taking—in steel and automobiles, in meatpacking and the garment trades. World War I had made the United States a creditor nation, its banks, factories, and troops having turned an unspeakably brutal conflict in favor of the Allies. With Europe exhausted and reeling, American finance and industry dominated the world stage.

New York City stood at the center of it all. Its population of 5,650,000 was twice as large as second-place Chicago. Wall Street was the undisputed king of capital transactions, and midtown Manhattan, a few miles to the north, headquartered 75 percent of the nation's four hundred largest corporations. The Woolworth Building, the Metropolitan Life Insurance Tower, the Bank of Manhattan, the soon-to-be Chrysler and Empire State Buildings—all symbolized the city's economic clout. "The American does not realize what a shock New York can be to a European who has never before seen a building higher than ten floors," a British writer marveled. "The effect is bewildering."

It wasn't simply the skyscrapers. The shock value of New York City came in many forms. The splashy wealth, jam-packed streets, and immigrant enclaves spoke to one part of it; the cultural tone to another. "The parties were bigger . . . the morals were looser and the liquor was cheaper," F. Scott Fitzgerald wrote of Roaring Twenties New York in *The Great Gatsby*. Though his vision hardly compared to that of mere mortals, few would deny the excess, escapism, and lawlessness that permeated city life. Many blamed it on rural attempts to counter urban "immorality" through repressive measures like Prohibition, the constitutional amendment that banned the manufacture, sale, and transportation of alcoholic beverages starting on New Year's Day 1920. Opinion polls showed most Americans coming to loathe and openly flout its provisions, nowhere more than in New York City, where thirty thousand speakeasies cropped up to dispense illegal alcohol, much of it foul-tasting, some of it deadly. Over time, Prohibition would be blamed for the birth of organized crime, thousands of fatal poisonings, and the resurgence of Tammany Hall led by "wet" politicians like James J. "Jimmy" Walker, the aptly named "nightclub mayor." Jazz Age New York had become America's "city on a still."

Prohibition changed Bellevue as well. The flow of illegal whiskey not only taxed the hospital's emergency rooms, it also fueled a curious new specialty, developed in Bellevue's pathology labs, to provide a scientific explanation for the manner in which a person died. Its founders called it forensic medicine.

Every so often, following a sensational exposé of municipal corruption, the New York state legislature would rise up and pass a well-meaning bill in response. One such moment arrived in 1915 when Leonard Wallstein, New York City's fastidious, anti-Tammany commissioner of accounts, published his investigation of the local coroner's office. In scathing terms, Wallstein described it as a sinkhole of "favoritism, extortion, and malfeasance," adding that crimes of "infanticide and skillful poisoning" routinely went unpunished because the prosecutor's office received "no adequate medical data whatever."

The main problem, Wallstein noted, was the political nature of the beast. Coroners were elected officials, meaning that most were "absurdly ignorant" of medical matters but remarkably well versed in the petty graft of Tammany Hall. According to Wallstein, the list of coroners since 1898, the year of New York City's consolidation, included "eight undertakers, seven politicians, six real estate dealers, two saloonkeepers, two plumbers, a lawyer, a printer, an auctioneer, a wood carver, a carpenter, a painter, a butcher, a marble cutter, a milkman, an insurance agent, a labor leader, and a musician." Occasionally, an actual doctor would be elected—a dependable hack plucked from the ranks of "medical mediocrity."

With the report in hand, the state legislature abolished the old system. There would be no more elections for coroner in New York City. All future hiring would be done by a "chief medical examiner" selected from a pool of "skilled pathologists [holding] the degree of M.D. from an approved institution of recognized standing." Mayor John F. Hylan wasn't thrilled by the change. "We have had all the reform that we want in this city for some time to come," he fumed. Hylan tried to subvert the process but the Republican governor intervened. The new post went to Dr. Charles Norris, the director of laboratories at Bellevue Hospital and a professor of pathology at NYU Medical School.

Standing well over six feet, the hard-drinking, goatee-sporting Norris came from money and privilege, his ancestors having founded Norristown, Pennsylvania. A graduate of Yale and the College of Physicians and Surgeons, Norris had traveled to Europe for further study in pathology and bacteriology—treading the same path as William Welch, whose laboratory research he deeply admired. Arriving at Bellevue in 1904, as plans for a new pathology building were under way, Norris took an early interest in forensic medicine. Among the improvements he helped oversee was the expansion of the city morgue, making it the largest such facility in the world. When his job offer arrived in 1918, Norris had been teaching and researching at the hospital for more than a decade. He demanded, quite logically, that the Office of Chief Medical Examiner be headquartered where "the greatest activity resided," and that meant Bellevue. It took some hard lobbying, but Norris got his way.

By law, the new Medical Examiner's Office was responsible for investigating all cases in which a victim died "from criminal violence, or suicide, or suddenly when in apparent good health, or in any suspicious or unusual manner." Given that more than 25 percent of New York City's fatalities fell into one of these categories, the workload was daunting. Was the body in the river a simple drowning or something more sinister? Was the gunshot wound the work of a murderer or perhaps self-inflicted? Had the victim died of natural causes or had she been poisoned?

By all accounts, Norris welcomed the challenge. His fiefdom covered several floors of the Bellevue pathology building, from the basement morgue to the laboratories and animal quarters housed directly above. "It would be imprecise to say that Dr. Charles Norris loved the job of chief medical examiner," a writer noted. "He lived it and breathed it. . . . He gave it power and prominence and wore himself into exhaustion and illness over it." His faculty position at NYU provided another advantage. Norris couldn't fire all the holdovers from the previous system; that was politically impossible. But he could bring in fresh blood to run the new laboratories he created—the most important addition being a young NYU chemist named Alexander O. Gettler.

It proved a spectacularly good hire. Born in Austria to Jewish parents who emigrated to Manhattan's Lower East Side, Gettler had attended public schools before entering the City College of New York, which accepted students based on grades and a competitive exam, and, best of all, was free. Spending his nights as a ticket-taker on a ferryboat, Gettler got a doctorate in chemistry from Columbia, where his reputation for creativity earned him an instructorship at NYU Medical School, which welcomed Jews, and a laboratory slot at Bellevue. It hardly mattered to Norris that the young man lacked a medical degree. No one knew more about the adverse effects of toxins on the human body—or how they got there—than the brilliant, irascible Alexander Gettler.

Superficially, at least, the two men were polar opposites: Norris the physically imposing, Yale-educated, old-stock American living luxuriously on Manhattan's Upper West Side; Gettler the diminutive product of immigrant neighborhoods and public education living modestly in the outer reaches of Brooklyn. What bound them together was an abiding faith in laboratory research. Forensic medicine had yet to emerge as a legitimate pursuit in the United States. The very idea of a medical examiner's office in an American city—much less one pro-pelled by serious science—was striking in itself.

Skepticism abounded. For most of the 1920s, the Medical Exam-iner's Office would get far less funding than the old coroner's system had received. Money was so tight early on that Norris used his entire $6,000 annual salary, and sometimes his personal fortune, to meet the department's basic needs. "All new equipment purchased in 1921 had been paid for by Norris himself or by his staff; every test tube, every scalpel, a new scale to weigh tissue samples, a small brass microscope to study tissue damage. All of it."

The results were nothing short of remarkable. Starting from scratch, Norris and Gettler devised ways to examine semen stains on clothing, trace the trajectory of a bullet, detect minute levels of different poisons in the system, and then determine the body's exact tolerance for each one of them—the so-called lethal dose. In the 1920s and 1930s, these two men didn't simply revolutionize the field of forensic science, they *were* the field.

Riding the freight elevator between the basement morgue and his fourth-floor laboratory, Gettler would return with vials of blood, tissue samples, and body parts to examine. When working on a particularly difficult case—a rare or unfamiliar toxin—he'd visit his local butcher, buy a few pounds of raw meat, "spike it with the substance involved, and then determine how efficiently he could recover the substance and how conclusively he could identify it."

Gettler's experiments relied heavily on animals, especially dogs. One high-profile case involved a woman who had bled to death in her doc-tor's office from a bungled abortion. Her autopsy showed suspiciously high levels of chloroform in her brain, leading prosecutors to charge her doctor with performing the (then illegal) procedure himself, which he vigorously denied. The abortion had occurred elsewhere, he swore, adding that the woman had come to see him shortly afterward, and that he'd done everything possible to save her life.

Gettler had his doubts. After completing the woman's autopsy, he injected ten dogs with varying amounts of chloroform to observe their behavior. Then he sacrificed them to measure the level of chloroform in their brains. His conclusion was unambiguous: the victim couldn't possibly have walked into the doctor's office under her own power. The chloroforming—and thus the operation itself—must have been done there. A jury agreed, and the doctor went to jail.

Gettler also used dogs to test his theories regarding drowning and intoxication. Determining whether a body that washed ashore had fallen drunkenly from a pier or been dumped into the water already dead was always guesswork for the coroner, who generally took the word of the police. Gettler wanted more evidence. Knowing that water in the lungs enters the heart's left chamber before circulating through the body to reach the right chamber, he correctly assumed that one could differentiate between a suicide or an accident, where the victim was still alive in the water, and a homicide, where the victim was already dead, by comparing the contents (especially the salt level) in the two chambers. A major difference would imply the former, because the victim had survived long enough to pump the blood from one chamber to the other; no difference would likely mean murder. Gettler drowned a fair number of dogs before declaring his research a success.

His intoxication studies demanded both a test group and a control group. In one experiment, Gettler gave the test group—a dozen dogs—a mixture of water and alcohol to drink, while the control group—another dozen dogs—got water alone. It took some doing. Because dogs dislike the taste of alcohol, Gettler denied the test group all liquids until they became so thirsty that they welcomed anything put before them. Soon they were lapping down a concoction equivalent to 100-proof whiskey and behaving like "common drunks" as they "staggered about the laboratory . . . howled in lieu of weeping or singing [and] sometimes . . . even hiccupped."

Gettler next provided equal amounts of alcohol to both groups— his *"habitués"* and his "abstainers"—to measure their tolerance. Not surprisingly, the "abstainers" became inebriated more quickly, with lesser amounts, than the *"habitués."* After destroying the dogs, Gettler discovered why: the organs of the *"habitués"* contained lower levels of alcohol, meaning "they oxidized it at a faster rate." With further study, he provided some of the key measurements of the modern sobriety test, such as the concentration of alcohol in the blood.

There were objections to experiments like this one—less from fellow researchers than from antivivisection groups that had begun targeting Bellevue's pathology labs for their liberal use of animal subjects in the Norris era. The trigger had been the publicity surrounding the suicide in 1920 of a longtime lab worker named Ernest Goetz, a favorite of Norris, who had retired after forty years at Bellevue, a span in which he'd done almost every menial task the hospital had to offer, from shoveling coal to washing glassware to caring for the animals in the pathology building. At seventy, badly hobbled and almost blind, Goetz was found dead while on a periodic visit to the hospital's animal quarters. His body lay on the floor with the gas jets turned on.

The press had a field day. Headlines like "TOO OLD TO CARE FOR PETS, TURNS ON GAS" accompanied stories hinting, not too subtly, that Goetz had been tormented by visions of his beloved Bellevue animals being destroyed. It reached the point where a furious Charles Norris felt obliged to "set forth the true facts" in a letter to the *New York Times.* Goetz hadn't committed suicide "out of deep sympathy for white mice," Norris fumed. He'd taken his life because he was desperate and depressed at having to live on a city pension of less than a dollar a day following four decades of loyal service—a proud man, barely able to walk or to see, found dead with 45 cents in his pocket.

The criticism faded quickly, overwhelmed, in part, by news of Gettler's successes. Flattering features in *Time* and *Harper's* called him the "Test-Tube Sleuth" and "The Man Who Reads Corpses." Years later, a forensic expert claimed that Gettler "sent more criminals to the electric chair through his tests than any police detective applying all of the police department's methods of investigation." This wasn't hyperbole. Gettler averaged close to fifty court appearances a year, rarely on the losing side. In one case, he nailed a killer by tracing the grass and soil in his trouser cuffs to the terrain at the murder scene. In another, he linked a piece of string on a dead woman's body to the upholsterer doing work in her apartment. (Both men were found guilty and executed.) Gettler's methods became the gold standard for detecting intoxicants, barbiturates, and poisons. He even testified for the "radium girls" in a celebrated civil suit, settled in 1928, which revolutionized occupational safety laws, demonstrating that years of swabbing wristwatch dials with a luminous radium-based paint had caused an assortment of deadly cancers. The women won, though few of them lived long enough to collect the settlement. The press called it "The Case of Those Who Were Doomed to Die."

His office bulged with memorabilia. Among the exhibits on display were the charred remains of the captain of the ill-fated *Morro Castle,* a cruise ship that had run aground on the beach at Asbury Park, New Jersey, in 1934, following a fire that took more than 130 lives. Many of the survivors had been rushed to Bellevue by ambulance, a two-hour drive, suffering from burns, exposure, and smoke inhalation. Also delivered by police car was a metal plumber's box containing the ship captain's remains. With rumors flying that he'd been fatally poisoned, and the fire deliberately set to cover up the crime, public attention turned to the medical examiner's investigation.

A banner headline perfectly captured Gettler's dilemma: "WILL-MOTT ASHES IN POISON TEST." There was reasonable suspicion of foul play, but precious little to work with. Captain Willmott had been incinerated—the plumber's box contained no bone fragments, no clothing fibers, just ash.

It was, in the days before modern chromatography and DNA testing, an impossible task. Since volatile poisons burn off quickly, only the milder ones could be detected. Gettler did find traces of lead, copper, and barium, but that meant little because the captain's quarters contained piping and wiring that had probably contaminated the ash. Put simply, there was no way to determine the cause of death or the time it had occurred. That is why Gettler kept the captain's remains in plain sight until the day he retired: not as a reminder of failure, but of the work that lay ahead.

No one was ever indicted for the *Morro Castle* fire. It remains an open book, though suspicion later pointed to the chief radio operator, George Rogers, who had a criminal record, a history of mental illness, and a grudge against the captain. (He was convicted of murder in a separate incident and died in prison.) Ironically, Rogers spent several weeks recovering at Bellevue, just a building away from the laboratory where Gettler was examining the captain's remains. "I recall that one victim, the ship's radio operator, was specifically assigned to the Third Medical Division and to my ward," a Bellevue intern recalled.

"I came to know him very well. As a result of having imbibed large amounts of seawater, he arrived in a very edematous condition [but] was restored to good health. Some years later . . . we heard the arson was committed by an aggrieved member of the crew, the ship's radio operator." Where else but at Bellevue? the intern remarked—"the most exciting hospital in the world."

In 1926, *The New Yorker* ran a piece on the current "liquor market" in the city, noting that the price of good gin and Scotch in the midst of Prohibition was "up slightly after a post-holiday drop." This was more than simple supply and demand, the article said. It reflected the preference of discerning consumers for spirits of guaranteed quality—foreign brands like Cutty Sark, Dewar's, and Haig & Haig. Why drink American "squirrel whiskey" that "makes men talk nutty and climb trees" when finer (if costlier) blends could be had?

There was another advantage to foreign distilleries. Their products were safe. The "hip-flask, fur coat" crowd could drink their gin martinis and whiskey sours without worrying about the hidden dangers of the booze. Later that year, the *New York Times* captured the reality of Prohibition for those unable to afford a case of Dewar's or Cutty Sark. "23 DEATHS HERE LAID TO HOLIDAY DRINKING," the headline screamed. "89 ILL IN HOSPITALS."

The culprit was poisoned whiskey. When alcohol sales were legal, few had questioned the safety of the main ingredients—corn, grain, hops, and grapes—or the final product itself. Starting in 1906, however, the federal government had mandated two categories for processing alcohol—one for human consumption, the other for industrial use—to ensure that sales of "potable spirits," a key source of federal revenue, were properly taxed. And to enforce this separation, the government required that industrial manufacturers "denature" their alcohol with additives that made it unpleasant, even poisonous, to drink.

When Prohibition began in 1920, the supply of drinking alcohol dried up. With domestic breweries and distilleries now shuttered, bootleggers took to producing spirits with whatever was at hand—mainly denatured alcohol bought on the black market or stolen from factories. The larger bootlegging operations were able to remove some of the poison by redistilling it. Others added sweeteners to soften the taste. Many did nothing. The profits were so large, and enforcement so lax, that illegal stills cropped up everywhere. Barely a month went by during Prohibition without an explosion in a New York City tenement caused by the mixing of "bath tub gin."

Despite the risks, millions of Americans continued to drink. Federal officials had to do something—but what? Ignoring the problem would enrage the anti-liquor forces responsible for Prohibition, yet stepping up enforcement was expensive and guaranteed to fail. Instead, the government decided to scare the public into compliance by *increasing* the levels of poison in the denatured alcohol produced for industrial purposes but now being used in illegal whiskey as well. If more Americans got horribly sick or died—well, that choice was theirs to make.

The *Times*'s "holiday drinking" headline well described the result. Bellevue's emergency department overflowed that Christmas with the casualties of Prohibition. According to Charles Norris, the Medical Examiner's Office had discovered three new poisons added by federal chemists to the denatured alcohol commonly used by bootleggers. The government, he charged, was poisoning its own people.

Protected by his wealth and Social Register contacts, Norris had no concerns about the liquor he personally imbibed. But Prohibition offended him as both a health catastrophe and a misguided crusade reminiscent of Mark Twain's popular adage: "Nothing so needs reforming as other people's habits." Before long, Norris had found a kindred spirit in Mayor Jimmy Walker, who viewed Prohibition much the same way. When Norris proposed to investigate the full impact of poisoned alcohol on New Yorkers, Walker told him to go ahead and send the results directly to City Hall.

The Norris Report of 1927 became a medical bible for the anti-Prohibition forces. Official deaths from alcohol poisoning in New York City had jumped from 47 in 1919 to 741 in 1926—a likely undercount because many doctors were loath to embarrass the families of their private patients. Norris claimed that alcohol poisoning was the greatest health menace currently facing the city, and he wasn't shy about saying so: "The mortality rate from this cause, in my opinion, is larger than the vehicular accidents and the illuminating gas poisoning cases combined."

And, he warned, it was going to get worse. A close study by Gettler's laboratory of more than a dozen bootleg whiskeys showed each one of them to be contaminated with deadly substances. Some reeked of shellac and antifreeze; all contained denatured alcohol. In addition, there'd been "a striking increase" at Bellevue of patients suffering from "alcoholic psychosis" marked by hallucinations and delirium tremens. Gettler attributed this to the enormous *potency* of the bootleg liquors he'd tested, some reaching 140 proof. The stuff not only was poisonous, it was astonishingly strong.

Who was most at risk? The answer was self-evident. The rich needn't worry, Norris told the press. "No one having good wines, beers, and whiskeys is going to drink denatured alcohol." Small wonder that the city morgue was overflowing with the bodies of poisoned New Yorkers "from the poorer classes," alongside bullet-riddled corpses of thugs from the ranks of organized crime.

Some political leaders, including President Calvin Coolidge and soon-to-be President Herbert Hoover, had described Prohibition as "a noble experiment." Norris thought them delusional. Prohibition hadn't stopped the consumption of alcohol; it had simply made it deadlier. "It is common knowledge that at least all the people who drank before Prohibition are drinking now," he said, "provided they are still alive."

Though Norris was correct in addressing the dreadful toll of poisoned alcohol caused by Prohibition, he was wrong—perhaps even disingenuous—in claiming that drinking remained as popular as ever. Indeed, statistics from his own hospital showed that the number of alcohol admissions had dropped from 11,307 in 1910 to 2,091 by the end of 1920, the year Prohibition officially began. These numbers would rise again at Bellevue during the 1920s—to about 6,000 annually—but only because Mayor Walker, first elected in 1926, refused to enforce the law.

Some Bellevue staffers actually saw an upside to Prohibition. Mary E. Wadley, the hospital's director of social work, insisted that it had lowered alcohol consumption in immigrant neighborhoods across the city—a claim that turned out to be true. Historians of this era are virtually unanimous that most Americans resented Prohibition as a violation of their rights, and that millions of them simply ignored its provisions. But all agree that drinking went down by as much as 30 percent across the country during the 1920s, and probably more.

Wadley didn't take issue with Norris regarding the dangers of poisoned alcohol. But she did view Prohibition as something of a savior for New York's poorer classes, when enforced, by providing social benefits that followed naturally from lower drinking rates. "We almost never see now a pile of furniture on the sidewalk with a starved, dispossessed family sitting on it," she wrote, with some hyperbole. "Instead the children are decently clothed, the men are keeping their jobs better and paying their bills. They do not have to pass the inviting door of the corner saloon on payday."

Prohibition ended early in 1933, with the Twenty-first Amendment to the U.S. Constitution repealing the Eighteenth. The carnage in New York City would stretch into the final months of the ban, one late headline reading: "16 KILLED IN 4 DAYS BY POISONED LIQUOR." That same year, Charles Norris established the nation's first academic department of forensic medicine at NYU, staffed by his Bellevue colleagues, including Alexander Gettler. It would blossom into an elite training ground for generations of medical examiners, turning a once primitive pursuit into a rigorous scientific discipline.

In an odd way, Prohibition had strengthened the bond between Bellevue and City Hall. Mayor Walker had relied heavily on Norris and Gettler to document the fatal consequences of bootleg alcohol. And Walker had become particularly close to Dr. Menas S. Gregory, the longtime director of Bellevue's Insane Pavilion, who'd been relentless in publicizing the severe brain damage caused by Prohibition whiskey, despite the falling numbers of alcoholics in his wards. In Jimmy Walker, Bellevue had found an ally of convenience.

Gregory had an agenda. A relentless sort, he'd been lobbying one city administration after another to move forward with plans for the new psychiatric building envisioned by McKim, Mead & White in 1904. And he'd hit a brick wall until Walker took office and vowed to make the project a reality. The bond between the psychiatrist and the mayor would produce a remarkable edifice—the largest single structure on the Bellevue grounds—though each would resign in disgrace before it became fully operational.

15

THE SHOCKING TRUTH

The checkered career of Mayor Jimmy Walker is an enduring part of New York political folklore. No urban history is quite complete without a description of his lightning rise to power and breathtaking fall. The son of an Irish-born Tammany Hall ward leader, Walker gave up a budding career as a songwriter to enter politics at his father's insistence. Elected to the New York State Senate, he became a protégé of Governor Al Smith, the first Catholic to run for president, who cleared the way for Walker's mayoral election in 1925. Handsome, witty, immensely charming, Walker "seemed to be New York brought to life in one person," the columnist Ed Sullivan marveled—someone equally at ease in an immigrant barroom or a suite at the Waldorf. As mayor, Walker pushed the Tammany line, which included social programs for the poor and massive building projects for the city. Above all, he worked tirelessly *against* the enforcement of Prohibition, which he considered a bigoted assault upon the cultural habits of urban America. And that, in turn, served only to increase his standing among the masses.

Walker governed New York City at the height of the Roaring Twenties. Times were prosperous, on the whole, and personal excess seemed more a virtue than a hindrance for the mayor, whose playboy lifestyle became daily fodder in the press. His elegant wardrobe, extensive vacations, and relentless womanizing offended few, it appeared, beyond the ranks of political reformers and the cardinal of New York.

"During his first two years in office," an observer noted, Walker spent "143 days" visiting London, Paris, Rome, Hollywood, Bermuda, and other far-flung destinations. When the fawning City Council raised his salary from $25,000 to $45,000 a year—almost quadruple the pay of a U.S. senator—Walker quipped: "That's cheap! Think what it would cost if I worked full time."

There was another side to the mayor, however. While reveling in the image of someone too busy enjoying himself to bother with the humdrum details of governing a city, Walker ran a tighter ship than he cared to let on. In regard to Bellevue's future, he had created a citywide entity, the Department of Hospitals, to oversee the eighteen public institutions spread over the five boroughs, a move that centralized control in the mayor's office. And he regularly relied on leading physicians from the medical colleges to advise him on policy matters that didn't restrict the business interests of Tammany Hall. In fact, Walker had a soft spot for Bellevue. His friends and relatives had been patients there, and he viewed the hospital as an unfinished project, ripe for completion. Among his medical advisors was Dr. Menas S. Gregory.

An Armenian refugee, Gregory had fled to America to escape the Turkish genocide that slaughtered much of his family. After earning a medical degree and interning at various state asylums, he arrived at Bellevue's Insane Pavilion in 1902 as an assistant "alienist" and became its director the following year. It was a job no one else wanted. The wards were absolute bedlam, a staffer recalled—"despairing persons of both sexes and all ages" packed together like cattle in "a never-ending kaleidoscope of human misery."

Gregory had big plans for Bellevue. He quickly substituted "Psychopathic" for "Insane" in the Pavilion's title—hoping, he said, to make the patients appear curable—and had the iron bars removed from most of the windows. Those who visited the wards saw more substantial changes: less reliance on narcotics and physical restraints. Appalled by the ignorance of fellow physicians about mental illness, Gregory lobbied to place psychiatry on par with other specialties in training medical students and interns. Close to half of the total admissions at Bellevue were patients suffering from alcoholism, blackouts, dementia, depression, drug psychosis, epileptic confusion, and other mental conditions, Gregory remarked. "Is it strange that the average physician's knowledge of psychiatry is almost as crude as the layman's?"

In truth, Gregory had opinions on just about everything, few of which he kept to himself. Eminently quotable, he claimed that weight loss in women caused nervous breakdowns (he preferred the "plumper" variety), and that "twilight sleep" produced by anesthesia led to cases of insanity. From addiction to delinquency to the works of Sigmund Freud, a judgment would be rendered. Even when not seeking the spotlight, which was rare, Gregory seemed unable to avoid it. In 1925, he was assaulted and almost killed in a bizarre incident near the doctor's midtown apartment. "LUNATIC WITH A PISTOL CHASES DR. GREGORY," a headline screamed. "He Dodges Among Motor Cars After Bullet Grazes His Cheek." Gregory was "put to bed" suffering from "severe mental shock." His patient, "knocked senseless by the police," was remanded to Bellevue for observation.

Gregory's crowning achievement came in 1926, when City Hall allotted funds for a six-hundred-bed psychiatric building on the Bellevue grounds. It followed an intense lobbying campaign by Gregory, including a well-scripted tour of the old pavilion by Mayor Walker, who declared: "I wouldn't send my dog there." At the groundbreaking ceremony, Walker grandly described the five-foot-tall psychiatrist as "perhaps the greatest little man in the world." Another dignitary turned to Gregory and said, "The dream of your life is being realized."

It didn't come cheap. McKim, Mead & White, the firm most intimately connected to Bellevue, was now a shell of itself. All three founders had died—Stanford White, the key figure, having been gunned down in spectacular fashion over an affair with a deranged millionaire's wife. Instead, the city chose a rival group led by architect Charles B. Meyers, a favorite of Walker's who, by happy coincidence, had just designed the luxurious Tammany Hall headquarters in lower Manhattan. Within a year, the cost overruns at Bellevue had reached $3 million—the work slowing to a crawl when the lead contractor took his sizable advance and fled to Europe.

Mayor Walker soon followed him there. On the eve of his landslide reelection victory over reformer Fiorello La Guardia in 1929, the stock market crashed. Within months, the country slid into the worst economic depression in its history, with New York City, the financial engine, especially hard-hit. Suddenly, Walker's extravagant ways didn't seem nearly as endearing. Critics, emboldened by the crisis, accused the mayor of lining his pockets with kickbacks from contractors seeking business with the city. Even the Catholic Church weighed in, disgusted by Walker's very public extramarital affair with actress Betty Compton. When a State Senate hearing validated most of the corruption charges, both Al Smith and sitting governor Franklin D. Roosevelt urged Walker to step down. In September 1932, the mayor tendered his letter of resignation and boarded an ocean liner for Europe with Betty Compton, whom he later married. No criminal charges were filed, though Walker remained abroad for several years until the threat of prosecution dissolved.

Walker's final legacy—the Bellevue Psychiatric Building—opened in 1933. Standing eight stories tall, it looked more like a fine hotel than a mental institution (if one ignored the high cement wall with wrought iron spikes on top). Mired in controversy—the Italian Renaissance facade didn't quite match the somber mood of the Great Depression—it had taken seven full years to complete. "It was a big graft job; they made fortunes on the contract," a Bellevue psychiatrist recalled. "If they had anything that was expensive, they just put it into the [place]."

He wasn't exaggerating. The building seemed a throwback to the grandest days of McKim, Mead & White. Jimmy Walker had rewarded Dr. Gregory—and City Hall's favored contractors—in his notoriously overstated way. Why a mental facility needed "cinquecento porticoes, Michaelangelesque stairways, carved pediments, and fluted cornices" was, indeed, a mystery, wrote one perplexed observer, adding: "It appears to have been based upon a misapprehension of the Villa Medici."

Before long, however, its beds were full. Hard economic times meant more patients seeking free medical care—not just in Gregory's building, but across the hospital. By 1933, close to a third of New York City's adult labor force was out of work, with one public school student in five suffering from malnutrition. Shantytowns dotted the land from Red Hook to Central Park, where twenty thousand people now lived, many evicted from their apartments. Studies showed a fair share of those seeking government aid to be "first-time charity recipients" who had seen their well-paid employment disappear. There even was a name for them: "the new poor."

"For many New Yorkers," a historian noted, "the economic catastrophe of the 1930s became a health catastrophe as well." With so much hunger, emergency room doctors took to admitting patients just to get them a hot meal or two. Orthopedic departments noted a spike in foot problems because so many of the unemployed couldn't afford a subway ride or a new pair of shoes. At Bellevue, an average day had the feel of an epidemic. One journalist likened it to "military hospitals after a great battle." An immigrant patient, writing in Yiddish, recalled the "titanic task" of those who supervised her ward, where beds stretched into the corridors and out onto the balconies. Bellevue, she marveled, "is indeed a gigantic factory where healing is brought to mortal flesh."

Many entering Bellevue during the Depression had never been there before. Barely able to pay for food and rent, much less a private room at New York Hospital or Mount Sinai, they came knowing they wouldn't be turned away. Meanwhile, the private hospitals were half full and teetering on bankruptcy. In the words of S. S. Goldwater, the city's chief health officer: "There was a time when people feared the evil reputation of Bellevue. That has changed now." The Depression had taught the middle classes what the lower classes knew all along. "Bellevue stands as an institution that can compare favorably with any in the world."

Even the upper-crust *New Yorker* seemed to agree. For decades following the Great Depression, its stories would juxtapose Bellevue's fine medical care with its bare-boned environment—like getting a five-star meal at the local delicatessen. In one (nonfiction) piece, the writer takes a cab ride up First Avenue. Coming upon Bellevue, he claims that he'd recently been rushed there by ambulance after suffering a heart attack. "They treated me first-rate," he tells the cabbie, who replies: "Now that's a funny thing. My wife's brother said almost the same words. Said he met some fine people in there, and the treatment he got from everybody was real good." Surprised by his own candor, the writer notes: "I had to laugh at myself a little for having said 'Good Old Bellevue!' to a stranger. Yet that is the way I feel whenever I chance to pass the place—almost as if it were a school I had attended as a youth and could not let slip lightly from my mind. Indeed, it *is* almost that way—like an alma mater."

In 1933, Dr. Gregory was entering his fourth decade at Bellevue, appearing secure, close to indispensable, in his role. As admissions climbed past twenty thousand per year, he hired a new crop of psychiatrists to handle the patient flow. Many were European Jews fleeing the Nazi rise to power. At NYU, psychiatry was one of several departments that employed them. Privately, Currier McEwen, NYU's medical school dean, partnered with Albert Einstein to provide "at least 20 life-saving appointments to German/Austrian medical scientists"—a list that included Nobel laureate Otto Loewi.

Before long, Gregory's junior staff was filled with recent medical school graduates and political refugees. Younger and better educated than the typical "alienist" at Bellevue, they defined themselves largely by the research they did, which put them at odds with Gregory, who viewed patient care, not article writing, as the sole imperative in the current economic crisis.

Gregory wasn't opposed to research per se. He'd indulged it in the past when the prospects for success—and good publicity—outweighed the inconvenience. When Jimmy Walker wanted a study done on the deadly consequences of Prohibition, Gregory had been more than willing to oblige. When a well-connected scholar requested confidential patient records for examination, Gregory provided them. In one notable instance, he opened his files to researchers studying whether Jews had a higher incidence of mental illness than other groups, which many psychiatrists believed to be true. Earlier works on the subject, bearing ominous titles like "The Insane Jew," claimed that centuries of persecution had produced a "hypersensitive race" with unique "psychogenetic" disorders. Living apart, barred from the more physical trades, Jews had survived by their wits in the mercantile world—a tense and sedentary existence favoring "overstimulation" of the mind and "underdevelopment" of the body, a combination ripe for "serious mental disease."

The study, endorsed by local Jewish leaders, compared the records of thousands of Jews and non-Jews at Bellevue between 1914 and 1926. It concluded that Jewish psychiatric patients (especially men) suffered more from anxiety and depression than non-Jews, but less from alcoholism and drug addiction. The authors, who were Jewish, didn't seem especially optimistic about the future. "We expect," they noted, "a continuous growth in the number of Jewish patients."

The first refugee psychiatrist to arrive at Bellevue was Dr. Paul Schilder, a star pupil of Sigmund Freud. He was followed, in short order, by European-trained psychiatrists Walter Bromberg and Fredric Wertham, and the Romanian-born psychologist David Wechsler. All would leave their mark—Schilder in psychotherapy, Bromberg in drug addiction, Wertham in forensic psychiatry, and Wechsler in human intelligence testing—the popular Bellevue-Wechsler scale. All saw themselves as members of a modern profession in which reputations were forged by attending prestigious conferences and publishing in specialized journals. It was a new generation that looked down on Dr. Gregory, who believed that the cause of most mental disturbances could be traced to the stresses of modern life upon temporarily overwrought people, not to their buried neuroses. Good food, rest, and a reassuring manner would solve all but the most difficult cases, he believed, along with counseling and medical attention for those suffering from drug and alcohol withdrawal.

A collision was inevitable. In 1934, a group of Bellevue psychiatrists sent a withering memo to the city hospital commissioner titled "Gross Defects in the Management of the Psychopathic Division." The memo took direct aim at Gregory, describing him as a tyrant who spent his time dispensing "special favors" to his Tammany friends. As an example, it claimed that "a niece of the former Commissioner Donahue was treated for 4 months in a suite of two rooms while other patients were sleeping on the floor of crowded wards." Even worse, the woman was an outlander—"a resident of the state of New Jersey."

Mostly, though, the memo painted Gregory as someone whose time had passed. It mocked his "disgraceful ignorance" of new psychiatric methods and condemned his "failure to adequately encourage the staff in the scientific work [and] publication of papers." Little wonder, it concluded, that "younger physicians and interns" were now looking elsewhere for jobs.

Subordinates took to calling him "Mean Ass Gregory." "We rarely saw him except when he wanted to bawl us out," a junior colleague recalled. Discipline was enforced by example, as when Gregory fired an intern who had overslept and arrived late on the ward. In another case, he terminated a recent hire for taping a patient's mouth closed. "She was screaming, 'Oh My God they are killing me' and people were gathered out in the street . . . wondering what was going on," the doctor explained. "I did it purely as a therapeutic measure, as an emergency procedure . . . and I beg you to reconsider. . . . To err is human, to forgive is divine." Gregory didn't budge. The doctor left in a rage.

Theories abounded as to the root cause of this behavior, with Gregory's "startlingly diminutive stature" usually winning out. He did, after all, wear elevator shoes, lecture from a raised platform, and confide to a colleague that he never married because he feared having children no taller than himself, though rumors of homosexuality also circulated among the staff.

Once, Gregory might have brushed off these critics, but times had changed. His political support had collapsed with Jimmy Walker's demise; the Tammany chiefs no longer provided cover. Indeed, Walker's bitter rival, Fiorello La Guardia, was sitting in the mayor's chair. And La Guardia's choice for hospital commissioner, S. S. Goldwater, held a deep grudge against Gregory from battles long past.

Calling Gregory a Tammany hack, Goldwater demanded his resignation. "The alliance between the director of the psychiatric division and the political organization under which he rose to power was a sinister one," Goldwater said. Bellevue deserved better.

If Goldwater had any evidence, he never supplied it. Even the *American Journal of Psychiatry,* no friend of Gregory's, called the offensive against him "crude, stupid, and heartless." Years later, one of the conspirators described the "coup at Bellevue" as a generational clash reflecting the changing standards of the medical profession. What most bothered him—in retrospect—were the methods employed in tossing Gregory aside. "Almost overnight," he recalled, "residents, junior physicians, and psychologists grouped together against [his] administrative oppression. Charges and countercharges flew. Clandestine meetings were held. . . . A kind of minor hysteria developed." The irony was that Gregory had hired every one of these conspirators in his quest to fill Bellevue with the best young talent he could find.

Gregory's ordeal was not quite over. A crushing final indignity awaited. In past years, Gregory had testified at dozens of high-profile criminal trials. His track record rivaled those of his Bellevue colleagues Charles Norris and Alexander Gettler—the three men sometimes appearing together in court. Whenever an insanity plea was raised in a high-stakes proceeding, one could count on Gregory's presence. In 1915, he had attested to the sound mental state of Father Hans Schmidt, the only Catholic priest ever to be executed on American soil following Schmidt's conviction for killing his lover and throwing her dismembered body into the Hudson River. The following year, Gregory had debunked the insanity defense of a fellow physician, Arthur Waite, who was found guilty of butchering his wealthy in-laws in what the *New York Times* called "the swiftest trial of a sensational murder case in years." In 1934, Gregory had helped shred the insanity claim of the prominent banker Joseph Harriman, convicted of embezzling close to a million dollars by describing the defendant as "quite intact mentally." Hardly a year went by without a banner headline reading: "Court Orders Delay Until Dr. Gregory Finishes His Examination" or "Dr. Gregory Finds [Defendant] Apparently Normal." Then, in 1935, came the case of Albert Fish.

The details were revolting. The previous year, Fish had sent a letter to the family of Grace Budd, a ten-year-old girl who disappeared from her Brooklyn apartment in 1928. Confessing to the crime, Fish couldn't resist torturing Budd's parents with the hideous details. "First I stripped her naked," he wrote. "How she did kick—bite and scratch. I choked her to death, then cut her into small pieces so I could take my meat to my room, cook, and eat it. How sweet and tender her little ass was roasted in the oven. . . . I did *not* fuck her tho I could have had I wanted. She died a virgin."

Fish, a sixty-five-year-old house painter, wasn't simply a cannibal, but a serial killer as well. Once in custody, he admitted to molesting dozens of children and murdering at least fifteen. The press dubbed Fish the "Brooklyn Vampire"; many believe him to be the model for the grotesque Hannibal Lecter in *Silence of the Lambs*. "What I did must have been right or an angel would have stopped me," Fish explained. Given the graphic confession, the only issue facing the jury was the defendant's state of mind—whether to declare him insane and send him to a mental institution or to find him sane and send him to the electric chair.

Much of the trial centered on Bellevue's responsibility for what had transpired. Indeed, the one thing that the prosecution and the defense could agree upon was the hospital's egregious negligence in allowing a violent lunatic to freely walk the streets. "Oh, you'll hear plenty about Bellevue before this trial is finished," said the scornful district attorney. "Yes, Bellevue has a lot to answer for," replied the lawyer assigned to Albert Fish by the court.

At issue was the discovery that Fish had twice been committed to Bellevue for observation in the years between the kidnapping of Grace Budd in 1928 and his arrest for her murder in 1935. In both instances he'd been examined for sending obscene letters through the mail, and in both instances he'd been declared "harmless"—and released. Under withering cross-examination, the now-retired Dr. Gregory claimed that the records on Fish were "not voluminous" because Fish himself was "not an insane person." When asked why no one had taken the time to seriously examine the writings of someone whose family history was studded with madness, Gregory blamed the workload imposed upon his staff. "If I had more help, I could have gotten a lot of interesting things from a psychiatric point of view," he said, adding that Fish was "just one of many sent to us from the courts."

Things went further downhill for Gregory when Fredric Wertham, one of the discontented refugee psychiatrists he had hired, took the stand for the defense. Given free access to Fish in the weeks before the trial, Wertham laid out a narrative so eerily repulsive that one could only marvel at Gregory's use of the words "harmless" and "not insane." Here was a man who burned himself with hot pokers, engaged in bloody episodes of self-flagellation with a nail-studded paddle, and repeatedly stuck metal objects into his rectum. (X-rays taken following the arrest showed twenty-nine rusted needles lodged near his pelvis.) "I always had a desire to inflict pain on others, and to have others inflict pain on me," Fish matter-of-factly told Wertham. "I always seemed to enjoy everything that hurt."

Wertham seemed to relish the chance to embarrass his former boss, whom he clearly despised. His answers ranged from contempt to amazement as he wondered aloud why Gregory hadn't bothered to take a detailed history of the defendant or to read his letters carefully enough to appreciate their unmistakable depravity. Albert Fish was a virtual encyclopedia of deviant behavior, Wertham concluded. "However you define the medical and legal borders of sanity, this certainly is beyond that border."

Two psychiatrists joined Wertham at the trial to support the insanity plea; two others joined Gregory to insist that the defendant understood right from wrong. The low point came when one of the prosecution's psychiatrists described Fish as "a psychopathic personality without a psychosis," and therefore "sane," leading the baffled defense attorney to inquire whether the cannibalistic murder of a child didn't point to some sort of abnormality. "Well," came the deadpan reply, "there is no accounting for taste."

The death sentence was hardly a surprise. A number of the jurors supported it while also believing Fish to be insane. Their logic, quite simply, was that the crime itself was too demonic to be punished by anything less than the electric chair, regardless of the defendant's state of mind. Albert Fish saw no reason to protest. "Thank you, Judge," he said, with a wave of his hand. How thoughtful of everyone to provide the greatest gift one could imagine: unspeakable pain. Getting electrocuted, said Fish, "will be the supreme thrill of my life."

The trial would be Menas Gregory's professional swan song. Humiliated by his junior colleagues, forced into retirement by La Guardia's allies, he took on some private patients and added a few hobbies to his suddenly uncluttered days. The final headline bearing his name appeared to sum it up well: "DR. GREGORY DIES ON GOLF LINKS: Noted Psychiatrist Stricken [on] Second Tee of Tuckahoe Course."

If one had to pick the ringleader of the coup against Gregory, it most likely was Paul Schilder. Arriving in America in 1928, Schilder had lectured at Johns Hopkins before coming to Bellevue as its first director of psychiatric research. His prime interests were psychotherapy and what he called the "mind-body connection," with a strong emphasis on child development. "It was extraordinary how under Schilder's encouragement almost every clinical encounter on the wards became grist for the research mill," a colleague noted. Schilder attracted those who would form the core of the anti-Gregory revolt, a group that included Lauretta Bender, a recent medical school graduate who became Schilder's research collaborator—and then his wife.

Their marriage proved tragically short. Among Schilder's many quirks was a disdain for traffic lights, which led him to cross major thoroughfares "with books piled to eye level" and an arm extended to halt speeding cars. In 1940, he was run over and killed outside Bellevue after visiting Lauretta and their week-old baby in the maternity ward. He was fifty-four years old.

Schilder's death appeared to end two promising careers—his and Bender's. Married only five years, the couple had published extensively together in the psychiatric journals. Whether Bender could survive professionally without him was doubtful, given the low regard for women in medicine and her duties as a single mother. Her colleagues expected her to cut back her schedule; some even urged her to retire. But Bender, then forty-three, had other plans. She would honor Paul Schilder by continuing their research, she told friends, and her three children would be just fine. "She may not have been home to give us milk and cookies, but there was never [neglect]," her son recalled. "She did everything the men were doing in medicine while also raising a family and running a house."

Bender's own childhood had been chaotic. Her father, a restless sort, had moved the family from one town to another before putting down roots in rural Iowa. And her mother, barely nineteen when Lauretta was born, grew more depressed with each coming child. "She loved her infants as infants," Bender wrote in her unpublished autobiography. "But once they were out of her arms, there was nothing she could find in her background or limited experience that made her ready or willing to meet their needs."

Lauretta's needs were many. She repeated first grade three times and didn't learn to read until she was nine. Spelling, grammar, and penmanship remained elusive for years. In fact, Bender was dyslexic—a condition she would study in great depth later on. Had a close relative not been in charge of her elementary school, she recalled, "I doubt that I would have graduated."

Spending painful hours each day on the basics of her education, Bender became the valedictorian of her high school. From there she attended the University of Chicago and earned her medical degree at Iowa State. She chose medicine "because of the scientific subjects one could study, not in anticipation of becoming a practicing physician"—which led to a fellowship at Johns Hopkins, where she met Paul Schilder. "I knew immediately," she wrote, "that he was the man I had been looking for."

Bender followed him to Bellevue. Gregory's new psychiatric building had just opened, allowing patients to be separated by age, sex, and condition. There now were "quiet" wards for the least troublesome, "semi-disturbed" wards for the more difficult, and "disturbed" wards for the violent and suicidal. The hospital contained a children's ward, another for adolescents, twelve to sixteen, who previously were thrown in with adults, and yet another for prisoners, complete with holding cells, armed guards, and a courtroom to determine the patient's "mental capacity" to stand trial. "They flock to [us] by the dozen, mostly because they can get a bath, free food, and lodging," a Bellevue intern wrote in 1934, noting the impact of the Great Depression. "Our treatment of drunks [is] on the whole the noblest aspect of our psychiatric service—nowhere else are they afforded such a convivial welcome."

Bender took over the children's ward in 1934. Mayor La Guardia may have had little faith in her profession—disturbed people needed "more pasta and less psychiatry," he famously muttered—but no one was better at bringing federal relief dollars to his city. At Bellevue, funding poured in from New Deal agencies for all sorts of projects, most conspicuously the nine elegant murals in the hospital's main rotunda painted by David Margolis (at $26.50 a week) portraying "Agriculture," "Industry," "Research," and other stories of human progress. A steady flow of "aides" and "assistants" also appeared on Bender's ward, compliments of the Works Progress Administration. Bender favored aspiring artists, musicians, and dancers—those who might reach the children in novel ways. Her own struggles with dyslexia led her to develop the Bender Visual Motor Gestalt Test, which evaluated the "inner thoughts" of her patients by studying the ways they drew and interpreted different shapes. At times, Bender touched on questions common to the 1930s but harshly dismissed today, such as the role of race in determining behavior. In one instance, she wrote that the "two features which almost anyone will concede as characteristic of [Negroes]" are "the capacity for so-called laziness and the special ability to dance." These features, she thought, "may be an expression of specific brain impulse tendencies."

What most interested her, though, was childhood schizophrenia, a subject barely examined at the time. Her own definition was expansive, covering a wide range of disorders (including autism, which she studied decades before it became a popular diagnosis). "It was almost a pleasure to [see] a brain tumor, because you felt [it] could at least be treated," a Bellevue colleague recalled of psychiatry in the 1930s. "Before the vast bulk of our material we stood baffled, helpless and forlorn."

Then, from Vienna, came a ray of hope. A new treatment appeared to shock the brain of severely depressed and schizophrenic patients into "equilibrium" by inducing seizures akin to an epileptic fit. Researchers called it "convulsive therapy." Bender was intrigued.

The first wave of convulsive therapy involved insulin, discovered by Canadian researchers in the 1920s. Produced in the pancreas, insulin regulates glucose levels in the blood. A lack of insulin leads to hyperglycemia (high blood glucose), while a surplus results in hypoglycemia, a condition marked by convulsions and seizures when too little glucose reaches the brain. In the 1930s, a European psychiatrist named Manfred Sakel noticed that insulin-induced comas had a dramatic impact on those suffering from depression and schizophrenia. He began to induce these comas in his own patients, claiming that 88 percent of them showed fewer signs of mental illness, but warning that the long-term effects were yet unknown.

Other methods soon followed. From Hungary came word of a convulsive therapy using metrazol, a chemical stimulant known to cause "explosive seizures" when injected in high doses. Early studies showed it to be effective in treating schizophrenia. The downside was that the violence of the convulsions caused numerous broken bones and vertebrae fractures, though most were optimistically described as "hairline" or "innocuous."

Convulsive therapy made its American debut at Bellevue. One of the hospital's younger psychiatrists, Joseph Wortis, had witnessed Sakel's insulin comas while studying in Vienna. Amazed by the results, Wortis convinced Bellevue's new psychiatric director, Karl Bowman, to allow insulin shock treatment on patients in the "disturbed" wards. No one knew then—or knows for certain today—why a seizure restores a patient's mental faculties, or how it works. The therapeutic qualities of shock treatment remain one of the great mysteries of medical science. Wortis admitted as much in a speech to the New York Neurological Society. "It is not simply a shock . . . which accomplishes the result," he said. "It is something else; I do not know what it is, but my opinion is that it is something rather different."

The mystery of shock treatment proved no barrier to its use. "Our insulin wards now have 26 beds and I have been provided with two assisting physicians, ten nurses, and a secretary," Wortis wrote of his work at Bellevue. "We have had many visitors [coming] to learn the technique." He wasn't exaggerating. Four years later, the U.S. Public Health Service reported that more than 70 percent of the nation's mental institutions had experimented with, or were currently using, insulin shock therapy.

These experiments mirrored the shaky medical ethics of the time. At Bellevue, for example, Wortis never bothered to discuss the risks with patients undergoing insulin shock or to seek their consent. Nor did he explain that multiple treatments would be required, stretching over weeks and sometimes months. In a typical case, involving "an 18-year-old intelligent colored boy" with symptoms of "paranoid schizophrenia," Wortis admitted that the patient was uncomfortable with the early treatments and probably wanted them to end. The patient complained of headaches. His hands shook, his voice trembled, and he didn't see any positive results. Rather than stopping, however,

Wortis "gradually increased the doses of insulin" until "full epileptic seizures" were produced.

The patient improved. He no longer heard voices. "I don't feel confused. I don't feel afraid," he said. "I feel all right, like my old self." For Wortis, the end justified the means. "We can afford to wait for further results and observations," he wrote in a privately circulated memo, "but in the meantime we have every reason to welcome an important and invigorating new influence in psychiatry."

The optimism, though understandable, was premature. Insulin shock soon fell into disfavor. Hospitals found the treatment far too labor-intensive. The patient's heart rate, blood pressure, and respiration had to be carefully monitored, with a sugar solution at hand in case of trouble. Furthermore, the benefits of insulin shock seemed to wear off quickly, leading some to question whether the risks outweighed the rewards. The answer came in 1942, when a Bellevue patient died following an insulin-induced seizure. There would be no more.

Wortis was far from discouraged. Convulsive treatments hadn't disappeared at Bellevue; they'd simply taken a different form. "[Our unit] is now pushing electro-shock work and we expect to be started soon," Wortis wrote a friend in 1940. "[We're] already doing work on rats after electro-shock convulsions and the thing is full of interesting research possibilities."

"Electro-shock," known today as electroconvulsive therapy (ECT), also began in Europe. Its developer, an Italian psychiatrist named Ugo Cerletti, got the idea by watching pigs being stunned with an electric prod before they were slaughtered—the jolt caused pronounced convulsions. At his laboratory in Rome, Cerletti worked to find the "margin of safety" that human experimentation required. What constituted the proper amount of electricity? How long should each shock be? And how many were needed to produce the desired result?

ECT had its advantages. There were no toxic reactions, and the convulsions were less violent—thus fewer broken bones. Cerletti claimed that schizophrenic and severely depressed patients responded well to multiple sessions of ECT, appearing more relaxed, coherent, and self-aware. There seemed to be no medical complications beyond temporary memory loss—nothing, in Cerletti's words, which "could damage the nervous system." Observers who flocked to his Rome clinic were duly impressed. Within months, the procedure had spread across Europe, and on to the United States.

The biggest hurdle to ECT is one that still haunts the treatment today: its disturbing resemblance to the fictional experiments of Mary Shelley's Dr. Frankenstein. When an American psychiatrist first proposed a demonstration at the prestigious New York Academy of Medicine in 1940, he got nowhere. "What? Pass an electric current through a patient's head?" a colleague shouted. *You* must be crazy.

There were fewer qualms at Bellevue. One had only to visit the "very disturbed" ward to grasp the problem, a psychiatrist wrote: patients "shrieking and screaming, restrained in straight jackets with only amytal sodium or wet packs available to quiet them temporarily." Perfect or not, ECT offered hope.

It also reached America at a moment when an even more controversial treatment was being employed, making it seem almost tame by comparison. Called a "lobotomy," the rival process involved snipping the nerve fibers that connected the frontal lobe to other parts of the brain, causing irreversible change. No one doubted that a lobotomy could turn an unruly patient into a docile one; the problem, according to several Bellevue psychiatrists who witnessed it, was that those undergoing the procedure emerged as "amiable vegetables." How many were performed at Bellevue is unclear, though the number appears to be small.

The pioneers of electric shock at Bellevue included Joseph Wortis, David Impastato, and, most surprisingly, Lauretta Bender in the children's ward. Impastato administered the first ECT treatment in the United States in 1940, using a clumsy apparatus with precise, if somewhat frightening, instructions:

1) Place a generous amount of electrode jelly on both sides of the patient's head.
2) The electrodes should be applied in the frontal-temporal region with firm pressure.

3) The large knob marked "SET TO DESIRED VOLTAGE" should be turned counter-clockwise.
4) Plug the electrode connecting cord into the stimulating unit.
5) Turn the knob marked "RESISTANCE" until it is opposite the white dot.
6) Set switch marked "SHOCK DURATION" to 0.10.
7) Throw the "TREAT" switch from "A" down to "B" position. As this is done the patient will receive the shock.

Above all, it warned, "NEVER ADMINISTER ELECTRO-SHOCK IN A METAL BED."

Thousands would undergo ECT at Bellevue in the coming years—many of them children. Indeed, few units employed it as systematically as Dr. Bender's. The tragic death of her husband in 1940 may have played a role in her decision, as she grew closer to Karl Bowman, her boss, who strongly favored its use. Whether Bowman encouraged Bender, or whether he simply acquiesced, is lost to history. What is clear is that he didn't say no.

Bender would soon be running one of the more questionable experiments in Bellevue's history. A few years earlier, the leading child psychiatrist in France, Georges Heuyer, had raised eyebrows by using ECT on a handful of "depressed" adolescents. But no one had thought to lower the bar even further—until Dr. Bender in 1942.

Over a period of eight years, more than a hundred children in Bender's Unit (PQ6), some as young as four, would undergo ECT on a regular basis. In an era before medical science demanded random controls, double-blind studies, or informed consent, the experiment nonetheless stood out for the age of its subjects. There was nothing clandestine about it. Bender received generous funding from the U.S. Public Health Service and shared her findings in the leading psychiatric journals. Publicly, she spoke of electric shock as an effective method for treating serious mental disorders. Privately, she described it as the last hope for previously "unreachable" children. "If you were confronted by the cross-section of patients at Bellevue [that I deal with]," she told a

British colleague, "you would do everything to try to make life easier for [them] and their families."

By the mid-1940s, Bender's ward was dangerously overcrowded. Children came from every direction, dropped off by parents and relatives, by other hospitals, and by social service agencies. The beds ran out; patients routinely slept on cots in the halls. Bender estimated that 75 to 85 percent of her cases had severe behavior problems resulting from broken families, learning disabilities, and "organic brain disorders." Those "under observation" spent thirty days at Bellevue before being sent home, or to foster care, or to a state institution. Those receiving "intense therapy" stayed for sixty days and more. The latter group, containing the tougher cases, became candidates for ECT.

Bender's goal wasn't to make life simpler on the ward by taming unruly children. Nor did she view ECT as a permanent "cure." Her belief, after seeing the results of electric shock on adults, was that it would allow her most disturbed patients to respond more effectively to other treatments—psychotherapy, counseling, music, puppetry, and dance. Bender helped establish a public school at Bellevue to teach remedial reading and language classes. And at a time when many psychiatrists, led by her former colleague Fredric Wertham, were blaming comic books for causing "juvenile delinquency" and "sexual perversion"—Wertham insisted that Batman and Robin were secret lovers—Bender encouraged her older patients to read them as a form of "mental catharsis." Her personal favorite was Wonder Woman, who, she believed, taught girls that they, too, could be heroic, powerful, and just.

In pushing shock therapy, Bender may also have been reacting to the views of several prominent neurologists at Bellevue, who argued that "severely defective" children were beyond saving. Indeed, the department chair, Foster Kennedy, had recently lectured the prestigious American Psychiatric Association on the subject. "We have too many feeble-minded among us," he said, adding: "I *am* in favor of euthanasia for those hopeless ones who should never have been born— Nature's mistakes." Bender was appalled.

Each of her subjects received an "extensive neurological examination" before and after ECT. The procedure mimicked the one for adults:

twenty shocks in all, one per day, with 95 to 130 volts "until a grand mal convulsion was produced." In a follow-up study, published in 1947, Bender claimed that while "the essential schizophrenic process [did] not appear to be modified by the treatments," the subjects seemed "less disturbed" and thus "better able to accept teaching or psychotherapy."

There was some anxiety, Bender noted, especially among children "near puberty." The girls "clearly related the [shocks] to sexual intercourse and fantasy," while the boys feared "it was punishment or that they might not recover consciousness." Overall, however, the complications were "minimal." If anything, Bender concluded, "children can tolerate electric shock better than adults."

The first real criticism of Bender's experiments came in 1954. Two independent researchers using a national sample of ECT cases, the majority from Bellevue, concluded that the positive effects "were temporary and resulted in no sustained improvement in the patterning of behavior." Much of the evidence was anecdotal—provided by parents who believed that ECT had made things *worse* for their children. One boy had come home and tried to strangle his sister; a girl had beaten her infant brother; several had turned violent following minor disturbances.

The researchers didn't entirely rule out electric shock for children. It might be "justified," they wrote, when "all other measures have failed." But their study implied that Bender had ignored the potentially catastrophic risks. "It appears to [us] that one should be fearful of giving electric shock therapy to . . . those four or five years old," they concluded, "for we have no good understanding of [its] later effect . . . on the personality that is only in the developmental stage."

Though the parents in this study remained anonymous, they may have included the novelist Jacqueline Susann and her publicist husband, Irving Mansfield. In 1946—two decades before writing *Valley of the Dolls*—Susann gave birth to a son with severe developmental problems. His early words became shrieks and he seemed indifferent to affection. Alarmed, Susann took the boy to a specialist who suspected autism and recommended Dr. Bender, an obvious choice.

Bender didn't believe that autism resulted from a lack of maternal warmth, as did other leading child psychiatrists of that era, including

Bruno Bettelheim and Leo Kanner. She suspected that it most likely was inherited. "I have never seen one single instance," she noted, "in which I thought the mother's behavior produced autism in the child." Bender met with Susann and Mansfield and proposed electric shock. The couple reluctantly agreed.

The treatments didn't work. "I think they destroyed him," Mansfield recalled. "He came home with no expression, almost lifeless." Whether electric shock worsened the boy's condition is impossible to say. He was sent to a private mental facility, where he remained for the rest of his life.

The most disturbing parts of the critical 1954 study were the interviews with the children who had received ECT. Many displayed emotions that Bender hadn't commented upon: anger, humiliation, and pain. One child wanted to "kill" the doctor who shocked him. Another had tried to hang himself in order to stop further treatments, saying he was "afraid of dying and wanted to get it over with fast." A third was so furious at his mother for consenting to ECT that he assaulted her and then tried to leap from an apartment window. Numerous children recalled the throbbing headaches that followed each session. And few claimed to be better off. "I don't think they did me much good," an eleven-year-old told the investigators in a typical comment. "I couldn't do any school work so good any more."

The most detailed recollections of ECT at Bellevue would come decades later from an attorney named Ted Chabasinski. Born to an unwed mother with a history of schizophrenia, Chabasinski was living in foster care when a social worker, noting signs of mental illness (which Chabasinski disputes), had him committed to Bellevue for observation. The year was 1944—the height of Bender's ongoing ECT experiments—and the six-year-old Chabasinski became a subject. "On the mornings when I was going to get the shock treatment, I didn't get breakfast, so I knew what was going to happen," he recalled. Three attendants would drag him, kicking and biting, to the treatment room, where a rag was stuffed into his mouth and the electrodes fastened to his head. "And that was the last thing I would remember, until I woke up in a dark room somewhere. . . . I had learned to try to memorize my name . . . so I would remember it after the shock. . . . I would cry and realize how dizzy I was."

Chabasinski described the children's ward as an unspeakable place where the attendants abused and raped him. He also recalled Dr. Bender as an austere presence, cold as ice. "Sometimes she would pass very close to me, looking at me but not acknowledging me, as if I didn't exist."

Following the requisite twenty sessions, Chabasinski was returned to foster care but removed shortly thereafter and sent to a state mental facility, where he spent the next ten years of his life. "The little boy who had been taken [to Bellevue] to be tortured didn't exist anymore," he wrote. "All that was left of him [were] a few scraps of memory and a broken spirit."

Chabasinski's narrative is as complicated as it is painful. Written more than sixty years after the experience, it had a larger purpose in mind: to abolish what Chabasinski and his supporters see as the barbaric practice of electric shock. But the people who worked alongside Bender in these years hold very different memories. The children's ward they describe was hectic and overloaded, on the one hand, but caring and professional, on the other—staffed by an army of skilled psychiatrists, nurses, social workers, teachers, and volunteers.

Their perceptions of Dr. Bender border on the reverential: a brilliant woman, a devoted mother, a fearless pioneer. "She brought her children to the unit so often that this became an unremarkable event," wrote the renowned psychiatrist Stella Chess. "Clearly, the warnings I had been given that choosing a professional career ruled out marriage and motherhood need have no reality. . . . Lauretta Bender's greatest legacy was the group of leaders whom she bequeathed to the field of child psychiatry and who, in turn, trained others."

Bender left Bellevue in 1956 to become research director of the children's unit at Creedmoor State Hospital, a sprawling psychiatric facility in Queens Village, New York. If anything, her methods became even more controversial. At Creedmoor, she moved beyond electric shock to something with almost no experimental history in the medical world—LSD.

Bender was hardly a cultural rebel. She seemed driven, as before, by the so-called logic of default. If nothing presently exists to effectively reach those with "severe schizophrenia" (her definition of autism), the search must go on. Bender had seen a handful of adult studies on the liberating effects of LSD. She theorized that the drug, by arousing the "sensory stimuli" of autistic children, might breach their impenetrable defenses.

Bender began her LSD experiments in 1961 with few guideposts. (Even guru Timothy Leary had yet to be heard from.) She claimed to understand the dangers, recalling that "we were extremely cautious when first using the drug, even obtaining parents' consent"—a hint, perhaps, that she hadn't always bothered to consult them in the past. Eighty-nine autistic Creedmoor children, ranging in age from five to eleven, were given LSD between 1961 and 1965. Extreme caution soon disappeared; seeing "no serious side effects, no evidence of severe disturbances, or of toxicity," Bender tripled the dosage and accelerated the schedule from twice a week to once a day. Most of the children "became gay, happy, laughing frequently, especially early in the treatment program," she wrote in her preliminary report. "Nearly all of them were more alert, aware, and interested in watching other persons. . . . With some . . . there was a decrease in regressive behavior such as tearing clothes, smearing food and feces, and rocking and banging."

Hopes were raised. *The American Druggist,* a top industry publication, lauded the "beneficial results" of Bender's experiment, noting that Sandoz, LSD's sole manufacturer, was seeking "more studies" before committing to its "large-scale use in schizophrenic children." The problem, however, was that the few researchers who tried to replicate Bender's results were unable to do so. Their autistic subjects didn't improve on LSD, and the side effects were pronounced. The end came in 1965 when Sandoz, fearing the drug's potential for "recreational misuse," discontinued production.

Bender retired shortly thereafter, her reputation firmly intact. A survey of mental health professionals in 1982 described her as "the preeminent woman psychiatrist of the second half of the twentieth century," adding: "There is some justification for naming her the preeminent living psychiatrist in the world, period."

Bellevue, meanwhile, abandoned electric shock for children following Bender's move to Creedmoor, and then for all patients by the 1970s. It did so not because its psychiatrists believed it to be dangerous or ineffective—most felt just the opposite—but because of an intense anti-ECT campaign led by "medical rights" activists and fueled by the horrific portrayals of electric shock in movies like *One Flew Over the Cuckoo's Nest*. "Their violent attacks and even lawsuits intimidated [us]," a Bellevue psychiatrist admitted. The repeated claims of "barbarism" and "permanent brain damage" won the day.

Electric shock has made a dramatic comeback in recent years, with strong support from the pillars of mainstream medicine: the American Psychiatric Association and the National Institutes of Health. And the Bellevue legacy of Lauretta Bender has played a key role in this ongoing debate. Opponents of ECT often cite her as an example of the slippery slope of medical research, where a questionable treatment rides roughshod over ethical concerns. (Some anti-shock activists have gone a step further, describing Bender as a "child torturer" and the American twin of Dr. Josef Mengele.) More surprising, perhaps, are the growing number of child psychiatrists who insist that she was on to something important, and that her work, while deeply flawed by current standards, deserves a second look. "With appropriate checks and safeguards," five of them wrote recently, "modern researchers could do worse than follow the example of pioneers like Lauretta Bender."

Bellevue resumed electric shock on a limited basis in 2015. "We consider it the treatment of last resort, when medication and psychotherapy simply aren't enough," said Dr. Dennis Popeo, who came from Mount Sinai to restart the program. "Some of the hospitals in the area are using it on adolescents, with all the built in precautions, but the youngest patient at Bellevue so far has been twenty-two. We're not interested in controversy. We're taking it slowly. But the program thus far has been extremely effective."

16

SURVIVAL

In 1956, a Nobel Prize in Medicine came to Bellevue. The recipients, André Frederic Cournand and Dickinson Richards, were honored for their groundbreaking work in cardiac catheterization, a partnership that stretched back to the 1930s when the French-born Cournand was chief resident on Bellevue's famed Chest Service, and the American-born Richards ran a small laboratory there. Though the Nobel Committee had occasionally made a lackluster or head-scratching selection—such as the 1949 award to Portugal's António Egas Moniz, the father of lobotomy—the choice in 1956 was warmly received, and remains so to this day. "Just about everything modern medicine knows about the heart and lungs," wrote a breathless admirer, "was made possible by the work of [André] Cournand and Dickinson Richards."

The men were part of Columbia's First Division at Bellevue, which ran the Chest Service, the hospital's second-largest unit (behind psychiatry), with close to four hundred beds. Columbia had long viewed the Chest Service as a blessing and a burden—strong on public service, yet expensive to run. "Might I ask that [we] be consulted before any further assignments be made?" Columbia's perplexed medical school dean wrote the Bellevue trustees in 1916. "There seems to be an unwritten tradition that Tuberculosis should belong to the First Division . . . and it is not considered by Columbia an equitable assignment."

That tradition, however, would pay big dividends over time. Begun by James Alexander Miller in the early 1900s, the Chest Service quickly became Columbia's prized possession at Bellevue—a model for teaching and research. "At least six clinical studies will be published this year by various members of the visiting staff," the director reported in 1933. "[We] are engaged in very important anatomical and pathological studies [and] our chief resident is studying functional pathology by modern methods."

That chief resident was André Cournand. A graduate of the Sorbonne and the University of Paris, Cournand had served as a battlefield surgeon during World War I, earning medals for courage under fire. Reaching out to Dr. Miller, Cournand was offered an internship at Bellevue and told to look up Dick Richards about a position in his lab. "If you succeed, maybe we'll make something of it," Miller promised. "Are you willing to take a chance?"

Cournand and Richards bonded immediately. Both men were thirty-seven years old, decorated veterans of World War I, and devotees of the fine arts. Both agreed, moreover, that the future of their specialty lay in viewing the lungs, the heart, and the circulatory system as integral parts of a single unit. "Richards introduced me to all the techniques he had mastered in his early investigations," Cournand recalled. "He was a humanist; he was a scientist; he was a superb clinician and he was an outstanding gentleman." Together, they created the finest cardiopulmonary laboratory in the world.

There was no precise method at the time for measuring the heart's pumping power. The best tools were the trusty stethoscope and the electrocardiogram, developed in the early 1900s by Holland's Willem Einthoven, which won him a Nobel Prize. On a trip back to Paris in 1935, however, Cournand learned of an obscure journal article by a German researcher named Werner Forssmann, whose eccentricities had overshadowed his revolutionary ideas.

A few years earlier, Forssmann had performed the first human cardiac catheterization—on himself. Assisted by a nurse and some painkillers, he made an incision at his elbow and carefully threaded a thirty-inch rubber catheter—the kind used to drain urine from the kidneys—through a large vein in his arm. Upon reaching the shoulder blade, Forssmann walked down a flight of stairs to the hospital's X-ray room, the tubing still inside him, and got the technician on duty to record the moment when the outer point of the catheter touched the right chamber of his heart. Forssmann had not only done the medically unthinkable, he'd *filmed* it for posterity.

The first question, of course, was why? What good, if any, could come of it? Those who learned of Forssmann's experiment—and there weren't many—thought it a bad publicity stunt or, worse, a masked suicide attempt. Forssmann himself appeared vaguely interested in the possibility of delivering vital drugs quickly to the heart. Asked years later why he'd chosen to be the subject of his own procedure, Forssmann replied, as did many researchers of his era, that he had no choice: "I was convinced that when the problems in an experiment are not very clear, you should do it on yourself and not on another person."

In 1940, following numerous tests on dogs and a chimpanzee, Cournand got permission to catheterize a terminal cancer patient; the procedure failed, he noted, because the man had "extensive metastases to the lymph nodes of the [armpit], and Dick Richards [couldn't] get the catheter past them and into the right atrium." Still, a bridge had been crossed. Cardiac catheterization had been shown to be safe in animals—thus, human testing could proceed. Cournand never considered the path taken by Werner Forssmann—self-experimentation—and later regretted it. What bothered him most, Cournand admitted, was the judgment: "Well, he did it on other people, but not on himself."

Finding human subjects was a relatively simple matter at Bellevue, which had a long tradition of in-house research. And the timing couldn't have been better for Cournand and Richards, given America's entry into World War II. Desperate for information about battlefield shock, the government's Office of Research and Development funneled large grants their way for studies regarding cardiopulmonary blood flow. Early on, Cournand and Richards got their "clinical material" from the dozens of car crash survivors rushed to Bellevue's emergency room, but as wartime gas rationing cut down on automobile traffic, they turned to the victims of violent crimes, explosions, and fires. "We had . . . a surgical resident on call twenty-four hours a day," Cournand recalled. "I had my technicians in contact with me by phone and as soon as . . . a case [arrived] I would go to the hospital."

Through constant practice, Cournand and Richards became masters of cardiac catheterization—developing better needles, stronger nylon tubing, and safer ways to enter the heart without nicking a wall or causing dangerous arrhythmias. In 1947, Richards sent a memo to the Columbia administration citing the progress the two men had made. Cournand, he wrote, had perfected "the technique for which he is now known throughout the world of medical science—namely the successful passage of a catheter along the vein into the chambers of the heart." The procedure had opened a vital window into the causes of cardiopulmonary disease by allowing researchers to precisely measure the volume of blood pumped from the heart to the lungs. Stroke, shock, hypertension, congestive heart failure—all could be carefully studied now, leading to breakthroughs in cardiac care and the development of lifesaving drugs.

Nine years later, the Nobel Committee used similar language to honor the work of Cournand and Richards. And it awarded a share of the prize, somewhat controversially, to the little-known German researcher who had invented the procedure before joining the Nazi Third Reich as a physician and a propagandist: Werner Forssmann.

By war's end, Bellevue had become a magnet for cardiopulmonary research. "One rubbed neurons with the best and the brightest on a daily basis," a former student recalled. "Eminent physiologists from all over the world visited each time they came to the country for a meeting or a vacation." The laboratory hired staffers from Europe, Asia, Latin America, and Australia—a rarity in those days—and took pride in judging them on merit alone. "I don't know if it has anything to do with my being a Frenchman," Cournand once boasted, "but at Bellevue, from a very early time onward, I was always in favor of using the best talent I could find regardless of race, religion, or sex."

That talent did, indeed, include a large number of women and Jews. And Cournand, a man of no small modesty, claimed to have hired Bellevue's first African American secretary as well. While discrimination in medicine was still a serious problem—the profession being overwhelmingly white, Protestant, and male—the hospital had been a liberalizing force for change. Part of it was Bellevue's standing as the flagship of a largely immigrant city, and part of it was Bellevue's close relationship with NYU Medical School, which didn't have a quota system for Jews and was known for favoring a "female presence" in certain services, including Chest and Psychiatry, where many of the patients were adolescents and children. "Women always fared better at Bellevue," a pediatrician noted, "and this was very well known."

Though close to half the patients in Bellevue's sprawling Chest Service were children, it didn't have a formal pediatric unit until the 1920s, when Dr. Edith Lincoln took on the job. A graduate of Vassar and Johns Hopkins Medical School, Lincoln had arrived in 1918 as one of Bellevue's first women interns. It hadn't been easy. Assigned to take her meals with the nursing staff, Lincoln had demanded a seat at the intern's table, and won. (In retribution, she was warned for wearing her skirts too high.) There was no denying the quality of Lincoln's work, however, or the extremely long hours she put in. One of the reasons for hiring her, a male colleague admitted, was that she didn't have to worry about seeing private patients because her husband, a prominent New York physician, "earned enough . . . for Edith to devote herself completely to her work in tuberculosis."

By the 1930s, a tuberculin skin-patch test had been devised and X-rays could reveal the extent of damage to the lungs. But with no cure in sight, Lincoln could do little more than adopt a holistic approach to the disease, prescribing a good diet, rest, sanitation, and fresh air. Those who visited her wards were struck by the attention to the children's social needs as well—the donated books and toys, the musical instruments, typewriters, and sewing machines. Sulfa drugs raised hopes in the 1930s, but the promise quickly faded. Lincoln's pediatric unit recorded an annual mortality rate approaching 25 percent, and those who worked in the building were at heavy risk themselves. "Well, actually I had a little lesion when I left Bellevue, but it didn't amount to anything," an intern recalled of his all-too-common experience. Among the less fortunate was Walker Percy, the distinguished Southern writer, who abandoned medicine after contracting a near-fatal case of tuberculosis while doing autopsies in the Bellevue morgue.

Then, in the 1940s, came word of a miracle. Biologists at Rutgers

University revealed that a soil-based derivative had shown great potential in killing the tubercle bacillus. The laboratory's director, Selman Waksman, called it streptomycin, and the early trials, including those at Bellevue, were quite astonishing. Edith Lincoln's unit saw its mortality rate plummet to 5 percent. In 1952, Waksman would be awarded the Nobel Prize for discovering "the first effective antibiotic against tuberculosis."

At Bellevue, meanwhile, Dr. Lincoln was busy collecting data for one of the largest medical studies of that era—tracking close to three thousand TB "survivors" from the time they entered her unit until their twenty-fifth birthday. Popular culture at the time still tended to romanticize tuberculosis as the disease of tormented geniuses—Chopin, Chekhov, Kafka, Stravinsky, Stephen Crane, the Brontë sisters—or showed victims lounging at a plush retreat in the Alps or Adirondacks. But Lincoln's study reinforced what health officials and social reformers had known for decades: tuberculosis was a disease of the slums. The patients, almost without exception, "came from low socioeconomic backgrounds . . . poor, crowded homes [containing] tubercular adults." Nearly half these children were black and Puerto Rican at a time when their combined percentage in Manhattan, while climbing rapidly, was still below 20 percent.

Unlike Cournand and Richards, who had no trouble attracting the limited government funds then available for medical research, Lincoln relied on smaller grants from private sources like the popular Christmas Seals direct-mail campaign:

> Put this stamp with message bright
> on every Christmas letter;
> Help the tuberculosis fight
> and make this New Year better.

Her study proved a gold mine for policymakers, showing, for example, that age was a key factor in determining mortality: infants and the very young were at greatest risk, she concluded, recommending that medical resources be directed their way. But Lincoln's most vital data related to antibiotic use. They showed that patients given streptomycin in combination with certain other drugs did even better than those taking streptomycin alone. At Bellevue, the addition of the antibiotic isoniazid lowered TB mortality in the children's unit to 1.5 percent—a success rate confirmed in later trials by the U.S. Public Health Service.

Like Lauretta Bender, who became a role model for women entering child psychiatry at Bellevue, Edith Lincoln did much the same for women entering pulmonology and public health. "Word soon spread that [Lincoln's superiors] did not believe that women were necessarily an obstacle, and competent females began to flock to the service," a disciple of Lincoln's recalled. Some worked alongside Cournand, others were drawn to clinical work in the wards, especially pediatric TB.

Lincoln never got the acclaim of other researchers at Bellevue, though her studies of multidrug therapies would help reorient the treatment for tuberculosis—and later, some believed, for HIV/AIDS. Seeing herself primarily as a clinician, she took pleasure in watching her once jam-packed TB wards shrink to the point where the empty beds outnumbered the occupied ones, and inpatient admissions gave way to the outpatient service. For Edith Lincoln, that legacy seemed more than enough.

In 1947, Dickinson Richards was named director of Columbia's First Division. Judging from his correspondence, he ran it the same way he'd run his laboratory—warmly encouraging creativity and skewering those who didn't measure up. "I feel obliged to complain to you about the performance of Dr. Hutchinson," read a typical blast to one of his department chairs. "It is perhaps not necessary to give you every single instance upon which this complaint is based, since in point of fact he has not made a single presentation which has been satisfactory."

His most scathing criticism, however, was directed at the city. Bellevue—America's premier public hospital—seemed in serious decline, a victim of decades of municipal neglect. Its laboratories, once among the nation's finest, were now too cramped and antiquated to meet the sophisticated demands of medical science. "Our most serious limitation at the moment is that of space," Richards wrote his superiors. "[Our] rooms are small and not particularly well suited to the rather complicated research set-up. . . . Furthermore, there is practically no office space for Dr. Cournand, his desk being surrounded by filing cabinets, drawing boards, apparatus, etc., so that he has no privacy and is almost incessantly being interrupted."

That he and others lacked adequate lab space for cutting-edge research was discouraging enough; that more than a hundred adult TB patients were constantly stacked in the corridors awaiting a bed was, in his view, a moral outrage. When twenty-eight of the thirty-two Chest Service floor nurses threatened to quit, citing the high tuberculosis rate among the staff, Richards showed his solidarity by vowing to step down as division director and return to his lab. "We all wore masks, but they didn't do much good," a doctor recalled. "Working there was risky, with so many patients in such close quarters. Dr. Richards had a saying. He'd tell us: 'You don't get TB from those you know have it, you get TB from those you don't know have it.'"

Richards would threaten to quit with some frequency over the years, forcing Columbia to lobby for improvements on his behalf. "Dear Dick, I will tell you that . . . we have no intention of considering your resignation," his weary medical school dean wrote him following a periodic blowup. "Everyone is more than pleased with the way matters are developing at Bellevue Hospital and I know the city authorities are just as enthusiastic as we are. You are doing a wonderful job."

The news of the Nobel Prize in 1956 was a tremendous coup for Bellevue. Politicians lined up to praise the lifesaving research being done at a public institution serving the poor. But when the city rewarded the Cournand-Richards lab with a $30,000 gift, the response wasn't exactly what the mayor's office had in mind. Citing the "abysmal conditions" in the TB wards, Richards made his feelings abundantly clear. "I can win the Nobel Prize in Medicine," he told the press, "but I can't take care of my patients at Bellevue."

When Richards widened his scope to include the entire hospital, city officials angrily returned fire, calling his charges "exaggerated" and "largely untrue." But this back-and-forth only encouraged others at Bellevue to join the fight. A group representing the hospital's 450 interns and residents claimed that conditions were even worse than Richards had described. "A man can't even die in dignity in Bellevue," one physician lamented.

Feeling the heat, Mayor Robert F. Wagner, Jr., told reporters that he might "just walk in and take a look"—not "to make a circus of it," he said, but to judge the situation for himself. That Wagner had barely set foot in the hospital, despite two years in the mayor's chair and three years before that as Manhattan borough president, seemed a perfect example of what Richards had been saying: those with the power to improve things didn't seem to care.

Had Wagner taken that walk, he'd have seen a city within a city spread across eighty-four wards in fifteen buildings covering five full blocks—most built in the heady days of McKim, Mead & White, and barely touched since. On a typical day in the 1950s, Bellevue's population exceeded ten thousand, including staff, patients, and visitors. Its psychiatric building contained more beds (630) than all but four other hospitals in New York, and its Chest Service (382) ranked in the top ten. Designed when land along the East River was still inexpensive, Bellevue's horizontal layout contained seventy-five exits and fifty-five elevators, some so old that replacement parts were no longer being made. (A famous hand-lettered sign in the lobby read: "Ring Up For Down.") Travel among the buildings meant navigating a maze of dingy corridors and stairwells or, for the strong at heart, a labyrinth of rat-infested underground tunnels stretching the length of the hospital grounds. Stray cats roamed the basement where the doctor's dining room was located, easing the rodent invasion. Those who stopped in for leftovers—what the dead-tired house staff called "the midnight meal"—had a slogan for the spread: "chicken/rule out tuna."

Bellevue had no air conditioning. Surgeries were routinely canceled during heat waves because the operating rooms felt like saunas. The electrical system ran on obsolete direct current (DC)—a rarity in large complexes by the 1950s. Forty-bed wards were still the rule, with the sickest patients up front near the nurse's desk and a single open bathroom in the back. "If a patient needed privacy, say for a physical examination, screens were moved into place around the bed," an intern recalled. "This was also done when it was decided a patient was about to die." Cornell and Columbia had begun moving some of their laboratories off-site, and patience was wearing thin. There were rumblings that both might pull up stakes unless physical improvements were made. In a memo to the Bellevue administration, the division heads complained bitterly of the status quo: "It seems to us a sorry reflection upon the city of New York that the largest hospital in Manhattan, with its close affiliation with three of the leading medical schools in the country, should subject patients on the wards to such . . . miserable conditions of living . . . as now exist."

This was hardly a novel complaint. There'd been calls to tear down Bellevue during the typhus epidemics of the 1840s, the puerperal fever outbreaks of the 1870s, and the Great Influenza of 1918–19. Once again a chorus of staffers, led this time by a Nobel laureate, was portraying the hospital as a menace to those it served. Either fix it or build a new Bellevue, they demanded—one or the other.

The press quickly joined in. "NOBEL WINNER SEES BELLE-VUE IN SORRY STATE," warned the *Herald Tribune.* "For the sake of decency and pride, the city should take immediate steps to clean up the Bellevue mess," declared the *World Telegram.* Even the pugnacious *Daily News* took a sympathetic stand. "Bellevue is more than a city hospital; it is the very life beat and death rattle of the city. Bellevue is the city's people, fighting for their lives."

The *Daily News* got it right: Bellevue *did* mirror the "life beat" and "death rattle" of the city. An average of 2,600 babies were delivered at the hospital each year in the early 1950s—an eye-popping 8 percent of the recorded births in Manhattan—while thousands of bodies were autopsied in its morgue. As the region's premier teaching facility, Bellevue had trained more than 10 percent of the doctors currently practicing in the New York metropolitan area, with many still on staff. Peeling paint and obsolete elevators aside, the hospital remained a vital part of city life. As two journalists reported after a thorough survey in 1957: "the current uproar should not be allowed to obscure the fact that

Bellevue, despite its structural failings, is yet capable of providing the finest medical care to be found anywhere."

Dr. Salvatore Cutolo, the hospital's longtime deputy superintendent, saw better days ahead. "Contrary to popular belief," he wrote in 1956, Bellevue no longer catered to bums, drunks, addicts, felons, and lunatics. Seventy percent of its current patients came from "the city's respectable poorer classes." They were "decent individuals from tidy, if humble homes" who didn't need to be "deloused."

Of course, Bellevue administrators had been saying as much for two centuries. And, accurate or not, it seemed to miss the point. The hospital's future now depended less on the personal qualities of its patient population and more on its size. Following World War II, the number of New Yorkers using Bellevue began to decline. Where the Great Depression of the 1930s had seen an exodus of paying patients from voluntary hospitals into the free public system, the return of prosperity had reversed the flow. Even Bellevue's massive Chest Service had begun to thin out as new antibiotics took hold. With the exception of the Psychiatric Building and the Emergency Department, which never lacked for business, the hospital was seeing vacancies across the board. According to Dick Richards, Columbia's First Division in 1951 was running at barely 85 percent capacity. And it would have been far worse, he privately admitted, were not other city hospitals "referring their medical derelicts down to Bellevue."

New York City had built an enormous public system over the years—eighteen in-patient hospitals, seventeen thousand beds, and forty thousand employees. (Chicago, by contrast, had one public hospital, as did Boston and Philadelphia.) Providing this safety net was not just a tradition in New York, it was the law. The City Charter guaranteed it, stating: "The Department of Hospitals shall be primarily responsible for the care and treatment of the indigent sick." Those who could pay "in whole or part" were expected to do so, but rarely asked. Those who couldn't were welcomed on equal terms. At Bellevue, receipts from paying patients in a typical year accounted for about 2 percent of the hospital's operating expenses. Tax revenues picked up the rest.

The system worked well enough until the 1950s because expenses were low and the tax base was strong. Hospital workers, including nurses, were notoriously underpaid; the house staff—the interns and residents who did most of the day-to-day doctoring—cost next to nothing; and the attending physicians were paid by their medical schools. When Dickinson Richards complained about the dismal conditions at Bellevue, it wasn't hyperbole. Budgets were routinely underfunded, supplies were scarce, and repairs were slow in coming. Doctors freely admitted to hoarding bandages, tape, and ointment for their hospital rounds. Even with the usual "overhead" added in—padded civil service jobs, supplier kickbacks, employee theft—New York could afford to treat everyone who needed hospital care at a modest cost.

There is no exact moment when the gears locked and the system began to fail. In the 1940s, the city had optimistically floated $150 million in bonds to build five new hospitals and upgrade several others, with plans for a high-rise tower on the Bellevue grounds. But the following decades saw a steady outflow of working- and middle-class whites to the suburbs of Long Island, Westchester, and New Jersey, costing the city billions in tax revenue and consumer spending. As late as 1956, Bellevue's patient population was 80 percent "white" and 12 percent "Jewish." A decade later, these numbers were down by 50 percent and heading for the cliff. Part of the exodus was the appeal of better housing, greener space, and the lure of the automobile; the other part was about escaping the poor African Americans and Puerto Ricans now crowding into New York. The end result was a city with fewer financial resources and greater social needs.

Compounding the problem was the expansion of hospital insurance through third-party providers like Blue Cross. By 1960, more than half the families in New York City belonged to a group plan through the civil service, a labor union, or an employer-benefit program. Given the option, who wouldn't choose the comfort of a semiprivate room in a voluntary hospital over a bare-bones ward at Bellevue when the insurer was footing most of the bill?

Hospital costs, meanwhile, began to soar. It wasn't just expensive new technologies, though these, no doubt, played a role. By the 1960s, the care of patients had come to include a vast army of "allied health professionals"—therapists, dietitians, technicians, social workers, nursing specialists—who outnumbered the doctors ten to one. Many of them belonged to labor unions, and their example led hospital workers to demand the same collective bargaining rights as other municipal employees, which the city granted. Then came the embarrassing revelation that many of the foreign-educated interns and residents at public hospitals other than Bellevue had failed the AMA's screening exam, often more than once. To fix the problem, the city signed "affiliation contracts" with the better medical schools to give the likes of Harlem Hospital and Coney Island Hospital the sort of patient coverage that Bellevue already enjoyed.

It seemed like a good idea. Linking medical schools to public institutions could ideally help both sides—the former getting to train their students and house staff at city expense; the latter avoiding a loss of accreditation that might force them to close. But theory and practice, in this instance, rarely coincided. Without firm budget guidelines and regular audits, the affiliation contracts became an open piggy bank. "Double billing and false time sheets . . . were widespread," an observer wrote. "Money was diverted from life-saving equipment to buy office furniture and exotic research machinery. Doctors who were being paid to be in attendance refused to appear, leaving nurses to handle . . . delicate procedures." A program expected to run "a few million dollars or so" wound up costing the Department of Hospitals one third of its $300 million annual budget, with no end in sight.

Then, out of the blue, a lifeline appeared.

On the eve of his landslide presidential victory over Republican Barry Goldwater, Lyndon Johnson was asked whether a health insurance bill for senior citizens would be a priority in his administration. "Just top of the list," he replied. It seemed like typical campaign bluster, of which Johnson was a master, but in this case he meant exactly what he said. Health care for the poor and the elderly became a centerpiece of his Great Society. On July 30, 1965, Johnson signed the legislation that created Medicare and Medicaid, with former president Harry S. Truman, an early crusader for national health insurance, standing proudly at his side.

Medicare provided hospital and medical insurance for the disabled and those over sixty-five. Medicaid did the same for the poor, defined, most often, as those already on public assistance. The main objective was to allow these groups to receive health insurance without burning through what little income they had. Wilbur Cohen, the legislation's chief architect, described it as "perhaps the biggest single governmental operation since D-Day in Europe during World War II."

Initially, the American Medical Association warned against the bill, calling it "socialized medicine" and predicting the demise of the sacred doctor-patient relationship. "[We] cannot be restricted by decisions of untrained government employees on what services should and should not be performed in medical facilities," their spokesman declared. But it didn't take long for the AMA to come around. Medicare not only increased the number of patients seeking a doctor's care, it also guaranteed a healthy profit; federal guidelines provided reimbursement for "reasonable costs," which, as one student put it, "were whatever hospitals and physicians said they were." Few government programs would prove as popular—or harder to control.

Medicaid had less appeal. For one thing, it smacked of charity care. For another, the eligibility requirements varied from state to state, with reimbursements to doctors and hospitals often smaller than those for Medicare. Many physicians kept their distance, leading to the growth of "Medicaid Mills" in the nation's inner cities. The care, often provided by uncertified graduates of foreign medical schools, was seen as substandard and rife with fraud. Still, Medicaid touched millions of Americans who had rarely, if ever, been examined by a doctor.

If physicians were ambivalent about Medicaid, public hospital administrators were downright giddy. There'd be no more scraping and skimping, one of them predicted. "The chronic underfunding of municipal hospitals will come to an end."

That seemed especially true in New York. It not only was the nation's largest city, with a tremendous number of people on welfare, it also was among the most expensive places to live. For years, city officials had confronted the latter problem by offering free hospital care to the "medically indigent," a term used to describe those who weren't poor enough to be on relief, but who couldn't easily pay an unexpected hospital or doctor's bill. The city fully expected these people to be eligible for Medicaid, as defined by the state.

Initially, the legislature went along. Lawmakers agreed on a yearly income ceiling of $6,000 per family—the country's highest eligibility cap, actually *exceeding* the median national family income. One didn't have to be a welfare recipient to receive Medicaid in New York state, though that was the program's intent. The result was predictable: a veritable stampede occurred. "New York City launched a blitz of radio announcements, subway ads, and news stories urging eligible [residents] to enroll," one historian noted. "By 1967, more than two million people—about a quarter of the city population—had done so." Before long, New York state, with 10 percent of the nation's population, accounted for one third of the country's Medicaid recipients.

Trouble came quickly. Bellevue officials had anticipated a possible drop in admissions as voluntary hospitals competed hard for Medicare and Medicaid patients. This wasn't necessarily a bad thing, they assumed, because Bellevue would be handsomely reimbursed for those it did admit, and the city would soon have the money to build the patient tower that had been in the works for almost twenty years. What few foresaw, however, was the *steepness* of the patient decline in public hospitals, leaving their finances even shakier than before.

Worse still, the city found itself in the odd position of subsidizing this erosion because its share of Medicaid costs—split among Washington, the state, and the city—was about 25 percent. Which meant that each time a private hospital admitted a Medicaid patient, the city paid a large part of the bill. There was evidence, moreover, that some of these patients were being treated until their benefits ran out, and then transferred—or "dumped"—back into the public hospital system.

The patient shortage also affected the three medical schools serving Bellevue. How could they justify a continued presence when there were no longer enough cases to go around? Privately, Cornell and Columbia had been debating their commitment for years. Both were located some distance from Bellevue, while NYU sat right next door. Both had their own respected teaching hospitals to fall back on (New York Hospital and Presbyterian, respectively), while NYU had opened a hospital too small at this point to serve the needs of its students and trainees. By 1960, Columbia controlled fewer than 20 percent of the beds at Bellevue, with Cornell at barely 10 percent. For loyalists like Richards and Cournand, the shrinkage was alarming. "I have always been a Bellevue-Columbia man," Cournand asserted, as if the two parts were inseparable. Now they could only watch, Richards wrote a friend, as NYU "chiseled in . . . to progressively absorb the Cornell and Columbia services."

Both schools pulled up stakes in the fall of 1966, Columbia with greater regret. The crumbling facilities, the declining patient base, the city's apparent indifference to Bellevue's future—all made the decision a fait accompli. Cornell had been itching to get out for some time, held back, an official admitted, by the fear of being seen "in a bad light [for] abandoning its community responsibility." Columbia had a longer history with Bellevue and would be leaving more behind. But departing so close together gave each a bit more protective cover.

"One of the great strengths of Bellevue," a physician there noted, had been "the intramural competition [among] the three medical schools." Those days were over. But the school that remained seemed to be the best fit for the hospital. NYU, wrote its distinguished dean and medical writer Lewis Thomas, "was largely and traditionally populated by students from New York City itself, many of them from relatively poor families, most Jewish, some first-generation Italians, a few Irish Catholics, a very few blacks—a different student body from those at Columbia and Cornell. The school had turned out in the past some spectacularly famous people . . . but its solidest reputation was for its production each year of intelligent, soundly trained, above all *Bellevue* trained, physicians who formed the backbone of medical practice in New York City and its immediate environs."

Lurking in the background was an issue that Mayor Wagner had gingerly sidestepped during his three terms in office: the future of the city's public hospitals. Were they worth saving? Were there better alternatives? Should the public hospitals be modernized or simply retired?

The early optimism surrounding Medicare and Medicaid had begun to fade. The programs had proved a godsend for millions of newly insured Americans as well as the doctors and hospitals they chose to visit. Unfortunately, Bellevue and the other "publics" were rarely part of this equation—not just in New York but across the country. Cities from Philadelphia to San Diego were closing their public hospitals and sending the patients to voluntary or state-run facilities. "What better solution," wrote one cynic, "than to give the costly, troublesome, constantly complaining, unattractive, unloved brat to somebody else to rear?"

In 1965, New Yorkers elected a debonair political maverick named John Lindsay as mayor, the first Republican to hold office since Fiorello La Guardia, a man of similar liberal bent. Determined to fix the public hospital mess, Lindsay appointed a commission chaired by Gerard Piel, the publisher of *Scientific American,* to study the matter and find a solution. But the new mayor added a caveat: New York City's public hospital system must be preserved. "The most important reason," he said, "is that we have yet to come to the position where we can convince ourselves or anyone else that the private system, even if supported by Government money, would really look to the needs of the poor. It simply does not happen, and that is the danger."

Meanwhile a competitor to the Piel Commission emerged in the form of a legislative investigation of the city's hospitals chaired by Queens state senator Seymour Thaler. Described in press reports as a "leather-lunged loner . . . with an eye for the headlines," Thaler didn't disappoint. Barging into Bellevue for unannounced nocturnal visits, he compared it to "the worst slum building in New York City . . . a crumbling ruin that must be seen to be believed."

Warming up with some preliminary hearings on waste and theft in the hospital affiliation contracts, Thaler moved on to the issue that interested him most—patient abuse in the city's research hospitals, especially Bellevue. Showmanship aside, Thaler had been an early critic of unregulated human experimentation—an issue casually dismissed by many in this era as a needless obstacle to scientific progress. Having already proposed one bill to require the "informed written consent" of those participating in such studies, and another to get a court order before allowing minors to take part in experiments "not related to their illnesses," he now accused Bellevue of turning indigent patients into "human guinea pigs."

The examples, presented at a raucous press conference, were pure Thaler—some true, some false, most impossible to pin down. He claimed, among other things, that an NYU virologist, Saul Krugman, was feeding live hepatitis virus to severely handicapped children at the Willowbrook State School on Staten Island in order to test a vaccine—a charge, true on its face but lacking in context, that would reverberate for years. And he alleged that a thousand unnecessary liver biopsies had been performed on alcoholic patients at Bellevue without their consent, five of whom had died.

Clearly caught off guard, city hospital officials denied Thaler's more damaging charge—the death of five patients—while conceding, almost matter-of-factly, that hundreds of "Bowery derelicts" had been biopsied at Bellevue without their knowledge for a "diagnostic study." Though Thaler vowed to provide further details on the deaths, he never did. The closest he came was to insist that a "competent medical authority" had assured him that for every one thousand patients undergoing a liver biopsy, "four or five" would die. Surprisingly, Thaler made no mention of the human experiments that might have given him the banner headlines he craved—Lauretta Bender's use of electric shock treatment on children in the hospital's psychiatric wards.

Thaler's career soon unraveled. On the eve of his election to the State Supreme Court in 1971, he was indicted for selling stolen U.S. treasury bills. Found guilty and sentenced to prison, he died of a heart attack shortly thereafter. Why Thaler chose Bellevue as his whipping boy, claiming it had consistently abused its patients, "most of them Negroes and Puerto Ricans," is a mystery. Whatever the motive, his charges stained the hospital's cherished narrative—care for the weak and the underserved—at a vulnerable moment in its history.

The Piel Commission took a more measured approach. The problem, its members understood, was that New York City's generosity to the poor had created a dual hospital system: one public and failing; the other voluntary and thriving. Since both relied heavily on the same funding for their support, the commission recommended the creation of a "quasi-public" body to oversee the distribution of all government monies pouring into the city for hospital care. Ideally, a more equitable use of Medicare and Medicaid dollars would improve the public hospitals while making the "voluntaries" more accountable to the community.

The idea wasn't new; Lewis Thomas had been floating a similar plan for several years. Most everyone agreed on two points, he wrote: first, the city had done a perfectly miserable job of running its hospital system because the bureaucracy was maddening and the civil service untouchable. Second, almost no one trusted the "voluntaries" to act responsibly on their own. The best solution, therefore, was a corporation independent from the bloated inertia of City Hall, on the one hand, and the selfishness of the well positioned, on the other.

It didn't quite work out that way. In 1969, following months of intense lobbying, the New York state legislature created a "public benefit corporation" vaguely similar to the one proposed by the Piel Commission and Dr. Thomas. To pacify City Hall, the law gave the mayor's office almost full control in choosing the corporation's board of directors. To get the labor unions on board, it continued civil service protection for most hospital workers and kept all collective bargaining agreements in place. And to win over the private sector, it limited the corporation's oversight of third-party payments—Medicare, Medicaid, Blue Cross—to the public system. In the end, the new body seemed little more than a mildly streamlined version of the cumbersome Department of Hospitals it had replaced. The biggest plus was the city's promise to spend an additional $175 million each year to help keep the failing "publics" afloat.

On a warm June evening in 1971, six people arrived at Bellevue's emergency room with cuts and bruises sustained at an open forum on health care, held in the hospital's auditorium. Civility at public events had become something of a rarity in the Vietnam era, and this one was no exception. Scattered throughout the overflow crowd that night were members of the Maoist Progressive Labor Party, neighborhood activists chanting "Hire More Workers, Lay Off the Bosses," and radical young Bellevue physicians demanding a "general strike" to improve conditions. Fists flew as protesters battled for control of the microphones. The featured speakers never got a chance to discuss the current state of public hospitals or their plans for the future. Facing a steady barrage of insults and profanity, they simply gave up.

Thus ended one of the first public meetings of New York City's star-crossed Health and Hospitals Corporation.

For the moment, though, the public system had survived. For all its weaknesses, HHC represented New York's long-held belief that serving the medically indigent (generously defined) was a civic duty best left in public hands. Earning a degree of independence was a goal the corporation might not be able to achieve. But maintaining a medical safety net for the poor was priority number one, and high on that agenda, it turned out, was the construction of Bellevue's twenty-five-story patient tower—a project decades overdue.

The decision reflected the tireless efforts begun by Dick Richards and his supporters. But the timing seemed odd given the large expense, the declining patient rolls, and the shaky economic times. The late 1960s had seen major cutbacks in Great Society programs, partly to finance the Vietnam War. To rein in Medicaid, Congress had lowered the contribution for "non-welfare patients," and New York state had followed suit, reducing the family income cap from $6,000 to $5,000, which cut 700,000 people from the roles. Even more surprising, the ribbon-cutting for the "new" Bellevue in 1973 coincided with a national recession that hit New York City especially hard, many blaming City Hall for years of reckless spending on union contracts and social programs for the poor. When the White House rejected a bailout to prevent a disastrous default in 1976, the *Daily News* ran one of the most quoted headlines of the era: "FORD TO CITY: DROP DEAD."

In truth, Ford never uttered these words; he would shortly sign legislation providing federal loans to the city. This vital infusion, coupled with several billion dollars borrowed from union pension funds, reversed New York's rush to bankruptcy—but at a cost. A wave of layoffs followed, with thousands of city workers losing their jobs. The subway fare, just raised from 20 to 30 cents in 1970, jumped to a half dollar, while the guarantee of free tuition at the city's college system, the social escalator for generations of immigrants, disappeared. The new Bellevue, costing close to $200 million by most accounts, had made it just under the wire.

The project had consumed more than two decades. Guiding plans of this size through the maze of city bureaucracy became a nightmare of "picayune nitpicking." Much like the experience with McKim, Mead & White in the early 1900s, city officials kept cutting the height of the building—from thirty-two stories to twenty-five—and complaining about the expensive "frills," such as phone jacks and reading lights at the patients' bedsides. But the biggest dispute concerned the definition of a "semi-private room." It was clear that Bellevue's traditional ward system, the relic of a bygone era, had to go. The initial design called for two patients to a room, but city officials demanded six, infuriating the project's chief planner. "I resolved that . . . every element which smacked of the attitude that it is good enough for the poor or the medically indigent would be [opposed]," he wrote, adding that six patients to a room was to "semi-private" what a six-month pregnancy was to "semi-virgin." The deadlock was broken by the passage of Medicare, which defined "semi-private" as no more than four patients to a room. Desperate for federal revenue, the city reluctantly caved in.

Dickinson Richards died a few months before the building opened, but André Cournand was there to see the vision come to life. With the top floors still unfinished, Bellevue's psychiatric patients remained in the garish, decaying edifice built during the Jimmy Walker years. Each floor in the new building ran to an acre or more, with twenty elevators in operation. "The corridors are clean, wide, and glossy," a critic remarked. "Neat signs direct the visitor to spacious rooms that yield stunning views of the river or the Manhattan skyline." Lewis Thomas called it "a spectacular building"—a fitting home, he said, for "the most distinguished hospital in the country, with the most devoted professional staff."

Still, a feeling prevailed that, new building or not, Bellevue's eccentricities remained. As William Nolen, the distinguished surgeon, put it upon learning that the plans had actually gone through: "She resists improvements as her bacteria resist antibiotics. . . . So let the city fathers . . . do their damnedest to destroy her personality and make her a replica of every other white, cold, sterile and efficient citadel of healing. . . . I'm willing to bet that when the last new building has been built, the last technician hired, the last dollar spent, there will still be no scissors on Ward M5."

17

AIDS

In November 1980, a man arrived at Bellevue with a fever and shortness of breath. He was given a chest X-ray, which showed "a little haziness, nothing dramatic," and then a lung biopsy. "Surprise is too weak a word. We were floored," Dr. Fred Valentine recalled. "The guy had pneumocystis pneumonia."

An infectious disease specialist, Valentine had treated one other case of pneumocystis pneumonia (PCP) in recent years: a malnourished child with leukemia whose immune system had collapsed. The Bellevue patient was a thirty-four-year-old homosexual. A bluish purple blotch soon appeared near his shoulder blade and his T cell count—measuring the body's defenses against microscopic invaders—plummeted. He fell into a coma.

Valentine prided himself on having seen it all. There wasn't much, medically speaking, that didn't pass through Bellevue. But a few days later, while treating a drug addict with a heavy cough and a fever, Valentine received the same laboratory results: "pneumocystis pneumonia with profound cellular immunodeficiency." This was more than a coincidence, he thought: two apparent strangers, the same obscure diagnosis. Both men would soon be dead.

A few blocks north at NYU's Dermatology Clinic, the nation's largest, another mystery was unfolding. A man had come in with colored blotches on his feet. He'd recently been treated at a local hospital for swollen glands and an enlarged spleen. The dermatologist on duty, Alvin Friedman-Kien, did a biopsy. It revealed Kaposi's sarcoma.

The natural response was to dismiss the case as an anomaly. Some things happen to the body that can't be explained. Kaposi's sarcoma (KS) is a skin cancer seen mostly in elderly men of Mediterranean descent and transplant patients on immunosuppressant drugs to prevent organ rejection. Its frequency among cancers is barely a blip.

But then a second case appeared at the clinic—a gay actor in his thirties with a purplish spot on his nose. "I suddenly began to take sexual histories, something nobody ever taught me in medical school," Friedman-Kien recalled. "Asking about one's personal sex life? I mean, [I'd] never asked anybody those questions. Nobody, not even a prostitute."

A check of the NYU Cancer Registry showed only three cases of KS in the 1970s, none at Bellevue. Now they were streaming in by the week. On July 3, 1981, the *New York Times* ran a piece about the growing cluster—"Rare Cancer Seen in 41 Homosexuals"—by Lawrence Altman, one of the few science reporters with a medical degree. Relying heavily on the work of Friedman-Kien, Altman suggested a sexual link, reporting that many of the victims had engaged in "multiple and frequent" hookups in the city's gay clubs and bathhouses. That same day, the CDC issued an alert regarding the spread of "opportunistic infections associated with immunosuppression in homosexual men."

Among the patients Friedman-Kien examined was Gaëtan Dugas, the French-Canadian flight attendant later described as "patient zero" in the bestseller (and HBO movie) *And the Band Played On* by San Francisco journalist Randy Shilts, who, himself, would die from AIDS. The claim turned out to be false; Dugas didn't bring AIDS to North America, though his boast of engaging in unprotected sex with hundreds of unsuspecting partners in dozens of different cities very likely was true. "I once caught him coming out of a gay bathhouse, and I stopped my car and said, 'What are you doing there?'" Friedman-Kien remembered. "And he said, 'In the dark nobody sees my spots.' He was a real sociopath. . . . [After that] I refused to see him. I was just so angry."

Was this the tip of an iceberg? Friedman-Kien believed so. Joined by Bellevue oncologist Linda Laubenstein and others, he published the results of a study involving sixty homosexual patients: one group showing clear evidence of KS, PCP, or both; the other group symptom-free. "The variable most strongly associated with [these illnesses] was a larger number of male sex partners per year," the authors concluded: the first group averaged sixty-one partners, the control group twenty-six. The first group also reported a higher incidence of herpes, syphilis, and enteric parasites. As the weeks passed, gay men began arriving at Bellevue with cancers of the mouth, tongue, larynx, retina, colon, penis, and rectum. All clinical indicators pointed to a devastating new disease.

Fred Valentine also feared the worst. In March 1982, city health officials compiled a list of the latest "surveillance figures" showing close to 160 people already hospitalized with rare infections and badly damaged immune systems. All but six were gay men. At the bottom of the page were two handwritten notations. The first, "amyl nitrate," referred to a drug commonly used by these men to enhance the sexual experience. Perhaps it played a role. (It didn't.) The second, "IVDU," was shorthand for "intravenous drug user," a category that would grow dramatically over time.

At first, medical researchers used the term "Gay-Related Immune Deficiency," or GRID, to describe the cluster of symptoms, while the media dubbed it "Gay Cancer." But as cases mounted among heterosexuals—Haitians, drug addicts sharing needles, hemophiliacs receiving blood transfusions—the condition was renamed Acquired Immunodeficiency Syndrome, or AIDS. No one yet knew how these disparate groups were connected, if at all. In 1982, New York City reported 543 new cases. The only constant, at this point, was the mortality rate. The victims seemed all but certain to die.

When the American Medical Association was created in 1847, the sorry spectacle of doctors refusing to treat epidemic victims—or worse, running away—was common literary fare. In his eighteenth-century novel *A Journal of the Plague Year,* Daniel Defoe had written: "Great was the reproach thrown upon those [London] physicians who left their patients during the sickness . . . they were called deserters." Image and principle required a forceful stand from the infant AMA, and the result was a Code of Medical Ethics imploring its members "to face the danger [of pestilence] and continue their labours for the alleviation of the suffering, even at the jeopardy of their own lives."

As research advanced, the worries of contagion receded. Vaccines, wonder drugs, and better sanitation tamed the worst outbreaks of the past, making medicine a much safer profession. The AMA revised its Code of Medical Ethics in the 1950s to reflect this reality, leaving doctors "free to choose whom to serve . . . and the environment in which to provide medical care," barring unspecified "emergencies." Then, out of nowhere, came AIDS. The comforting bubble of medical protection seemed to burst overnight.

Old questions resurfaced. What was required in perilous times? Should the stricter Code of Medical Ethics be revived? The AMA thought not. In a hairsplitting 1986 statement, its Council on Ethical and Judicial Affairs described AIDS in terms so uniquely threatening as to give hesitant colleagues what amounted to a free pass. "Not everyone is emotionally able to care for patients with AIDS," the statement read, and no one should be forced to do so, despite medicine's "long tradition" of facing epidemics "with compassion and courage." Should a doctor choose to opt out, it added, "alternative arrangements for the care of the patient must be made."

Actually, few physicians faced this dilemma because the vast majority of AIDS cases would be treated in the public hospitals of cities with large homosexual and drug-abusing populations. As late as 1990, almost a decade into the epidemic, a New Mexico workshop on strategies for treating AIDS attracted a single physician—one of 1,300 invitees. Even in liberal New York City, the Gay Men's Health Crisis could find barely fifty doctors in private practice willing to put their names on a referral list for those with the disease.

Finances no doubt played a role. AIDS patients were often poor, and "private doctors won't take people who don't have health insurance and can't pay upfront," an activist complained. But studies showed safety concerns and personal prejudice to be even more important. "In refusing to deal with such patients," a bioethicist wrote, "many physicians seem not merely to be saying, 'Why should I risk my life?' but rather 'Why should I risk my life for the likes of homosexuals and intravenous drug abusers?'"

Doctors were hardly alone. Stories appeared of funeral directors refusing to embalm the bodies of AIDS victims and EMS workers ignoring calls in gay neighborhoods. A number of state dental associations recommended that nonroutine procedures for AIDS patients, such as bridgework and root canal, be postponed. And a poll of 350 New York City dentists showed "100 percent" of them opposed to treating someone with the disease—a major blow since several of the early warning signs of AIDS, including thrush, a fungal mouth infection, and leukoplakia, a colony of lesions along the gums and tongue, are easily flagged during a routine oral examination. For their part, dentists claimed to be especially vulnerable to dangerous viruses like hepatitis B, which they attributed to a diseased patient's saliva. Why take a chance with something far more deadly?

In issuing its statement on AIDS, the AMA had assumed that two exceptions applied: first, an AIDS victim must never be denied treatment in a medical emergency, such as an automobile accident; second, the nation's public hospitals would continue to admit AIDS patients, emergency or not. And nowhere were these exceptions more relevant than in New York City, which accounted for close to one third of the country's AIDS cases by the mid-1980s, and where the disease would become the leading cause of death among men between the ages of twenty-five and forty.

As New York's flagship public hospital, serving both the gay neighborhoods of Greenwich Village and the drug-plagued streets of the Bowery and the Lower East Side, Bellevue became the epicenter of the spreading epidemic. (St. Vincent's and St. Clare's, two Catholic hospitals in Manhattan with large gay populations, also provided essential AIDS care, with the consent of Cardinal John J. O'Connor.) The problem, early on, was the dearth of information. Nobody knew what precautions to take or how long the epidemic would last. "It had no name, no journals referenced it, no textbooks described it," an intern recalled, adding: "we thought it would go away."

With so many victims and so few facts, a sense of dread swept the hospital. Staffers balked at delivering food to AIDS patients, cleaning their rooms, and removing their waste. A nursing supervisor noted the pressures put upon her Bellevue colleagues by their own families. "They'd say, 'You're going to get AIDS'; or 'Take a shower before you come home.' Or 'Wash your uniform there: don't bring it home.'" One had only to pick up a local newspaper to read of "deadly germs" escaping the hospital and putting the entire city at risk. "JUNKIE AIDS VICTIM WAS HOUSEKEEPER AT BELLEVUE," screamed the *New York Post*.

Of all the potential dangers, however, none compared to a "needle stick" from the blood-filled syringe of an AIDS patient, a not uncommon event. Statistics would show that the odds of acquiring the virus this way were quite slim—about 1 in 275 incidents, according to the Centers for Disease Control. Still, those who accidentally jabbed themselves faced months of uncertainty. "In an instant," a nurse recalled, "all I could feel was a wave of fear."

Reporters on the "AIDS beat" came to rely on frontline NYU/Bellevue doctors for clues to the medical mystery playing out. Whenever a major article appeared, a telling quote from Fred Valentine or Lawrence Friedman-Kien or Linda Laubenstein was likely to be in it. Laubenstein already counted close to one hundred AIDS patients in her private oncology practice, while Friedman-Kien's dermatology clinic would diagnose its one thousandth case of Kaposi's sarcoma in 1987, a marker no one could have imagined just a few years before.

Laubenstein's role was particularly bittersweet. A polio survivor, paralyzed from the waist down, she'd graduated from Barnard College and NYU Medical School before doing her residency at Bellevue and accepting an NYU faculty position in 1983. Assigned back to Bellevue, a place she adored, Laubenstein would whiz through the halls on a motorized scooter, terrorizing staffers she suspected of "short-changing" her patients. "By the speed of the buzz, one could tell if Linda was on the warpath, and [we'd] duck into closets, or under desks or counters— anything to escape [her] wrath," a resident recalled. Plagued by asthma and a heart condition, Laubenstein insisted on making house calls long after the practice had gone out of style. Friends would see her on a city bus, a doctor's bag in her lap, crutches at her side, "sicker than most of her patients," but always looking out for them.

At times, Laubenstein clashed with colleagues who thought her approach to AIDS "overly aggressive." She made no apologies for employing medicine's full arsenal, including chemotherapy, a controversial treatment for those with dangerously weakened immune systems. "She took wonderful care of her patients," said Friedman-Kien. "But we disagreed; we fought a lot about the fact that as an oncologist everybody got chemotherapy. . . . When we looked at an autopsy, she looked from her wheelchair and said, 'No KS.' I said, 'Yeah, but Linda, he's died of every opportunistic infection; we bumped him off.'"

What the two *did* agree upon was the devastating role of promiscuous, unprotected sex in spreading the disease. Laubenstein would soon be leading the charge to close down the city's gay bathhouses—a move resisted by Mayor Ed Koch and resented in much of the homosexual community. But among her strongest allies was the playwright Larry Kramer, whose searing 1985 play about gay life in New York City, *The Normal Heart,* included a character named Emma Brookner, a brilliant, wheelchair-bound physician specializing in AIDS care and safe sex for gay men.

Laubenstein admired Kramer's activism, but hated the script. "Someone suggested it might be because there were so many other doctors at [NYU/Bellevue] who were taking care of [AIDS] patients. And by singling her out, she felt I might be exploiting her because she was in a wheelchair, and hence more dramatic," Kramer said, adding: "I confess to being guilty of this. I wanted to make a parallel with her . . . overcoming such a physical liability as a yardstick for the guys getting sick to see what courage can really be."

Over the years, Emma Brookner would be played by Julie Harris, Barbara Bel Geddes, and Ellen Barkin (who won a Tony Award for Best Actress in the role). Hearing that Barbra Streisand had optioned the movie rights, intending to play the part herself, Laubenstein scornfully told a friend: "She'd better clip her damn nails if she's going to do a rectal." Laubenstein died of heart failure in 1992, at age forty-five, never having seen *The Normal Heart* on Broadway and not living long enough to grasp the impact of her pioneering work. In 2014, a movie version finally appeared on HBO, with Julia Roberts, not Streisand, in the lead. For those unaware of the history of AIDS in New York City, Kramer announced that "the part of Dr. Emma Brookner is based on Dr. Linda Laubenstein," and "will, I hope, enshrine her legacy forever."

—

Those who trained at Bellevue in the 1980s knew exactly what to expect: Bellevue meant AIDS. Dr. Saul Farber, NYU's iconic chief of medicine, insisted that none of the 1,500 yearly applicants for the hospital's seventy-eight prized residencies had ever expressed the slightest concern about the disease. On the contrary, they seemed eager to tackle it. Farber's words are part of the familiar narrative of the AIDS crisis at Bellevue: a place where doctors went the extra mile, as was the creed, to serve the most vulnerable and despised patients, whatever the cost to themselves. When others flinched or turned their backs, Bellevue stayed the course.

There is much truth to this. The challenge of battling AIDS held a strong appeal to those steeped in the Bellevue tradition, as well as those hoping to become part of it, including members of the gay community. At the same time, it warned off those who thought the battle too dangerous or depressing or simply not for them. Medical students are "canny planners," an intern noted. "Over and over [they] mentioned to me their intentions to lie low, ride the epidemic out. 'I wanted to go to New York, but I never even applied,' said one. 'I couldn't stand to see so much AIDS.'"

For many who did come, reality set in quickly. A survey of 250 interns and residents at four New York City hospitals (most from Bellevue) revealed "a substantial degree of concern about acquiring AIDS" and a deep ambivalence about what to do. Twenty-four percent of the sample believed that "refusing to care for AIDS victims was not unethical," while 34 percent felt they should be allowed to make this decision for themselves. Dr. Nathan Link, the study's lead author, worked at Bellevue. "The view that doctors may refuse care to patients appears to undermine the tacit social contract that has long existed between physicians and their communities," Link declared. "Whether these views reflect trends that will compromise the level of medical care . . . available to AIDS patients remains undetermined."

Having stuck himself more than once with a contaminated needle, Link knew the emotions at play. A terrifying disease with an irreversible outcome had put everybody on edge. "We all felt it on some level," a chief medical resident recalled. "There was a lot of talk going around about AIDS and the 'Four H's'—the homosexuals, heroin addicts, Haitians, and hemophiliacs. We thought of ourselves as the 'Fifth H'—the house staff."

While an open refusal to treat AIDS was rare at Bellevue or neighboring NYU Hospital, it did occur. "I've actually seen attending physicians take stances of clearly preferring not to, to the point of refusing to, take care of [AIDS] patients," said Dr. Roger Wetherbee, NYU's director of infection control, in 1985. "I've never seen this before with any other disease." For Wetherbee, the emotional toll of AIDS was even greater than the fear of contagion. "I'll tell you very frankly," he said, "that I've managed, either accidentally or somehow intentionally, to not care for more than one or two patients at any one point in time."

Implicit in these remarks was the matter of covert resistance— a problem almost impossible to gauge. "The AIDS patient who never quite gets visited on morning rounds 'because there's nothing more to say,' 'because all the students upset him,' 'because [someone] will come back and talk to him later' is all too familiar," an intern wrote of her Bellevue experience. "So is the thin, feverish young man who waits somewhat longer than his turn in the emergency room."

Frustration played a role. Medical school had emphasized the life-saving miracles of medical science; AIDS revealed the horrors of an illness no one could figure out, much less contain. "I mean this is a place where people who had their legs chopped off in an industrial accident come, and we're the first people to put them back on," said an intern, referring to Bellevue's world-class emergency services and microsurgery department. "We're used to miraculously helping people." Worse yet, the victims now flooding the hospital were mostly the same age as the medical staff assigned to treat them. "Every third admission seemed to be a patient in his mid-20s who looked as if he'd arrived from Dachau or Biafra," a Bellevue resident confessed. "Witnessing your own generation dying off is not for the faint of heart."

Was medical training compromised in a climate of such relentless gloom? Did seeing so many AIDS patients stunt one's professional growth? Was there too much focus on a single disease? Publicly, at least, such questions were quickly brushed aside. "AIDS is so very complicated that it teaches you a great deal—from immune infections to cancer," Dr. Farber told the press. "AIDS is the study of medicine and everyone who treats it deserves the Silver Star Medal."

Privately, though, Farber had his doubts. Bellevue already had one albatross around its neck as the quintessential "snake pit" or "crazy house" of Hollywood lore. Would it now be known as America's AIDS hospital as well? Ideally, Farber wanted these patients quarantined in well-equipped state institutions, relieving Bellevue of another headache it couldn't afford.

As for AIDS as a teaching tool, the verdict was decidedly mixed. The origins of the disease were still a mystery, after all, and the illnesses it triggered were exotically rare. To train at Bellevue in the 1980s meant seeing more cases of Kaposi's sarcoma than breast cancer, more obscure parasitic infections than the common flu. When one faculty member asked his students to keep a list of the diseases they'd observed in their eight-week rotation, half the logs contained "pneumocystis pneumonia." A third-year student described his morning rounds this way: "One woman has rampant diabetes; another has belly pain. A young Hispanic male complains of a chest infection, which in any other hospital might suggest ordinary pneumonia. Here at Bellevue . . . we think of AIDS."

The problem, which Farber acknowledged, was that students might learn some valuable lessons about compassion, but precious little about how to put the vast toolbox of modern medicine to good use. Where were the moments of satisfaction that came from achieving a positive result? The life of an AIDS victim might be extended for several months by treating a secondary infection, but the end result was the same. "They all die on you," a young doctor lamented. "It's intense, low-tech care."

Some struggled to put the experience into words. A resident who'd come to Bellevue to "serve the underserved" found herself "buried alive" in a world of endless plague. "AIDS had saturated our training . . . ," she recalled. "Every day felt the same—legions of feverish, emaciated patients admitted from the emergency room. . . . There was a Third World feel to our existence, a soul-numbing tedium of affliction and despair."

At times, the frustration boiled over. Friedman-Kien recalled a grand rounds talk he gave on Kaposi's sarcoma at which Farber himself stood up and said, "Thank you for this very nice lecture, doctor, but why does NYU have to be the *Titanic*?" Though offended by the remark, Friedman-Kien understood the consequences for everyone in the room. His own practice had begun to suffer, as longtime private patients drifted away. "We know how involved and dedicated you are to AIDS," they told him. "Would you refer us to a doctor who's less busy with those problems, so we don't have to interfere with your function?"

In 1986, Bellevue's Dr. Robert Holzman toured the much touted AIDS Unit at San Francisco General Hospital with a group of colleagues from New York. The differences were striking. "Almost everything in San Francisco was geared to the gay patient," Holzman recalled. "There were only a handful of drug abusers in the AIDS Unit, and they seemed just about invisible."

The contrast spoke volumes about the two cities. Most every San Francisco AIDS victim in the 1980s was white, male, and gay. That once had been true in New York City, but no longer. The majority of AIDS cases now included heterosexual black and Hispanic drug addicts, their partners, and children. San Francisco also boasted a gay rights movement with the clout to get things done. And that was due, in large part, to the well-educated, middle-class backgrounds of those with the disease. While New Yorkers were angrily debating calls for needle exchanges, free condoms, and housing for AIDS victims ("Not on *my* block" became the rallying cry), San Francisco was opening clinics, group homes, and hospices for the terminally ill. Small wonder that the average stay for a typical AIDS patient at Bellevue was about three times longer than at San Francisco General, and that virtually all of Bellevue's cases were readmissions, sometimes for the fifth or sixth time. All too often, the patient had nowhere else to go.

There is never a good time for an epidemic to strike a city, but some moments are surely worse than others—AIDS in New York being a prime example. Still reeling from the financial woes of the 1970s, City Hall had slashed a number of department budgets, with public hospitals suffering more than most. One reason was simple arithmetic. Institutions like Bellevue had seen their occupancy rates drop in the years before the AIDS epidemic. Another was simple politics. When the Comptroller's Office asked the various community boards to list their top priorities, police, fire, schools, garbage collection, parks, and transportation topped the list. "We came in about 47th out of 50," said Dr. Jo Ivey Boufford, president of the Health and Hospitals Corporation. Public charity patients remained among the least popular constituents—a perception that only hardened with the coming of AIDS.

Almost every state beyond California would waste years ignoring the epidemic. New York governor Mario Cuomo was reluctant to fund AIDS projects early on, saying the money wasn't available, while Deputy Mayor Victor Botnick insisted that New York City had "no AIDS crisis" as late as 1985—by which time 20 percent of Bellevue's patients were HIV-positive, and 3,766 AIDS-related deaths had been recorded citywide. In Washington, meanwhile, President Ronald Reagan had carefully distanced himself from it all—partly because of the promises he'd made to slash domestic spending, and partly to mollify supporters who saw AIDS as divine retribution for sinful behavior. Why focus on a preventable disease that appeared unlikely to spread beyond the confines of unpopular groups whose perverse habits had caused the problem in the first place?

Even parts of New York's gay community opposed a full mobilization against AIDS out of fear that their rights to privacy and sexual expression would be trampled in a public health crusade reminiscent of the forced quarantine of "Typhoid Mary" in the early 1900s. The internal battles over whether to close down the bathhouses or support mandatory AIDS testing served to mute a powerful voice when it was needed most. It all made for a perfect storm of delay and neglect.

Statistics showed that 5 percent of the public hospitals were treating 50 percent of the nation's AIDS patients by the mid-1980s—most located in California and, especially, New York. And that put enormous pressure on an institution like Bellevue—the largest admitting facility, by far—which housed more than a hundred cases on an average day. Reaching its jam-packed emergency rooms meant inching through corridors lined with cadaverous young men strapped to gurneys or slouched in wheelchairs. For the first time in anyone's memory, ambulances bringing in stroke and heart attack victims were diverted to other hospitals. Each AIDS patient at Bellevue meant more nursing hours, more specialists, more CAT scans, chest X-rays, respirators, and pricey drugs.

Who would foot the bill? Private health insurance was always a rare commodity at Bellevue, and those who held a policy before the epidemic started—mostly gay men with a job and a permanent address—rarely got to renew it. Insurance companies took to weeding out homosexuals by flagging the zip codes of neighborhoods like Greenwich Village and, in one instance, scrutinizing "single men without dependents whose jobs entailed no physical exertion." This left Bellevue to limp along with funds cobbled together from erratic state and city programs bolstered by Medicaid coverage for the indigent. It was never enough.

On returning from San Francisco, Holzman and several colleagues wrote a memo describing Bellevue's problems and needs. "Over 60 percent of our [AIDS] patients are drug abusers," it began. Some were prisoners from Rikers Island; many were homeless and mentally ill; most had horrific multiple infections as well as HIV. Resources were slim, staff morale dangerously low. A "pervasive fear of contagion" had taken hold at Bellevue, compounded by "depression due to therapeutic impotence"—the inability to heal. Two words described the current mood of the hospital: "stressed" and "overwhelmed."

Some remedies were easy. It didn't cost very much to serve AIDS patients their meals on paper plates with plastic utensils or to give the cleaning staff galoshes to mop up the excretions. Gowns, face masks, double gloves, and goggles became standard gear for those on the front lines, with each ward getting a special ventilator (or Ambu-bag) to replace the S-shaped mouth-to-mouth devices commonly used—and feared—by staffers in AIDS-related crises. "It wasn't just a 'better safe than sorry thing,'" Holzman explained. "It was about making people feel secure enough to do their jobs."

The centerpiece was a special AIDS unit to provide "short-term intensive primary care nursing for selected patients." Beginning as a ten-bed operation, it quickly expanded to twenty, then thirty, then forty—the unit segregated on account of sanitation (the huge volume of vomit and diarrhea) and patient protection (the extreme vulnerability to hospital germs). Known as "17 West" for its location, the unit was soon treating a third of Bellevue's AIDS cases, which eased the load in other parts of the hospital. Those in the final stages of the disease, the "actively dying," were moved to a group of single rooms on "12 East" to spend their last days in relative peace. It was perhaps the closest one came to hospice care in mid-1980s New York City, where terminal AIDS patients had few options beyond the generosity of friends, a homeless shelter, and the proverbial park bench.

Treating these patients was either a nightmare or a point of pride, depending on the teller. "Imagine somebody completely miserable, covered with lesions, maybe scary-crazy," a former intern recalled. "Now picture somebody right out of medical school, five feet tall and maybe a hundred pounds, poking at him with gadgets and needles, and you get a tiny sliver, minus the God-awful smells, of what it felt like to walk into the place."

Others, though, seemed grateful for the chance. AIDS was humbling. It taught one humility and perspective. A resident spoke of returning home each night to his wife's edgy command to shower before touching anything. "I can't blame her. It's a bit unsettling," he said. "But, on the other hand, working with the acutely ill . . . you cut out the superficial, the bullshit. . . . It deepens your humanity."

One thing was certain: the AIDS Unit wasn't about saving lives. Five years into the epidemic, there was no cure in sight. And that put a premium on greater patient comfort and care. According to the nursing supervisor, AIDS offered a prime example of what her profession did best. It was, she said, "a nurse's disease" rather than "a doctor's disease"—not just because nurses spent more time with patients, but because their skills were better than anything "a doctor can prescribe." The evidence ranged from a device the nurses designed that allowed those with painful mouth sores to chew their food more comfortably to the simple kindness of allowing the patient's partner to stay beyond visiting hours. "It may sound corny," an AIDS nurse added. "But when you're caring for someone who knows he's going to die, you know he needs you. . . . All that's left are two human beings."

Fittingly, no one ever complained about the block letter sign taped above the nurse's station on 17 West:

THE ONLY THING BETWEEN THIS PLACE AND THE TITANIC—THEY HAD A BAND!

Given the large number of AIDS-related cases at Bellevue, troubling legal and ethical issues were bound to arise. "It's different from other diseases," a doctor explained, in that every patient knows "he'll be dead within two years, weighing perhaps 65 pounds, incontinent, in severe pain [and] experiencing mental changes." Sooner or later, a decision had to be made to stop treatment and let the person die. But how far along did that person have to be, and who would decide? Could he designate a friend or family member to make his wishes known if he were unable to do so himself? Must the instructions be written out, and, if so, how precisely? Could a hospital get involved without subjecting itself to a lawsuit—and serious financial loss?

This was virgin territory in the 1980s. While New York state no longer contested the right of a competent adult to refuse medical treatment, complex issues surrounding the "right to die"—especially living wills and health care proxies—were just beginning to emerge. One of the key early struggles, largely forgotten today, involved a patient at Bellevue in the final stages of AIDS.

In the summer of 1987, Thomas Wirth, a gay artist from Greenwich Village, was admitted to the hospital with toxoplasmosis, a parasitic brain infection. Having watched a close friend suffer horribly through the final stages of AIDS, Wirth had left written instructions to withhold "life-sustaining procedures" when there was "no reasonable expectation of recovering or regaining a reasonable quality of life." The document gave Wirth's friend, John Evans, the power of attorney in the event that Wirth could no longer speak for himself.

Within a week of his admission to Bellevue, Wirth fell into a coma, leading Evans to demand that nothing further be done. The hospital quite naturally objected. Sidestepping the larger issue of AIDS, it described toxoplasmosis as a condition often successfully treated with antibiotics—and not, therefore, a death sentence. With drug therapy, Wirth might at least regain consciousness and tell his doctors how he wanted to proceed. Without it, he had no chance at all. "The situation could resolve itself," a Bellevue spokesman explained. "He could come out of [his coma] next week and say, 'I don't want any more treatment,' and we would have no problem with that."

A lawsuit quickly followed. Evans claimed there was nothing complicated about the wording of the document or the wishes of the writer. Thomas Wirth was now suffering the very horrors he'd hoped to avoid. "He wanted to die with dignity," Evans asserted. "What he didn't want to happen is happening."

The hospital responded that the document didn't apply because Wirth had a "reasonable expectation of recovery" from the condition *currently* threatening his life. And several Bellevue doctors took the stand to insist that keeping an AIDS patient alive as long as possible made good sense in a world where medical research was rapidly advancing. "The treatment . . . changes every six months," one of them stated. "Regularly, new therapies become available."

The court decided for the hospital. Accepting the claim that Wirth's brain infection might not be fatal, Judge Jawn A. Sandifer found "no clear and compelling evidence" that the patient was "not without hope"—a tortured pronouncement, to be sure. "There is nothing more precious than human life," the judge declared in ordering Bellevue to continue the treatment for toxoplasmosis, which it did. Wirth died the following month without regaining consciousness.

Though *Evans v. Bellevue* wouldn't rival the more spectacular right-to-die cases of that era, its impact was substantial. In 1985, Governor Cuomo had formed a task force on "Life and the Law" to help patients and hospitals find common ground. And two years later, in the weeks following *Evans,* the task force endorsed the concepts of the "living will" and the "designated proxy"—the first to provide "specific instructions" regarding life-sustaining treatment; the second to "protect the wishes and interests" of the incapacitated patient.

The irony, of course, is that Wirth had little in common with the typical Bellevue AIDS patient. Well-educated and middle-class, he'd exhausted both his health insurance and his bank account, forcing him to "spend down" into poverty, where a public hospital bed awaited. Drug addicts didn't normally plan ahead for medical emergencies, and gay patients of that era often hid their illness, refusing to be tested for AIDS or to tell their families for fear of being shunned. As a result, the great bulk of these end-of-life decisions fell to the hospital.

At Bellevue, the general policy for comatose patients who hadn't made their wishes known was to employ life-sustaining measures. Not wanting the ominous words "Code Blue" blaring over the loudspeakers all day, the hospital used a series of innocuous terms like "Airway Team" to alert staffers of an emergency without alarming other patients and visitors. Once in the room, the attending physician or resident took charge. In most cases, a serious attempt was made to keep the patient alive.

But not always. Staffers cited examples of what is known today as the "slow code"—treating a hopelessly ill patient in cardiopulmonary failure at a pace that encourages death to naturally occur. Whether hesitating to put a tube down the throat, or to hook up the ventilator, or to put the paddles to the chest—the result is the same. A "Code Blue" is a supercharged and sometimes dangerous event. People are tense and packed together. It's a time when the most needle sticks and careless accidents occur. "This wasn't cowboy medicine. Nobody tried to play God," a Bellevue doctor recalled. "These people were unbelievably sick, they had no chance of getting better, and they were going to keep suffering until the minute they died."

AIDS today no longer drives the debate over living wills, health care proxies, slow codes, or "Do Not Resuscitate" orders. And that alone is notable, marking its turn from a death sentence to a manageable condition. The vital work of identifying the Human Immunodeficiency Virus (HIV) that triggered AIDS took place in the laboratories of the National Cancer Institute in Rockville, Maryland, and the Pasteur Institute in Paris, while a group of academic medical centers, including NYU, played key roles in researching aspects of the disease. NYU focused on Kaposi's sarcoma and other cancers, the maternal-fetal transmission of the virus, mathematical models for measuring HIV levels in the bloodstream, and human trials for new drug therapies.

By 1990, NYU had two groups running independent trials: one at Bellevue led by Dr. Fred Valentine; the other at the Aaron Diamond AIDS Research Center directly across First Avenue headed by Dr. David Ho. Each group, working with different pharmaceutical houses, tested a multidrug therapy designed to suppress HIV in already infected patients. And both showed remarkable results. The viral loads of the subjects dropped to almost undetectable levels and stayed there as long as the routine was faithfully followed. The therapy produced some uncomfortable side effects. It was expensive and complicated, and had to go on indefinitely because the virus had not been fully eradicated—just kept in check. Still, a watershed had been reached in the containment of a once fatal disease.

Dr. Ho published first. The response was volcanic. Plucked from obscurity, he became an instant media star at thirty-six, a modern-day Jonas Salk. *Time* named him "Man of the Year," and articles appeared predicting, prematurely, the end of the plague. But for the millions fortunate enough to receive these therapies, the nightmare had passed. "I have begun to believe that I will live a normal life," wrote the critic Andrew Sullivan. "I don't mean without complications. I take 23 pills a day—large, cold pills I keep in the refrigerator, pills that, until very recently, made me sick and tired in the late afternoon. But normal in the sense that mortality . . . doesn't hold my face to the wall every day . . . that life is not immediately fragile; that if I push it, it will not break."

By the year 2000, Bellevue saw far more AIDS patients in its outpatient clinics than on its wards—patients with the same garden-variety illnesses as everyone else. And in 2012—with the disease no longer among the top ten killers of young men in New York City for the first time in thirty years—the hospital shuttered its AIDS (or Virology) Unit, a once unthinkable move. Looking back to a time when Bellevue was choked with bodies, "all dying, some rapidly, most slowly," Fred Valentine called the move "astounding." A momentous chapter in Bellevue's history had closed—perhaps for good.

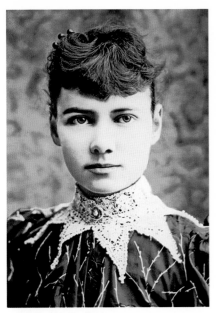

Posing as a mentally disturbed young woman, Elizabeth Jane Cochran, using the pen name Nellie Bly, wrote a scathing exposé of conditions in two of the city's leading psychiatric facilities—Bellevue and the Octagon on Blackwell's Island. Published first in Joseph Pulitzer's *New York World* and then in a book titled *Ten Days in a Mad-House,* Bly's writings cemented the connection between Bellevue and insanity that endures in the public imagination.

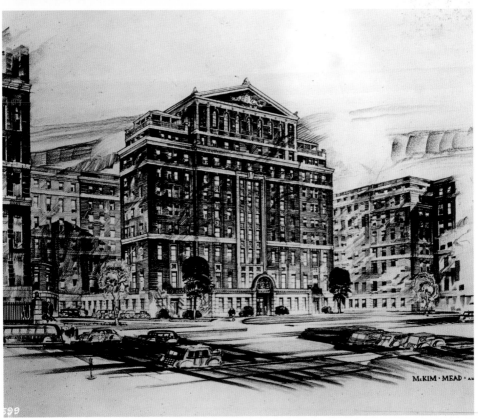

In 1904, with immigration from Europe at its height and concerns about public health (especially the spread of tuberculosis) growing rapidly, the city hired one of the nation's leading architectural firms, McKim, Mead & White, to provide plans for an expanded Bellevue on the current hospital grounds. The plans would be scaled back, and the final structures completed almost four decades later, but some of the buildings remain in use today.

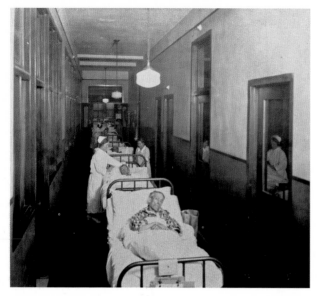

In times of medical crisis, Bellevue's wards teemed to overflowing. During the 1918–19 influenza pandemic, which killed upward of fifty million people worldwide, patients at Bellevue slept in corridors, in closets, and on beds of straw on the floors. No one was turned away.

Menas S. Gregory ran the psychiatric division at Bellevue for the first third of the twentieth century. A devoted reformer, he minimized the use of narcotics and restraints, and had the bars removed from the wards inhabited by all but the most violently insane. In 1933, Gregory's grand vision, a massive psychiatric building, opened on the Bellevue grounds. Gregory would be fired shortly thereafter amid charges that he mistreated his staff.

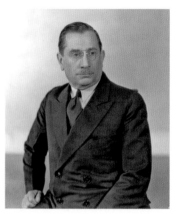

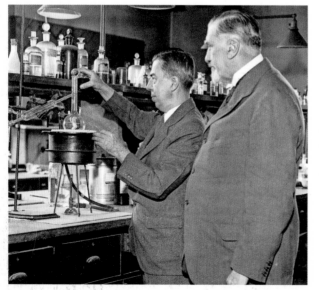

In 1918, New York City created the post of medical examiner to replace the inept and scandal-ridden coroner system then in place. The first medical examiner, Charles Norris (right), a professor of pathology at NYU, demanded that his office be run out of Bellevue, where his laboratory was situated. With the aid of Alexander Gettler, a brilliant chemist, Norris turned the infant field of forensic medicine into a vital professional discipline.

Opened in 1933, the eight-story, six-hundred-bed psychiatric building was the largest and most recognizable structure on the Bellevue grounds. In 1985, the hospital's psychiatric patients were moved to the upper floors of the newly completed Bellevue patient tower, and the psychiatric building, now a crumbling relic, became the city's largest shelter for homeless men.

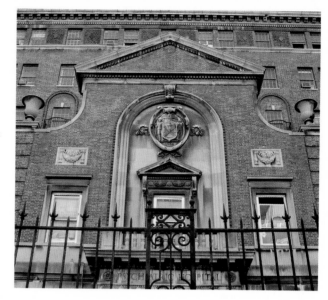

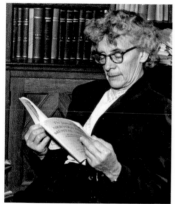

Lauretta Bender, the director of Bellevue's pediatric psychiatric unit from the mid-1930s through the mid-1950s, was a pioneer in the study of childhood schizophrenia and autism. Consistently ranked as one of the leading psychiatrists of her era, Bender became an extremely controversial figure because of her use of electroshock treatment on children.

As members of Columbia's Chest Service at Bellevue, André Cournand (right) and Dickinson Richards shared the 1956 Nobel Prize in Medicine for their groundbreaking work in cardiac catheterization. Both men believed deeply in Bellevue's mission as a medical safety net for the poor, and both worked tirelessly to improve conditions at the hospital.

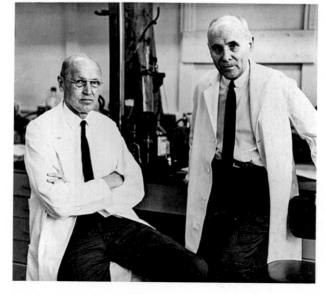

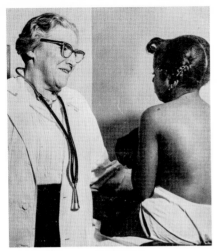

A graduate of Johns Hopkins Medical School and one of the first women to intern at Bellevue, Edith Lincoln created the pediatric Chest Service at Bellevue, which became the nation's key research center for childhood tuberculosis. Lincoln's greatest contribution involved the development of multidrug therapies, a concept used later in treating HIV/AIDS.

In 1973, following thirty years of planning and delays, Bellevue opened a twenty-five-story building for inpatient care along the FDR Drive bordering the East River.

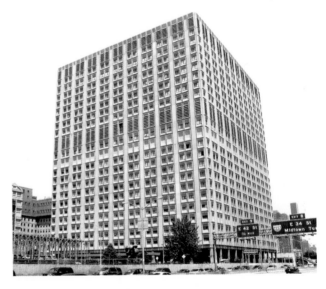

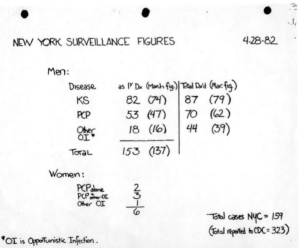

NEW YORK SURVEILLANCE FIGURES   4-28-82

Men:

Disease	as 1° Dx (March fig.)		Total Dx'd (Mar. fig.)	
KS	82	(74)	87	(79)
PCP	53	(47)	70	(62)
Other OI*	18	(16)	44	(39)
Total	153	(137)		

Women:

PCP alone	2
PCP other OI	3
Other OI	1
	6

Total cases NYC = 159
(Total reported to CDC = 323)

*OI is Opportunistic Infection.

Bellevue infectious disease specialist Fred Valentine saw several of the first AIDS cases. His files include some of the earliest recorded surveillance figures in New York City. Nobody at this point knew anything about the disease, beyond the fact that gay men were appearing in growing numbers with extremely rare conditions, including Kaposi's sarcoma (KS) and pneumocystis pneumonia (PCP).

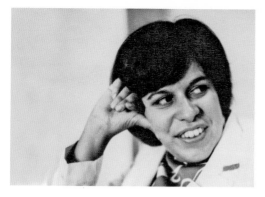

NYU/Bellevue oncologist Linda Laubenstein, a polio survivor, specialized in treating AIDS patients at a time when many doctors refused. Laubenstein offended some in the gay community by campaigning to close the bathhouses, which she correctly saw as transmission points for the disease. Larry Kramer's *The Normal Heart,* a searing account of gay life in New York City, includes a main character modeled upon Laubenstein—a wheelchair-bound physician devoted to AIDS care and safe sex for gay men.

In 1989, a thirty-three-year-old pregnant pathologist named Kathryn Hinnant was raped and murdered in her Bellevue office by a homeless man in stolen doctor's scrubs who had been living in a machinery closet inside the hospital. Her death triggered an angry debate over security at Bellevue, which abutted the largest men's homeless shelter in New York, as well as the hospital's unique relationship with the city's indigent population. Dr. Hinnant is buried in her native South Carolina.

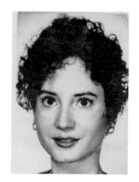

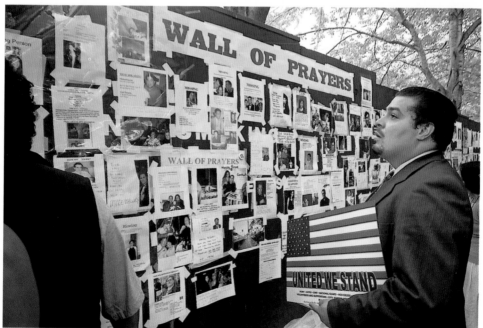

In the days after 9/11, the city was blanketed with notes and flyers seeking information about missing friends and family members. Makeshift message boards went up at Grand Central, Penn Station, the Port Authority, and dozens of other places. The largest one, stretching for several hundred yards along a construction fence at Bellevue Hospital, was named the Wall of Prayers. Bellevue abutted the Medical Examiner's Office, where the identification of the 9/11 victims took place. The hospital had long been a gathering place for people seeking solace and information following a mass tragedy in New York City.

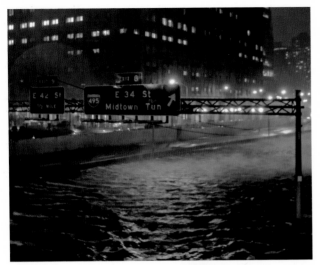

The FDR Drive, situated between Bellevue and the East River, began to flood minutes after Superstorm Sandy reached Manhattan in 2012. Primary electrical power at Bellevue (left) and lower Manhattan would be lost minutes later, following an explosion at a flooded Con Edison substation.

With no power and the basement fuel pumps flooded, dozens of volunteers—doctors, nurses, medical students, and Bellevue staffers—formed a human chain to haul five-gallon buckets of fuel up thirteen flights of stairs to the backup generators to keep the hospital functioning.

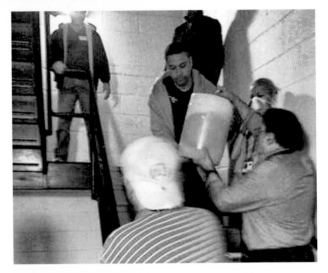

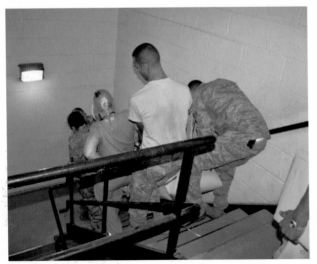

As conditions rapidly deteriorated, a decision was made to evacuate the hospital. With the elevators out of commission, hundreds of patients had to be taken down the semidarkened stairwells—some attached to IVs and monitors, some hand-carried, and others on portable sleds. The National Guard played an essential role in the evacuation. All the patients got out safely.

Dozens of ambulances lined the streets around Bellevue to transport patients to other facilities.

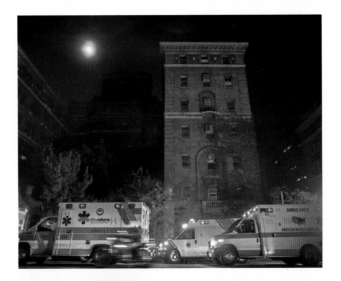

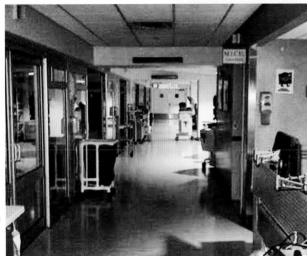

Following Sandy, Bellevue closed its doors for the first time in its history.

Bellevue staffers wore special protective clothing to treat the city's lone Ebola patient in the fall of 2014.

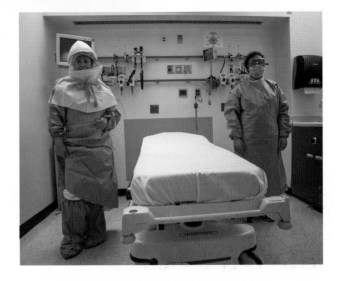

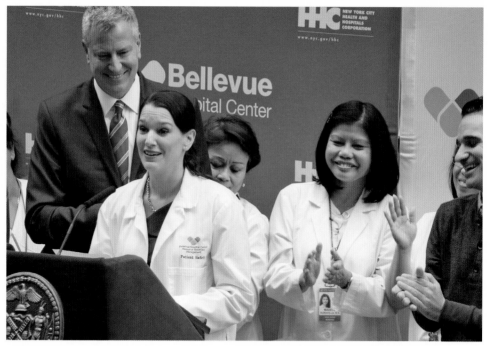

Dr. Laura Evans speaks at a celebratory press conference announcing the discharge of Ebola-free patient Dr. Craig Spencer, as Mayor Bill de Blasio (left) and Dr. Spencer (far right) look on.

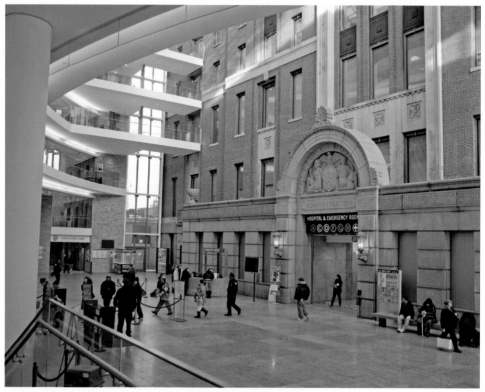

The glass-roofed Bellevue lobby designed by I. M. Pei, with the facade of old Bellevue on one side and four floors of outpatient clinics on the other.

18

ROCK BOTTOM

New York Hospital had long been a favored destination of celebrity patients seeking luxury, privacy, and top medical care. Relocated from lower Manhattan to the posh Upper East Side in the late 1920s with a $40 million gift from Payne Whitney, and modeled upon the Papal Palace at Avignon, it attracted the likes of Jacqueline Kennedy and the Shah of Iran. In the mid-1980s, however, New York Hospital suffered two devastating blows to its reputation, each involving the death of a patient under mysterious circumstances, and each raising doubts about the competence of senior physicians, nurses, and residents in training—in short, the entire medical staff.

Libby Zion, the eighteen-year-old daughter of a prominent journalist, had come to New York Hospital's emergency room in October 1984, with flulike symptoms compounded by emotional agitation. Eight hours later she was dead—the victim, a jury decided, of repeated errors by a poorly supervised and dangerously overworked house staff. Major reforms would follow, and a settlement be paid, but the bad news kept piling up. A series of high-profile malpractice suits would plague the hospital, followed by the death of pop artist Andy Warhol after routine gallbladder surgery in 1987, which officials blamed on cardiac failure compounded by indifferent nursing care. A withering exposé in the *New York Times* put it well: "A GREAT HOSPITAL IN CRISIS."

At Bellevue, meanwhile, an even darker tragedy was about to unfold.

It, too, would involve a death, though not of a patient, and put the hospital in the crosshairs of the media. The main difference was that the events at Bellevue would seem more plausible to the average reader, more in line with its reputation, than the events at New York Hospital. Where one narrative drew its strength from the element of surprise, the other read like an accident waiting to happen.

Kathryn Hinnant loved New York City. The daughter of a South Carolina stockbroker and a nurse, Hinnant had first come to Manhattan for an internship in pathology at Lenox Hill Hospital. "She was tough," her mentor recalled. "I have this vision of [a] young woman who looked like Audrey Hepburn, who weighed 100 pounds, doing autopsies, working in blood and intestines. Not only did she do it, but she was elected chief resident."

Following a brief stint at George Washington University Hospital, Dr. Hinnant returned to New York, lured by the museums, art galleries, and music venues she and her husband, a piano salesman, had come to adore. Specializing in cytopathology, the study of disease at the cellular level, she took a job on the NYU Medical School faculty as part of a research team developing a "thin needle biopsy" to reach "the deepest recesses of the body with great precision." It was a plum assignment, given the connection between rare cancers and AIDS, and her career was rapidly advancing. Her tiny fourth-floor office at Bellevue, a few doors down from the pathology labs and autopsy rooms, seemed perfect for her needs.

In the fall of 1988, Dr. Hinnant discovered she was pregnant. A decision loomed. Would she move back to South Carolina to raise a family and continue her research at a measured pace, or would she remain in the city, where daily life would be much more complicated than before? She and her husband agreed to put the question on hold.

On January 7, 1989—a bitterly cold Saturday—Hinnant went to her Bellevue office to prepare some slides for an upcoming lecture to medical students. The pathology wing, a building away from the patient areas, was completely deserted. "There ain't nobody there, especially on weekends," a housekeeper would remark. "You can holler as loud as you want; nobody can hear you." Because her office had no window, Hinnant left the door ajar to catch a breeze. She turned on her slide projector, and got to work.

That same day, a homeless cocaine addict named Steven Smith was wandering Bellevue in search of someone to rob. Smith had been admitted a few weeks earlier for swallowing rat poison and muttering about suicide. Released against his wishes, he ingested even more poison, which got him readmitted. Though Smith now spoke of killing others as well as himself, the psychiatrist in charge could find no "psychosis or depression." The patient was acting out, he thought, to get a warm bed and some personal attention.

Others were less certain. A female intern recalled Smith as a "threatening" presence, and avoided him when she could. Held a few more days for medical observation because rat poison can cause serious internal bleeding, Smith, nicknamed "Ratman" by the staff, was released again because the psychiatric wards were full. Refusing to leave voluntarily, he was escorted from the hospital by uniformed guards.

But not for long. Smith returned the following week by simply blending into the mass of homeless people—drug addicts, AIDS victims, psychiatric cases, emergency room arrivals—who poured into Bellevue as patients or who used the cavernous lobbies and rest rooms as part of their daily routine. But Smith went a step further: he *moved into* the hospital as a squatter, finding himself a machinery closet on Bellevue's twenty-second floor.

Dressed in stolen doctor's scrubs with a stethoscope, a beeper, and a security badge, Smith had free run of the premises. "He took great joy moving around and fooling people, looking like part of the scenery," the police commissioner recalled. That included taking some of his meals in the staff dining room and, according to Smith's account, watching an operation in progress. A nurse did alert security after seeing Smith steal a clock and a hypodermic needle, for which he was arrested. But since no one bothered to run a name check—and petty theft by the homeless was quite common—he was released. Feeling more comfortable, even out of costume, Smith visited the emergency department seeking drugs for "back pain." But the staff grew suspicious, and he retreated to his closet on the twenty-second floor.

When Smith came upon Dr. Hinnant's partly open office door on the afternoon of January 7, he peeked his head inside and said, as he later told police, "Can I talk to you for a minute?" He may not have seemed particularly threatening or out of place—a small man, five feet, six inches and 130 pounds, dressed in doctor's garb (though Bellevue had very few African American physicians on staff). By ghoulish coincidence, Hinnant and Smith shared a common bond: both had grown up in Columbia, South Carolina, and both had returned there just a few months before—Hinnant to celebrate her parents' wedding anniversary; Smith to track down and terrorize a former girlfriend, which had led to his arrest and a brief commitment to a mental hospital after he drank a bottle of liquid detergent. By his own estimate, Smith spent no more than twenty minutes in Hinnant's office. In that time, he beat her unconscious, raped and sodomized her, and strangled her to death with an electrical cord.

Dr. Hinnant's husband had become frantic when she failed to show up that evening and didn't answer her phone. Escorted to her office by a security guard, he found her battered, naked body on the floor. The slide projector was still running; her fur coat and pocketbook were gone.

"On a typical day in 1989," said the *Daily News,* "New Yorkers reported nine rapes, five murders, 255 robberies, and 194 aggravated assaults. Fear wasn't a knee-jerk reaction, it was a matter of self-preservation." Yet of all the homicides that record-breaking year, few grabbed the public's attention quite like Kathryn Hinnant's. Fifty police detectives were assigned to the case, which Mayor Edward Koch called "the number one [crime] to be solved." Smith was arrested a few days later at a homeless shelter with Hinnant's coat and credit cards in his possession. A search of Bellevue's twenty-second floor turned up evidence of his encampment. The man the newspapers called "The Beast of Bellevue" had been caught.

It would be hard to imagine a more chilling scenario: a young doctor, five months pregnant, brutalized in her office by a deranged man roaming a public hospital at will. Not only had the assailant been arrested and released a few days before, he'd apparently been declared harmless by the psychiatrist who examined him. Furthermore, a look at Bellevue's security log for the month before the murder showed "at least three reports of unauthorized persons living in the fourth floor locker room and at least five reports of persons sleeping in other common areas and in stairways around the hospital." Squatting at Bellevue, it appeared, was hardly an aberration.

To make matters worse, the murder had occurred at an institution well known for security lapses. Ever since the infamous Nellie Bly exposé a century before, the press had kept a running tally of Bellevue's blunders, some becoming the stuff of legend. In 1919, Captain Fritz Duquesne, a top German spy, had fled Bellevue's prison ward by sawing through the bars and scaling an eight-foot fence with "menacing spikes" on top. The incident became a global sensation—partly because of Duquesne's notorious exploits during World War I, and partly because he'd tricked Bellevue's medical staff into believing he was a "hopeless paralytic" with an incurable disease. Though New York's district attorney was certain Duquesne had bribed his way to freedom, no one at Bellevue was ever charged, and the elusive Duquesne went on to spy again, for the Nazis during World War II.

When Bellevue's massive psychiatric building opened in the early 1930s, space was provided for two secure prison wards—one for men, the other for women—each with fifty beds. But the wards filled up so quickly that male prisoners with medical problems were moved back to the main hospital, while those with psychiatric issues remained. Both buildings contained a courtroom to process the various cases, where the psychiatric staff assessed the suspect's competence to stand trial. And, as with Fritz Duquesne, the doctors had the unenviable task of distinguishing between a legitimate illness and the false symptoms of those hoping to cheat justice. Some cases proved easier than others; in 1941, for example, a prison psychiatrist recorded the intentionally bizarre behavior of two murder suspects "remanded to Bellevue for observation"—one "taking a banana, peeling it, throwing away the fruit, and eating the peel," the other "pouring out his soup, putting the bowl on his head, and wearing it." The suspects weren't insane, the psychiatrist testified; they were fakers clumsily trying to avoid the electric chair, which soon became their fate.

But such cases paled in comparison to the events surrounding William Morales, a leader of the FALN, a domestic terror group demanding independence for Puerto Rico, that had planted dozens of homemade bombs throughout New York City in the 1970s, including one that killed four people at historic Fraunces Tavern near Wall Street. While plying his deadly craft, Morales had accidently blown off his fingers and blinded himself in one eye. Tried and sentenced to eighty-nine years, he was moved to Bellevue's third-floor prison ward—D-2—for physical rehabilitation. Once there, he sued the police department for "illegally confiscating" his fingers as evidence rather than sending them to the hospital for "possible reattachment." Then he disappeared.

To this day, the breakout remains shrouded in mystery. Using a pair of fourteen-inch wire cutters, along with rolls of elastic bandage tied to his bedpost, Morales somehow removed the window grate and grabbed his makeshift rope, which quickly snapped under his weight, sending him tumbling down to a grassy patch below. Fortunately for Morales, a window air-conditioner broke his fall. He was met by fellow gang members, who whisked him to a safe house in New Jersey.

The *New York Post* broke the story in three perfectly scripted words: "HANDLESS TERRORIST ESCAPES." How, exactly, had a one-eyed man missing all ten fingers been able to pull it off? The Bellevue prison ward had armed corrections officers. Visitors were supposed to be searched. Who gave Morales the bandages and the wire cutters? Why had no one spotted a car full of strangers on the street below?

There were no answers, only theories. Investigators suspected that a member of Morales's legal team and a sympathetic doctor had provided the escape tools, while security personnel had been either complicit or astonishingly inept. Several officers were fired, followed by the city's corrections commissioner and key members of his staff. Meanwhile, Morales fled to Mexico and then to Castro's Cuba, where he was given asylum—and remains to this day.

While the Duquesne and Morales breakouts had raised fundamental security concerns, they lacked the emotional impact of the Hinnant murder, which left the entire hospital in shock. It was, said one observer, the difference between watching *The Great Escape,* on the one hand, and *Psycho,* on the other. If this could happen to a doctor, it could happen to anyone—a defenseless patient, a nurse making rounds, a visitor using the restroom. Hinnant's boss, Dr. John Pearson, spoke of two lives being taken that afternoon—his final memory of Kathryn bouncing into his office to announce that the results of her amniocentesis had just come back and everything was fine with the baby. "She was so loved," he whispered, "and so tiny."

Steven Smith was found guilty of first-degree murder and sentenced to life in prison. "We thought he was faking," a juror said of his insanity defense. Asked if he had anything to say, Smith mumbled. "I'm sorry . . . I didn't get what I expected I should have got"—meaning a death sentence. Following the trial, the city offered Dr. Hinnant's family $2 million to settle their much larger claim against Bellevue. The family refused, leading to a court battle that would ultimately absolve the hospital of negligence in the murder. "I don't think there is a juror who isn't angry about this occurrence, who isn't very disappointed with Bellevue Hospital," said one of the dissenting members. On appeal, a panel of five state Supreme Court justices dismissed the family's lawsuit in a 3–2 decision. The law did "not require a hospital security system to be flawless," said the majority. And no one could reasonably expect a place like Bellevue, whose population included a "high percentage" of violent, criminal, antisocial, and homeless patients, to be perfectly safe. Put simply, it had done its best with what it had.

On one level, it was hard to disagree. Budget cuts over the years had forced the Health and Hospitals Corporation to reduce security across the public hospital system. The gap was such that Columbia Presbyterian, a voluntary hospital with fewer beds than Bellevue, had three times the number of security personnel—250, as opposed to eighty. In addition, Columbia Presbyterian had installed card-reading machines that alerted authorities to anyone wearing a stolen identification badge. Bellevue, by contrast, could barely pay the salaries of its bare-boned security force. The average officer earned $23,600 after three years on the job, half that of a New York City beat patrolman, and carried only handcuffs and a nightstick. (New York City Corrections officers assigned to the male prisoners did have firearms, which were not allowed on the wards.) Derided as "toy cops," the Bellevue force spent much of the shift at fixed positions, rather than patrolling the halls and stairwells. Indeed, one of the first things that Steven Smith had told the police detectives who interrogated him was: "Bellevue security sucks."

There was more to the story, of course, than sorry policing. Steven Smith was on probation for a string of serious crimes, yet the justice system had completely lost track of him. He'd come voluntarily to Bellevue threatening suicide and homicide, yet he couldn't get himself admitted. And the reason, it appeared, had as much to do with overcrowding as with a botched diagnosis. At the time of Dr. Hinnant's murder, Bellevue's adult psychiatric wards were running at "103.9 percent of capacity." There simply wasn't room for another homeless addict with violent thoughts swirling in his head.

Public hospitals reflect the social ills of the inner cities that surround them. In the 1970s, as crime and drug addiction soared, Bellevue opened a Methadone Maintenance Treatment Center on the ground floor. Theft had always been a problem at the hospital, mostly by the staff. Now almost everything began to disappear—typewriters, adding machines, purses, drugs, needles, syringes, even the candlesticks from the Catholic chapel. "Clusters of men gather daily near telephone booths and elevators, lean not-so-casually against pillars and walls, linger near doors and stairwells," wrote a *New York Times* reporter under the headline "Intruders Find Bellevue an Easy Target." Asked why nobody tried to remove them, a security guard replied, "With what? What have we got to protect ourselves?"

In 1985, the city closed Bellevue's massive psychiatric building and moved the patients to the top floors of the main hospital, along with the prison wards. Though crumbling and in disrepair, the psychiatric building gained new life as an eight-hundred-bed men's homeless shelter, the city's largest, just a block from the Bellevue lobby and connected to the hospital by a guarded underground tunnel. Within weeks, the shelter had reached maximum capacity.

Some of New York City's homeless surge could be blamed on rough economic times. But the key factor, most experts agreed, was the well-intentioned but woefully misguided policy of moving state mental patients back into their neighborhoods for treatment, a process known as "deinstitutionalization." The belief was that successful new antipsychotic medications combined with group therapy in a familiar setting would be more humane and effective than "forced incarceration" in isolated, often brutal mental hospitals. With little planning and erratic funding, the policy flooded New York City with thousands of severely disturbed and ultimately homeless people.

Fearful that some might die of neglect, Mayor Koch authorized both a "cold weather alert," which protected the homeless when the temperature dropped below freezing, and the "involuntary hospitalization" of those "in serious danger of bringing harm to themselves within the reasonably foreseeable future."* Both plans relied on using newly designated homeless shelters and selected public hospitals with facilities already in place—Bellevue being the most prepared and welcoming destination. By the late 1980s, it contained four separate units for the homeless, split between the hospital and the adjoining shelter, to treat psychiatric issues, medical problems, and substance abuse. "With our traditional sensitivity to the poor and the indigent mentally ill," said Bellevue's chief of psychiatry, "we [now] accept our responsibility to the care of the homeless."

Each patient was given both a medical and psychiatric exam after being bathed and deloused. One day's "roundup" included a blind, feces-covered woman who spent her days on the Upper West Side

---

* Legal battles soon followed. A woman living on a midtown subway grate sued the city after being brought to Bellevue against her will for medical and psychiatric treatment, which she refused. "I'm not insane," said Joyce Brown, who went by the name Billie Boggs, "just homeless." Though virtually every psychiatrist who examined her disagreed, finding Brown to be a severe danger to herself, and incapable of functioning without powerful antipsychotic drugs, a judge released her. The Boggs case complicated an already difficult situation, since by New York state law, a patient cannot be held involuntarily for more than sixty days without a court order. At Bellevue, a courtroom set aside for that very purpose—Room 19E2—became a very busy place, with a steady stream of patients, including some with drug-resistant tuberculosis and other dangerous conditions, contesting mandatory confinement and treatment.

screaming epithets at strangers and a knife-wielding man who lived in a plastic bag in Central Park surrounded by rodents he claimed to know by name. A journalist studying New York's "Mole People"—those living in the railroad and subway tunnels beneath the city—watched an evening roundup in which six homeless men agreed to leave "after some cajoling and promises that they will be taken to Bellevue rather than the Fort Washington Shelter." It wasn't hard to see the appeal. Bellevue provided fine basic care; it was safer and cleaner, and in some cases brought about quick (if mostly short-term) results. "These people . . . you wouldn't believe what they look like," an advocate for the homeless explained. "Some have toilet paper wrapped around their heads because they don't want their ideas flying out or new ones flying in. And after a week in Bellevue, eating and sleeping [well], they go before a judge and they say, 'I don't know why I was brought here Your Honor, I just want to get out and get a job.'"

The alternative in this instance, the massive Fort Washington Shelter in upper Manhattan, housed a small unit for the mentally ill. A *Times* reporter described the sheer menace of Fort Washington after making an unannounced evening visit: "Noises arise in the darkness: the moans of men having sex with men, the cries of the helpless being robbed, the hacking coughs of the sick, the pounding of feet running through a maze of 700 cots packed into one vast room." While anyone willing to look could see the utter failure of these giant shelters, there were few ways to fix the problem because neighborhood resistance to small-scale group homes was simply too intense.

"Wintertime was the worst," wrote a devoted, if disheartened, young physician. "The cold weather drove the homeless into the hospital, and all of Bellevue seemed a fetid, overcrowded, wretched purgatory to which we were committed to the end of our residency . . . if ever that would arrive." She wasn't alone. Dealing with the homeless in such large numbers tested the most idealistic of souls. A third-year NYU medical student noted the emotional contradiction of Bellevue in these years—yearning to serve the underserved, yet facing the reality of what that entailed. "An acrid smell of cheese gone bad accosts me as I near his coat," he wrote of an all-too-common encounter. "This is awful. I feel I have to walk away, maybe find a toilet somewhere to vomit. Doesn't he know how bad he smells? How can he live with himself?"

The patient was homeless and drug-addicted, his arm "scabrous and pocked." A festering boil on his ankle looked "about to burst." There had been untold numbers like him in the past, but never in such heavy concentrations. "Please let me go home and get some sleep," the student silently pleaded. "And please God, please, do not make me touch [him] until he has had a shower."

Two months after Dr. Hinnant's murder, a survey taken by Bellevue's Department of Social Work classified 43 percent of the hospital's adult inpatient population as homeless, the figure rising to 70 percent in the psychiatric division. And a second survey of 298 patients brought involuntarily to Bellevue showed most to be single men with a history of schizophrenia who had been living on the streets for at least a year. A fair number were drug addicts, HIV-positive, and suffering from tuberculosis; fewer than 5 percent had families willing to accept them back into their homes. As a result, the average length of stay for a psychiatric patient at Bellevue rose from about ten days in the early 1970s to thirty-seven days by 1992. "[We've] changed from a receiving hospital to an intermediate and long-term patient care service," its psychiatric director admitted, adding: "We cannot [just] turn our patients out into the streets."

In truth, Bellevue had become hostage to circumstances it couldn't hope to control. The AIDS crisis, the crack cocaine epidemic, the deinstitutionalization of state mental patients, the adjoining men's shelter, the "cold weather alerts," the "involuntary" commitments—each took a heavy toll. "I hate to put it this way, but we're sort of the waste basket for the rest of society," said the head of Bellevue's psychiatric emergency service. "We take the people the other social agencies can't deal with, those who fall through the cracks."

But Bellevue, with the best of intentions, may have aggravated matters by the very nature of its social vision. On a given day, one could see a long line of semiconscious men on gurneys—what the staff called "the choo-choo train of drunks"—who had staggered in for a hot meal, an aspirin, and some free clothing from a veritable warehouse of goods donated by volunteers who distributed them to thousands of homeless patients each year. "We treat all the problems of society," a Bellevue social worker explained. "How can you send a person out in the cold without a coat?"

It was an admirable sentiment, but hardly problem-free. Was it wise to blur the line between homeless patients in need of medical and psychiatric attention, and those who looked upon Bellevue as a place to get warm, to be fed and to be used as a physical extension of the shelter next door? A homeless man in a wheelchair had been stabbed to death in the tunnel between the shelter and the hospital, and several Bellevue patients had been sexually assaulted, the last attack occurring a few months before Dr. Hinnant's murder. "Our security stinks," said Irwin Freedberg, the chair of dermatology, parroting Steven Smith's much quoted description to the police. He added: "The front lobby is a mess. I have never seen this hospital dirtier."

Could Dr. Hinnant's death have been prevented by better police training, a reasonable security budget, a stricter policy toward the homeless, or perhaps all three? Opinions varied. Some at Bellevue saw the murder as a rare tragedy that could have occurred in any public facility serving a diverse clientele. Of course, security must be improved, they agreed, but not at the expense of turning Bellevue into a less welcoming place. But others were left wondering whether the hospital they loved had begun to take on the look of a soup kitchen or a bus terminal. A young physician, noting that Bellevue had experienced three major security alerts on the day of Dr. Hinnant's murder—the other two being a hanging in a psychiatric ward and a drowning in the dermatology ward—vented his frustration to the press. "The risk of working in a place of such minimal security and an ever present criminal element is now constantly at the edge of our consciousness," he fumed. "We share a sense of violation and outrage, and many of us will never be the same."

Gerald Weissmann, the distinguished researcher and clinician who began his career at Bellevue in the 1950s, feared that a corner had been turned. Life was "less hazardous for young doctors in my day," he wrote. No one then could have imagined a scene in which "an unshaven derelict . . . in a scruffy scrub suit [and] a stethoscope around his neck . . . roamed around the hospital." For Weissmann, the presence of such deranged predators rested squarely with muddle-headed state officials who had closed the asylums with little forethought, allowing "the mad and violent to prowl the streets." But he wondered whether a conservative future historian "might find that we are unknowing accomplices in Kathryn Hinnant's death"—that she "died for our liberal creed."

19

SANDY

Shortly after Dr. Hinnant's death, a group of security experts held a workshop, "The Bellevue Murder: Could It Happen in Your Hospital?" Nothing remotely resembling a consensus emerged. Those from the private hospitals couldn't imagine a scenario in which a doctor would be killed under their watch. "It's hard for me to believe that someone could be living in a cubicle or storage room and not be noticed," said the director of security at New York's elite Memorial Sloan-Kettering Center. "We don't have an area of the hospital that's not monitored. . . . An ill-kempt person will stand out here."

Those representing the "publics" offered no such guarantees. Their hospitals faced "large numbers of homeless, an AIDS epidemic, increasing violence, the crack explosion, overcrowding, and tight budgetary restrictions." While not denying Bellevue's egregious security lapses, they noted that "unkempt" people were the rule at public institutions, and that Bellevue counted more than its share. Could the murder of Dr. Hinnant have occurred in any big metropolitan hospital? Of course—though the fact that it happened where it did was no great surprise.

Indeed, several weeks *after* Dr. Hinnant's murder, yet another squatter was arrested at Bellevue for criminal trespass. He'd been living in the hospital basement for at least two months, posing as a TV repairman and harassing patients. He was finally spotted carrying four trays of half-eaten food back to his subterranean quarters, where security guards found a stack of stolen visitor's passes. "We work hard and head off a lot of incidents," an official insisted. "But we have doctors who don't wear their IDs. We have people who tape locks open on the stairways so they don't have to wait for the elevators. We have employees who don't bother to report suspicious persons on the floors. Then they complain that security stinks."

The Hinnant murder began a decade of intense scrutiny for New York's beleaguered public hospital system. The early 1990s would see both an uptick in hospital crime and a cluster of wrongful death suits that reignited the debate over privatization. At Manhattan's Harlem Hospital, the body of a missing psychiatric patient turned up in an airshaft a few yards from his room. At Bronx Municipal Hospital, two patients died after one's cardiac monitor was disabled and the other received too much anesthesia. The most publicized case involved Yankel Rosenbaum, an Orthodox Jew attacked by a mob during the Crown Heights Riot of 1991. Rushed to Brooklyn's Kings County Hospital, Rosenbaum died in the emergency room. A review of his treatment showed that a poorly supervised intern had missed the stab wound responsible for Rosenbaum's death.

Medically speaking, Bellevue remained head and shoulders above these other institutions. Even those demanding privatization agreed that tampering with "the flagship of public hospital care in the United States may not be politically feasible." What set Bellevue apart, even in the worst of times, was its powerful connection to New York City's top medical schools. One had only to look at the near disintegration of Harlem Hospital under its affiliation contract with Columbia (P&S) to see the difference. Columbia had served Bellevue with distinction for generations before pulling up stakes in the 1960s. Now, however, its neglect of the Harlem partnership was so complete that its own dean conceded the point without a hint of embarrassment. "[We're] a big institution," he mused. "Certainly there are times when we'd have liked the university to pay attention to the Harlem affiliation."

Things were no better at Kings County, whose partnership with Downstate Medical School was described as "terrible" when it came to providing quality patient care. "I can't tell you now with a straight face that we get $475 million worth of service from the affiliates," the head of the Health and Hospitals Corporation admitted. The sad truth was that medical schools like Columbia and Downstate were taking large sums from the city without giving back much in return. The tradition of service—the sense of mission—that prevailed among physicians at Bellevue had been forged over centuries. NYU had been training its students and house staff there since before the Civil War, and a fair number of them, known as "Bellevue lifers," stayed on for their entire careers. While incidents like the Hinnant murder no doubt strained the NYU-Bellevue partnership, the institutions were too interdependent to think of parting ways.

By the 1990s, Harlem Hospital, Kings County, and Bronx Municipal were on the verge of losing their state accreditation. And a key reason, many believed, was the growing disconnect between the aims of the affiliated medical schools and the needs of the public hospital patient. The medical schools were moving more and more toward specialized training; the patients, lacking a primary physician, were most in need of a general practitioner. The inevitable result, a city official complained, was a style of medical care that had "little to do with the needs of the communities."

Bellevue's weaknesses lay elsewhere. According to the nonpartisan United Hospital Fund, the scourge of AIDS and homelessness—of patients "who are sicker, more difficult to manage, and sometimes more dangerous than in the past"—had taken a heavy toll on the hospital, which saw fourteen executive directors come and go in the years between 1983 and 1997. "We've had more Bellevue heads than [Yankees owner] George Steinbrenner had managers," a local assemblyman fumed. "It is beyond belief—a terrible embarrassment for the city."

There were many reasons for the exodus. One director was fired for covering up the embezzlement of an aide. Another was let go for refusing to make the budget cuts demanded by City Hall. "I will only run a hospital where I feel I could walk in and be a patient myself," she declared. Still another, recruited from Houston, took umbrage at the un-Southern hospitality. Having arrived with no place to live, he was housed "in an old, dreary, mice-infested section of the hospital that had been converted into an apartment" and then left to eat Thanksgiving dinner in a nearby coffee shop. "I don't need to subject myself to that kind of life," he announced upon heading back to Texas two weeks later.

The privatizers saw evidence of failure at every turn. That upward of $3 billion was spent each year to prop up a dysfunctional system surely spoke to the corrupting influence of labor unions and city bureaucrats. Cutting costs and raising standards were unrealistic goals; the system wasn't about to reform itself. The logical solution, therefore, lay in shuttering the worst of these hospitals and selling off the others, Bellevue being the possible exception. The poor wouldn't suffer—indeed, they'd be better off—because private hospitals would be more efficient in spending the government dollars set aside for their care.

Pushback from the unions and public hospital administrators was to be expected. But a blue-ribbon mayoral commission, chaired by the president of the New York Academy of Medicine, also raised objections. Twenty-five percent of the city's population lived below the federal poverty line, twice the national average; most came from minority neighborhoods where private hospitals were few and far between. New York's public system treated more homeless people and substance abusers, more AIDS, tuberculosis, and psychiatric patients, than any other provider in the country. Its emergency rooms and outpatient clinics served as primary care facilities for the city's huge underclass—a role that private facilities seemed unlikely to fill. Much like Mayor John Lindsay three decades before, the panel concluded that "the city should remain in the hospital business, because of . . . its social responsibilities in this area, including the necessity of assuring that care be provided to all who need it."

Privately, however, the committee chair was far less certain. The city's concern for the indigent sick was "a nice thing, a good thing, a proper thing," said Dr. Jeremiah Barondess. But those in charge lacked the knowhow to run a modern hospital system "in a world this complex politically, socially, [and] medically." Why, then, had his panel concluded otherwise? Barondess didn't say, but the pressure was intense. Community activists had demanded that the panel hold open sessions in minority neighborhoods, and Barondess reluctantly complied. Closing down the "publics" thus became a matter of race and class played out in an angrily divided city. Barondess honestly believed that privatization would remove the medical safety net for the most vulnerable New Yorkers, despite assurances to the contrary. But he also feared the ever-widening gap between a private system free to pick and choose its patients, and a public one left to treat the unwanted remainder. The wiser path, he thought, was to seek improvements in the status quo— and hope for the best.

Historically, Bellevue's Emergency Department is one of the crown jewels of the city system. Heart attacks and car wrecks, AIDS and crack cocaine overdoses, shootings and attempted suicides, poisonings and prison fights, frostbite and rotted feet—are dealt with at all hours, seven days a week. It isn't unheard of to treat a homeless man with a body temperature of 66 degrees—the equivalent of hibernation—or an immigrant with leprosy. Indeed, part of Bellevue's mystique lies in its handling of the sort of unusual cases that periodically light up the tabloids—the woman crushed by a construction crane in midtown, saved from certain death; the music student pushed under a moving subway, her severed hand miraculously reattached. "This is war zone medicine," a Bellevue emergency room doctor observed in 1990. "You'll never go anywhere in the world and see something we haven't seen here."

Hyperbole, though not by much. When word first reached Bellevue on September 11, 2001, that an American Airlines flight from Boston had crashed into the North Tower of the World Trade Center, the staff prepared for the worst. But to those familiar with Bellevue's history, the news had a familiar ring. In 1945, a fog-blind military craft bound for Newark Airport had flown into the upper floors of the Empire State Building, killing fourteen people and injuring hundreds. Bellevue's entire ambulance corps had rushed to the scene that summer morning; among those evacuated was an elevator operator named Betty Lou Oliver.

Occurring a week before the atomic bomb was dropped on Hiroshima, and two weeks before the Japanese surrender, her personal story still made the front pages. One of the plane's flaming engines had broken free and severed the cables of her elevator, parked without passengers on the seventy-fifth floor. The car rocketed downward, crashing through the shaft and landing in the subbasement. Miraculously, Betty Lou Oliver survived. "She was in a state of profound shock," a doctor recalled. "Her pulse was so weak, it was hard to tell whether she was dead or alive. She had a fractured spine, concussion of the brain, a broken kneecap, several other fractures, and multiple burns and abrasions." A priest performed last rites.

Oliver endured several months of skin grafts and surgeries. She was fitted with leg braces and taught to walk again—"put back together, almost piece by piece," in the words of a supervising physician. Oliver expressed her gratitude on the day she was discharged, saying, "This couldn't have happened at any other place but Bellevue."

September 11 also revived memories of 1993, when terrorists bombed the World Trade Center garage and Bellevue received the bulk of the wounded. After that, like other urban hospitals, it began to prepare for future attacks. In 1996, a journalist visiting Bellevue came upon a drill for a deadly sarin gas attack, like the one in Tokyo the previous year. "Oxygen tanks were piled by the door. Canisters of atropine, a drug used to control muscle spasms, were stacked in metal carts. Everyone donned blue plastic coats, masks with Plexiglas shields, rubber gloves and boot covers, then turned toward the emergency room door, waiting for the casualties to barrel through."

On the morning of 9/11, the smoke billowing from the North Tower was clearly visible at Bellevue, less than three miles away. "It's gonna be a big one," a nurse remarked. "They'll be coming in droves." Eighteen minutes later, the South Tower was hit and, as one doctor on duty put it, "the hospital shifted gears like I'd never seen in my twenty-five years working there."

The night staff, preparing to leave, remained in place. Routine surgeries were canceled to clear the operating rooms, and patients able to leave the hospital were quickly discharged. A physician's diary read: "The second tower falls. Alumni begin to arrive. . . . Twenty nursing students in green scrubs flock in. A group of residents in starchy whites ask what they can do." Outside, a line of volunteers snaked around the building, waiting to give blood.

"I've been thinking about something like this for twenty years," the hospital's chief trauma surgeon told a reporter. "We're ready to cope with whatever comes through our doors." Behind him stood a full medical army—"a sea of scrubs," a resident recalled, "gloved, masked and waiting." Rumors flew that scores of horribly injured victims were on their way. The minutes turned to hours. Where were they?

The most common memory of those on duty at Bellevue that day is the helplessness they felt. "Thousands of medical workers—doctors, nurses, medical students, technicians, orderlies, therapists, clerical workers—were poised [for action]," a staffer wrote, "but there were no patients . . . no one came." Records show that 169 World Trade Center victims were treated at Bellevue on 9/11, and twenty-five more in the following days. It's an extremely small number given the estimates of seven to ten thousand people in each tower that morning, even more so considering that most of those who did reach Bellevue were classified as "walking wounded" with injuries that didn't require admission, such as corneal abrasions, minor lung issues, and cuts and bruises.

The reason is painfully clear. Catastrophes of this scope tend to have three zones, a trauma expert explained. "The center zone is death on impact. The middle zone is gravely injured. The outer zone is minimal injury." The Twin Towers collapse had no middle zone. People either died in the buildings or walked away covered in soot but physically intact—too stunned, or relieved, or even guilty, to seek medical aid.

With so few victims arriving, some at Bellevue rushed to the scene. "Police cars barreled up and men and women wearing red scrubs clambered out," recalled a physician at Downtown Hospital, a few blocks from the fallen Twin Towers. "They were surgeons from Bellevue . . . who, despite our phones being down, had guessed where the patients were being taken." Minutes later, an intern arrived on a motorcycle, his backpack filled with supplies. Downtown Hospital, a 150-bed operation, treated more than a thousand people that day, most for superficial wounds. One rescue worker had a finger amputated after cutting himself on a piece of metal, and a severely burned woman was ambulanced to Bellevue because, as one doctor noted, "morphine was all we could offer her."

The Bellevue interns who reached Downtown Hospital were shocked by their assignments. Expecting trauma duty, they were told to search the smoldering wreckage of Ground Zero for body parts to be sent to the Medical Examiner's Office for identification. "We took heads, arms, legs, and labeled them and put them in the truck," one wrote of the assignment. "I thought I'd be able to handle it emotionally but . . . the amount of death that I saw was unbelievable."

All told, twenty-one operations were performed at Bellevue in the following days. Three of the final Twin Tower victims pulled out from under thirty feet of rubble required extremely delicate surgery, and two survived their wounds. The last person found alive, a Port Authority police sergeant named John McLoughlin, had led the rescue attempt in the North Tower moments before it collapsed. "Initially, I thought I had died," said McLoughlin, who spent twenty-two hours pinned under a girder. "I lost all sense. I had no sight. I had no smell. I had no hearing. Everything just went silent." Put into a medically induced coma, McLoughlin underwent thirty procedures over the next three months to remove dead muscle and tissue from his crushed lower body. His kidneys failed, forcing him to undergo renal dialysis, and he was placed on a respirator after developing a severe bacterial infection. But his recovery bore witness to the enormous skill of the medical teams left waiting for other victims to arrive. "So many lives were lost that day," one of the attending surgeons remembered. "At Bellevue and NYU, we were prepared to save more, if we only had the chance."

For weeks after the Twin Towers fell, the city was blanketed with fly-ers of the missing: "Has anyone seen Richard _____, 36, black hair, brown eyes, a firefighter; please contact his family at _____." Hundreds of them were taped to a two-hundred-foot-long construc-tion fence at Bellevue, which became a makeshift memorial covered in weatherproof plastic. What struck those who passed it each day were the strikingly personal images of the missing—at weddings and anni-versaries, receiving their diplomas, vacationing at the beach, wearing gowns and tuxedos. In one photo, a father is sitting on the grass next to his young daughter, the block letter words reading: "Have You Seen My Daddy?" As the flyers grew in number, so, too, did the length of the fence. New Yorkers named it "The Wall of Prayers."

It was the same as the ones that sprang up at Grand Central, Penn Station, the Port Authority, St. Vincent's Hospital, and dozens of other places—only larger. That was due, in some measure, to the fact that Bellevue abutted the Medical Examiner's Office, where the identification of the victims was taking place. One of the doctors who had rushed to Ground Zero recalled the enormous white coroner's tent that suddenly appeared below his office window. "I would look down during nights on call and see the constantly illuminated procession of trucks bringing remains for forensic analysis," he wrote. "I lost track of how many months they were there, but however long it was, the lights shining on the ceaseless work never turned off."

In fact, Bellevue had long been a gathering place for those seeking information after a catastrophe—partly because it housed the city's largest morgue, and partly because it treated so many of the wounded. Crowds had flocked there after the Civil War Draft Riots, the bloody Orange Day parades, the *General Slocum* disaster, the Triangle Shirtwaist fire that killed 146 garment workers in 1911, the Empire State Building plane crash, and the 1993 World Trade Center garage bombing. The Wall of Prayers remained at Bellevue for two months, with grief counselors on duty. In November 2001, a private memorial was held for the hospital staff as the Wall was taken down. Several hundred people attended; Protestant, Jewish, and Muslim religious leaders read prayers. The scribbled notes and photos that covered the Wall are preserved at the Museum of the City of New York.

Bellevue's role in 9/11 is ongoing. Its pathologists played a major part in identifying the victims, a painstaking process with 1,200 people still unaccounted for, though their death certificates were issued years ago. Its Chest Service partnered with other hospitals to treat the first responders who trekked through clouds saturated with asbestos, glass fibers, fuel ash, lead from pulverized computers, mercury from fluorescent bulbs, and toxins of all kinds. Today, Bellevue houses an Environmental Health Center staffed by NYU Medical School that screens neighborhood residents claiming a 9/11-related lung injury. While looking for the most telling symptoms—shortness of breath, a persistent cough, evidence of "WTC-derived particles"—the center, like Bellevue itself, turns no one away. Many patients come from low-income families without health insurance. Papers aren't required, and there are few out-of-pocket costs for treatment.

On the tenth anniversary of 9/11, a state-of-the-art "Simulation Center" opened at Bellevue to train first responders and hospital personnel in handling mass emergencies. At 25,000 square feet, the nation's largest, it contains mock operating rooms, a five-bed intensive care unit, and freakishly lifelike mannequins that can speak, bleed, sweat, moan, vomit, and even deliver a baby in response to computer-generated commands. Fittingly, the center occupies the same space as the old tuberculosis wards run by medical giants like Edith Lincoln, André Cournand, and Dickinson Richards—testament to the ever-changing priorities of urban hospital care.

Shortly after 9/11, a doctor who had been on duty at Bellevue that day jotted down the problems he'd seen. Poor communication topped the list. Like much of lower Manhattan, Bellevue's phone lines were overwhelmed and cell service was spotty. There weren't enough two-way radios, which are essential in such emergencies, leaving administrators to rely on medical student "runners" to relay critical information.

Next on his list was the possibility of a blackout. If the hospital's main power source went down, the survival of the most vulnerable patients would depend on a backup system of unknown reliability. Bellevue had dodged the problem this time, he wrote, but the legacy of 9/11 was that unthinkable catastrophes were now a fact of modern life. What would happen if the power cut out for several hours—or more? Was there a plan in place to deal with it? "Often, the capacity of emergency generators is unable to meet [these] demands," the doctor concluded. "Clearly someone should be assigned to control and conserve these resources."

Prophetic words, indeed.

In the realm of "emergency preparedness" at American hospitals, there really are two eras: Before Katrina and After Katrina. Until that point, attention had focused on treating mass casualties arising from a terrorist attack, a gas explosion, a highway pileup—what one expert called "disasters outside their walls." While there were a handful of previous wake-up calls—the massive Northridge, California, earthquake that buckled several local hospitals in 1994; the immense damage done to Houston's downtown medical complexes following Tropical Storm Allison in 2001—the danger to patients "inside their walls" seemed rather remote.

Katrina challenged that thinking. When the levees protecting New Orleans gave way in the summer of 2006, flooding the downtown hospitals, patients became casualties. It wasn't a big story at first, given the immense scope of the hurricane. But reports began to trickle out regarding the horrors that occurred in places like Memorial (formerly Baptist) Hospital, where more than thirty people died, most with suspiciously high levels of morphine in their system. Dr. Sheri Fink put it all together in *Five Days at Memorial,* a searing account of what happened when the backup generators failed, the water taps went dry, the food spoiled, the air-conditioning stopped, and critically ill patients lay in semidarkness and stifling heat. Isolated and exhausted, the medical staff took to making life-and-death decisions in an increasingly leaderless vacuum—the line between medicine and mercy killing so blurred that a doctor and two nurses were accused of euthanizing patients and brought up on charges of second-degree murder, which eventually were dropped.

In 2011, New York City faced its own mini-Katrina when Hurricane Irene roared up the East Coast. Fearing severe flooding, Mayor Michael Bloomberg closed the subway system and ordered the evacuation of all hospitals in Zone A, a low-lying area in lower Manhattan bordering the East River. NYU's Langone Medical Center, which includes Tisch Hospital, shut down, as did the Veterans Administration Hospital a few blocks away. But Bellevue, located just between these two hospitals, remained open to serve any emergencies that might arise.

Irene struck New York City a glancing blow, doing its real damage farther upstate. The dire warnings had proved false, leaving New Yorkers weary of preparing for violent storms that rarely seemed to materialize. From a hospital's perspective, an evacuation not only cost money, it also put the patients at risk by removing them from a secure medical environment. Weighed against the frightening but slim chance of a direct hit from a monster storm like Katrina, repeated evacuations seemed a heavy price to pay. New York City wasn't New Orleans—or so it appeared.

Bellevue did make one key improvement, however. Because its emergency generators were located on the thirteenth floor, while the fuel pumps that supplied them sat in the basement, the hospital's backup power system wasn't fully secure. Though it would take a massive storm surge from the East River even to reach the basement, the hospital, to be safe, encased the fuel pumps behind "submarine doors" of steel and rubber to withstand water damage from a future event.

In October 2012, a late-season storm named Sandy made landfall on the New Jersey coast. This time there was no glancing blow. Sandy would be the largest storm ever recorded in the Atlantic Ocean, with a diameter approaching one thousand miles. And it hit New York City full on, arriving at high tide on the night of a full moon. The damage from South Jersey to the eastern tip of Long Island was catastrophic, but the densely populated parts of lower Manhattan fared even worse. The storm surge of a major hurricane adds four to six feet to the East River; this one measured fourteen feet in Zone A, an unfathomable event.

On Sunday, October 28, with Sandy approaching, Mayor Bloomberg again shut down public transportation and strongly advised residents in low-lying areas to evacuate. But for reasons not entirely clear, the two major Zone A hospitals abutting the East River, Tisch and Bellevue, stayed open, a decision that remains controversial. (The neighboring VA hospital, under federal supervision, did evacuate.) Predictions of Sandy's storm surge varied widely, with city officials banking on the lower estimates. Dr. Thomas Farley, New York's widely respected health commissioner—and someone who had worked in New Orleans during Katrina—appeared confident that the rivers surrounding Manhattan would rise no more than six feet at high tide. It's also likely that the decision to "shelter in place" was colored by the false alarm of Irene: moving out patients prematurely might be more dangerous than keeping them in a well-stocked hospital with a secure backup power system. It certainly was more expensive.

Dr. Doug Bails, Bellevue's chief of medical service, arrived early on October 29 from his home in New Jersey. Knowing that the subways and commuter rail lines would shut down that morning, he packed a change of clothing and some extra food, expecting to spend the night on his office couch as Sandy passed through. The day began mildly, but by mid-afternoon the winds had reached tropical storm force, with severe damage reported along the Jersey Shore. At 5:45 p.m., Mayor Bloomberg held a press conference to deliver some very bad news. Sandy could well be "the worst storm of the century," he warned, and the time to evacuate had passed. Bails looked out his office window. It was raining hard, and the FDR Drive, a major north–south artery along the East River, had started to flood.

Just before 9 p.m., Bellevue went dark. "We were told it would take ten seconds for the backup system to kick in, so I began a silent count," Bails recalled. At nine, the lights came back on and the elevators started to move. An explosion at a flooded Con Edison substation several blocks away had left the southern part of Manhattan in full blackout. For the moment, Bellevue's backup power system was doing its job.

There was a problem, though. The hospital was taking in water—not in small puddles or isolated corners, but as one astonished worker put it, "like Niagara Falls." Millions of gallons had breached Bellevue's ancient retaining wall and flooded the 182,000-square-foot basement, much of it pouring in through the loading docks facing the East River. While the emergency generators were thirteen floors up, and therefore not in danger, the fuel pumps that supplied them sat directly in harm's way. If the floodwaters pierced the new doors protecting these pumps, the generators would soon run dry.

Two blocks north at Tisch Hospital, all power had been lost. With the basement fuel pumps already underwater, the backup system shorted out. "There was no electricity, and the IV machines were going haywire," a patient recalled. "I heard one nurse yell to someone: 'Don't use that water, it's brown.' I couldn't believe how fast things were failing."

Tisch had prepared for Sandy by calling in extra staff, stocking up on supplies, and discharging a quarter of its patients—standard procedures for "sheltering in place." Moreover, it had evacuated the building the year before during Hurricane Irene, giving it a feel for the process.

But this time was different. The storm had already begun, the hospital was dark, and the elevators were out. Frantic calls were being made to find nearby hospital beds and ambulances for transport. With the computers down, medical records had to be cobbled together.

There would be some bitter exchanges in the aftermath—the mayor's office claiming it had been misled about the hospital's vulnerable backup power system; Tisch officials responding that no one could have anticipated Sandy's record surge. What both sides agreed on, however, was the success of the evacuation. More than three hundred patients were brought down stairwells illuminated by medical students and residents holding flashlights and cell phones. Those who couldn't walk were carried on stretchers or wrapped in shielded plastic sleds— some attached to ventilators and IV drips. Dozens of ambulances lined First Avenue. "The patients started arriving at around 1:00 a.m.," a critical care doctor at Mount Sinai recalled. "First one or two came, then one or two more. Then 25 came all at once." Most had their paperwork in order. "I'm not sure how NYU managed to pull that off in a blackout," the doctor added, "but I give them a lot of credit."

Ironically, Ken Langone, the medical center's namesake and major donor, was a patient on the eleventh floor when the evacuation began. Interviewed several days later, he said: "The backup generators failed, it's as simple as that, but the story here is the magnificence of . . . the people. Just think of the effort to bring down [so many] patients, and they did it . . . all night long."

Asked if he ever felt himself to be in danger, Langone, the billionaire cofounder of Home Depot, replied: "Do you think they'd have kept me in there if they thought I was going to be unsafe?"

Bellevue faced a tougher set of problems. Larger than Tisch, it housed a more diverse population. In addition to its regular medical and surgical patients, there were prisoners in lockup, alcoholics and drug addicts, hundreds of psychiatric patients, and people detained under court order with highly infectious tuberculosis. Evacuating these groups would not be easy. Bellevue's best option, it appeared, was to ride out Sandy until the floodwaters receded.

This was nothing new. Bellevue had always "sheltered in place" during major storms. The drill was second nature—all hands on deck for staffers while shedding those patients who were able to leave. But Bellevue had an additional concern: an unusually large group depended on electric-powered ventilators, dialysis machines, intravenous drips, and aortic pumps to survive. "In the event of total power loss," recalled Dr. Laura Evans, director of critical care, "our limited resources would have to be allocated to the patients most likely to benefit from them." Presently there were fifty-six people in her intensive care units, who had to be ranked according to need. Evans knew the protocol; she'd compiled a similar list during Hurricane Irene.

On Monday evening, Evans formed a committee of ICU doctors and nurses plus a medical ethicist to review the patient charts. One of the key lessons of Katrina was that the main public hospital in New Orleans (Charity) had suffered far fewer deaths than Memorial, despite having many more patients, because, among other things, "the sickest were taken out first instead of last." At Bellevue, the committee looked at "severity of illness, need for life sustaining equipment, and likelihood of recovery." It was an eerie setting, Evans recalled, with cases being evaluated as the lights flickered on and off in the background.

At 10:30 p.m.—high tide—the storm surge overwhelmed the submarine doors protecting the basement fuel pumps. Barring a miracle, Bellevue's backup power would be gone in three hours, when the emergency generators exhausted the last drops of gasoline in their tanks. To make matters worse, the basement also housed the pumps that supplied wall oxygen to patient rooms and fresh water to the four fifty-thousand-gallon rooftop towers. Virtually everything needed to keep the hospital running was now disabled—or about to be. That meant no air-conditioning, no refrigeration, no flushing toilets, no laundry service, no wall oxygen, no blood work or laboratory results. Vacuum power was gone, forcing patients to be suctioned by syringe. All thirty-two elevators were out of service because the basement shafts resembled swimming pools.

Just after midnight came a reprieve. National Guard troops arrived, followed by a police tanker truck with 2,600 gallons of fuel. A call went out for volunteers to gather at the stairwell landings, and a bucket brigade quickly formed—guardsmen, doctors, nurses, medical students, technicians, secretaries—to pass five-gallon containers of gasoline hand to hand from the tanker to the backup generators on the thirteenth floor. "There was no division of labor, no complaints or hesitation, and no signs of stopping," a volunteer remembered. "No one said it, but the pressure was obvious. . . . If [we] stopped moving, patients' lives could end tonight. . . . This went on for hours, pushing . . . to dawn."

The bucket brigade staved off disaster. The backup generators provided just enough power to run selected outlets in the wards and keep the hospital from falling into complete darkness. Meanwhile, interns were dispatched with oxygen tanks to the bed of every ventilated patient in case the electricity failed and mechanical IVs were converted to "subcutaneous injection." In the pharmacy, prescriptions filled by flashlight were handed to medical student runners for delivery to the various floors.

At the hospital's command center on 17 West, a whiteboard took the place of computers. Emergency phone numbers were scribbled in Magic Marker, along with breakfast and dinner orders. "This being Manhattan," a staffer recalled, "deliveries of pizza and Chinese take-out food never flagged." Perhaps the oddest whiteboard notation read: "19 S East Stairwell (knock three times)"—the new code for entering the prison wards on 19 South.

On Tuesday morning, October 30, a mini-evacuation began. Infants were transferred out, along with ICU patients and those on ventilators and dialysis. The threat of a full power loss, compounded by fears of bacterial contamination, sealed the decision. It had become too dangerous to treat vulnerable and compromised patients in conditions like these. "I am caught behind a team from the Neonatal ICU," a social worker wrote in her diary of a stairwell trek. "One nurse who manages to seem stern, nervous, and commanding all at the same time, counts the steps. 'Step One . . . Step Two . . . Step Three.' She holds one of the babies . . . and five other nurses and doctors follow behind. They march in step . . . like soldiers down 16 flights of stairs."

By Tuesday afternoon, Bellevue seemed a hospital on the brink. Garbage was piling up, toilets were clogged, the stink was nauseating, the air insufferably still and warm. The staff had been on duty for two days and nights, and exhaustion was setting in. The hospitals on both sides—Tisch and the VA—were empty. What was taking so long? "I have to pee, but I really don't want to," a worker confessed. "With no running water, the bathroom situation has become intolerable." Hearing of a toilet with only urine in the bowl, she rushed over to use it. "Despite the many walks up and down the stairs," she added, "we attempt to drink as little as possible."

On Wednesday morning, October 31, the hospital was ordered to close. With lower Manhattan still blacked out, the danger of sheltering the remaining patients now outweighed the risks of moving them out. What followed was a "vertical evacuation" of unprecedented scope. Maneuvering hundreds of physically fragile and mentally ill patients through a maze of barely lit stairwells wasn't in anyone's playbook—Katrina notwithstanding. "All hospitals are required to do disaster planning," an official admitted, "but we've never had [a drill] where we carried patients downstairs."

It took a full day and most of that evening to complete the job. Working in teams, soldiers and staffers evacuated patients at the torturous rate of twenty-five per hour—some hand-carried, others on stretchers and sleds. Dr. Elizabeth Ford's unit was among the last to leave. "It's Bellevue, we're used to crisis, but this was different," Ford said of her criminal psychiatric ward on 19 South. "I don't think I ever panicked in my life, but I was starting to worry that we wouldn't get out." Some of her sixty-one patients, hearing of the flood, concocted fantasies of being drowned. Wearing orange jumpsuits, they were taken down in groups of six, chained together at the ankles and surrounded by a phalanx of police.

By Friday morning, only two patients remained. One was a 550-pound woman who couldn't fit into the sled to guide her down the stairs; the other was an elderly man with a ventricular assist device for a serious heart condition. Both had to wait until an elevator could be rigged to get them out.

More than seven hundred patients were in Bellevue when the storm hit and the power failed. All got out safely. Those transferred to other hospitals by ambulance were given handwritten discharge summaries, a list of their medications, and a doggy bag with a five-day supply. The rest—mainly homeless—were sent to local shelters. While the nearby hospitals were quite accepting of these transfers, the "patient handoff" could be trying, as Mount Sinai learned upon admitting a dozen Chinese psychiatric patients who spoke no English. Secure isolation rooms had to be found for the court-detained tuberculosis cases, and not all of the convicts were well enough to return to Rikers Island. Most of the evacuees wound up somewhere in the public hospital system. On Monday, November 5, 2012, Bellevue closed its doors for the first time in its history.

The travails of Sandy showed the hospital at its finest—its staff performing nobly in unimaginable conditions. Lives were saved because doctors and nurses, medical students and hospital workers, bonded together to protect their patients, and each other. And backing them at every turn was the National Guard—"our cavalry," said an admiring Doug Bails. A Bellevue resident put it this way: "I can recall the patient monitor going black from the power failure; the smell of gasoline in a stairwell, where people had spontaneously formed a brigade to fuel a backup generator on the 13th floor; and the physical exhaustion of safely carrying a patient down the staircase. I describe that night as the most rewarding experience of my career. . . . The visceral feeling of 'This is why I went into medicine' is my most powerful sentiment left behind from the storm."

Many shared his perception. But others couldn't help asking how it came to this. What had made Bellevue so vulnerable? Was it a freakish act of nature or a failure to shore up the hospital's primary defenses? And why did it take so long to evacuate, given the lessons of Katrina? With much of its infrastructure in ruins, its patients scattered to the winds, Bellevue faced an uncertain future. A disaster preparation expert put it well. "The amount of heroism that arises in situations like this one cannot be overstated," he said. But one has "to wonder why we needed so much heroism."

20

REBIRTH

In the days after Sandy made landfall, Manhattan became two distinct boroughs. There was life above 39th Street, where the storm caused little damage or inconvenience, and life below 39th Street, where the storm brought widespread misery and disruption. New York had experienced blackouts before, but never one this long. A full week without food stores and restaurants, subways and traffic lights, hot water and elevators, turned lower Manhattan into a ghost town. Residents scornfully dubbed it SoPo, for South of Power.

In the three hospitals along Bedpan Alley—the ten-block stretch of First Avenue housing Bellevue, Tisch, and the Manhattan VA—the storm surge not only damaged vital infrastructure, it left behind a toxic sludge of river waste, diesel fuel, leaking chemicals, and asbestos torn from pipes and walls. Early estimates of the repairs and cleanup topped $2 billion. There wasn't even a guess as to when these facilities might reopen.

The structural damage could be repaired. New medical equipment could be replaced. But some losses left a deeper void. One of the devastating consequences of Sandy was its impact on medical research. The storm surge that flooded the generators and elevator shafts drowned thousands of animals stacked in basement cages; the power outage that plunged these buildings into darkness ruined precious cell lines and specimens stored in laboratory freezers. Meanwhile, with the hospitals shuttered and the patients gone, future medical trials were put on hold.

The greatest damage occurred at NYU's Smilow Research Center, a few blocks north of Bellevue, where ten thousand rodents were housed. "Most of our knockout mice were destroyed," a scientist recalled. "They're the ones we alter by breeding out certain receptors to study disease. By the time we got down to the basement, only the top few rows of the cages were above water. The place stank of diesel fuel. It was dark and cold and the food was gone. Four years later, we're just getting back to where we were."

It was an all-too-common story. Genetically engineered mice are essential to research in arthritis, brain disorders, cancers, diabetes, and other diseases. "I felt an awful sense of despair for the suffering and loss of the animals, for the years of work lost and for the impact this would have on the people in my lab who had put their hearts and souls into their research," a biologist wrote of the carnage.

When the power failed, the laboratory freezers clicked off. Bags of dry ice and tanks of liquid nitrogen were hauled up five, ten, fifteen flights of stairs by volunteer bucket brigades. "We made a dash to retrieve our thawing specimens," NYU's chief of medicine recalled. "We rescued nearly all of the current studies, but lost some of our archives—samples obtained from villages and patients all over the world. . . . They were irreplaceable."

Instant decisions had to be made. One researcher got a frantic call from his department administrator. Electricians had just arrived to hardwire emergency lighting in the stairwells, he was told, and everybody in the lab could select one item to receive power. What would it be? The researcher picked his minus-80-degree freezer, which contained a career's worth of yeast samples, knowing that all else would be lost. "It was," he said, "like Sophie's Choice."

Bellevue had its own problems. A number of its labs were devoted to AIDS and drug-resistant tuberculosis. It wasn't simply a matter of saving precious research; some of the samples were hazardous if not properly contained. "We began packing up whatever we could in dry ice because my minus-80 degree [freezers] had warmed up to minus 49," the director of Bellevue's HIV/AIDS Trial Group recalled. "By the next day, they were at 4 degrees and all the remaining samples were lost." In some places, she said, "it was like walking through a giant slushy." But contamination was prevented.

The loss of so many animals and specimens raised the obvious question: Was it avoidable? And the somewhat surprising answer along Bedpan Alley was: probably not. Most researchers pinned the blame on nature, not on human error (or, perhaps, a combination of both). Only a freakish mega-storm of Sandy's size and violence could have flooded these buildings, they believed. And only a fortune-teller could have foreseen the catastrophic damage it left behind. "We knew that a hurricane was coming," a particularly hard-hit researcher explained. "We put things away and checked that the emergency power was on. The animal care people gave our mice extra water and food; we couldn't move the mice, because they had to stay in a germ-free environment to avoid infections, and there was nowhere large enough to put them." Everything that could be done *had* been done.

From a distance, however, a rather different portrait emerged. Animal rights activists skewered these facilities for leaving caged animals to die in the dark. "If you were one of the mice who drowned, it may have been more of a blessing," wrote one, referring to the "pain and suffering" inflicted by medical research. But criticism also came from those who had suffered similar losses in the past. In 2001, Hurricane Allison drowned tens of thousands of caged mice at the Baylor and University of Texas medical research facilities in Houston, along with dozens of monkeys, rabbits, and dogs. Five years later, Katrina killed thousands more living underground at LSU and Tulane. As a result, all four universities had taken steps to prevent a recurrence. "We will never place animals or critical equipment in the basement again," UT's president declared.

But few hospitals or universities followed suit. Even along Bedpan Alley, which rested on landfill abutting an ocean-fed river, a feeling of apathy—or false confidence—prevailed. Most of the buildings there predated Katrina, and moving heavy equipment to higher floors was expensive and gobbled up space needed for patient suites and state-of-the-art medical hardware. Put simply, infrastructure is invisible until the very moment it fails. As one expert put it: "People don't pick hospitals based on which one has the best generator."

Many researchers, moreover, preferred keeping their animals belowground. There were all sorts of rationalizations—it was cheaper space;

rodents thrive in low artificial light; the microbes they carry have less chance of escaping—but the desire to keep them hidden almost certainly played a role. "[Our] centers are the site of massive rodent slaughter . . . ," a researcher noted. "It's ugly work, even when it's useful and important."

Whatever the logic, the lesson was widely ignored, despite repeated warnings from those who knew best. "I talk about disasters all over the world," said a researcher who suffered through Hurricane Allison, "and I just tell them, 'Get your animals out of your basement.'"

Bellevue reopened in stages over the next ninety-nine days. First a few outpatient clinics and the pharmacy, then several more clinics and the Emergency Department—and, on February 7, the main hospital and its 828 beds. During this time, the staff faced a problem rarely seen, much less navigated, in the past: how to monitor the hundreds of patients who were evacuated and the thousands more who relied on Bellevue's multitude of clinics for their primary care. Tracking them became a logistical nightmare. Prescriptions had to be filled and operations rescheduled. X-rays, blood tests, dialysis, methadone—all had to be provided somewhere else. The crisis took on a name: the Bellevue diaspora.

Cooperation was essential. The hospitals that admitted the evacuees also provided space for the displaced Bellevue doctors and nurses. Glitches arose over things like record sharing and credentialing, but a rough kind of order soon emerged. "Hand-scrawled messages were taped to our cubicle," an internist recalled. "Psychiatry was at Metropolitan; the Cancer Center at Woodhull Hospital in Brooklyn. Dermatology was seeing patients in Manhattan, but only on Wednesdays and Thursdays. Dialysis was at Jacobi in the Bronx. . . . Each day a few locations were crossed out and new ones added."

If there was a silver lining, it was the recognition of how valuable Bellevue's services were, and how hard it was to get on without them. Doctors at other city hospitals were struck by the level of coordination and sophistication among the teams of Bellevue residents, nurses, and attending physicians who arrived to treat their evacuated patients. It was a level of care, some acknowledged, rarely seen at their own institutions. In the weeks after Sandy, moreover, the emergency room at Weill Cornell Medical Center, forty blocks to the north, was so jammed that the normal four-to-six-hour wait for a bed soon reached twelve to fourteen hours. The same held true for specialty clinics across the city—now forced to handle a surge of new patients, many of them foreign-speaking and uninsured. Bellevue averaged 500,000 visits a year. Its closing had proved a grim reminder of its worth.

In October 2014, exactly two years after the superstorm, a story aired on NBC News about the recovery efforts then under way. Titled "A Tale of Two Hospitals," it compared the paths of Bellevue and NYU Langone Medical Center, which included Tisch Hospital. Both had been forced to evacuate during Sandy and both had suffered catastrophic damage. Yet, standing just two blocks apart, their stories could not have been more different.

As the NBC report noted, NYU Langone had already received $1.2 billion from the Federal Emergency Management Agency (FEMA), the second-largest payout in the agency's history. And the money had come in one lump sum, rather than the usual approach of doling out funds piecemeal as repairs were made and bills submitted. On top of this, the National Institutes of Health had given NYU Medical School another $218 million for its research recovery plans, which included the construction of a new vivarium for lab animals on a higher floor.

Bellevue, meanwhile, had received only $117 million from FEMA to this point, and would be sharing just a fraction of the NIH largesse. Digging deeper, the NBC investigative team discovered that NYU Langone held an insurance policy to cover some of the storm damage—including $150 million for "research losses"—and that questions had been raised by FEMA officials about "using vast sums of money to bail out a private medical institution, especially one with ample private insurance."

While not explicitly crying foul, the NBC report dropped some strong hints about the lobbying clout behind the NYU Langone awards. The Medical Center's Board of Trustees read like a Who's

Who of Wall Street titans: JPMorgan Chase CEO Jamie Dimon, Goldman Sachs president Gary Cohn, and BlackRock CEO Larry Fink. And the center's namesake, Home Depot cofounder Ken Langone, had close ties to Republican House majority leader Eric Cantor and to New York's senior Democratic senator, Chuck Schumer, who publicly announced the awards. This stark difference in funding, said NBC, "raised uncomfortable questions about disparities in the way FEMA has treated the two hospitals in the wake of Sandy."

The report sparked more anger than surprise. Who didn't expect a well-connected private hospital to get preferential treatment in such circumstances? "When NYU has an army of wealthy donors, whilst Bellevue is consigned to treat the city's uninsured," there was no hope of equity, a critic wrote—though he, like many others, was startled by the "obscene" gap between the two awards.

There was more to the story, however. As a private operator, free of government red tape, NYU Langone put its FEMA proposal together within months of the storm. Bellevue, on the other hand, endured numerous inspections and estimates, while the city's final application to FEMA included three public hospitals besides Bellevue seeking relief. In truth, Schumer had fast-tracked the document when it finally arrived. Three weeks after the NBC story broke, he announced a FEMA commitment of $1.6 billion for New York City's storm-damaged public hospitals, with Bellevue receiving $376 million for projects that included a 3,200-foot-long wall to protect the hospital's perimeter and the movement of essential equipment to higher ground.

For some, the timing of these FEMA funds was hardly accidental. The NBC report played a role but so, too, did a global health alert that soon became the year's most terrifying news story. At the very moment Senator Schumer was making his announcement, the streets surrounding Bellevue were clogged with TV trucks and satellite dishes. A patient had just arrived with a deadly infectious disease. Fears of a pandemic were spreading, and few American hospitals appeared ready for what lay ahead. Bellevue, Schumer confidently declared, was one of those few.

—

In the summer of 2014, with Ebola tearing through the West African nations of Guinea, Liberia, and Sierra Leone, a group of Bellevue staffers began preparing for its likely appearance in New York. Selected for the role by state officials, the hospital seemed a natural choice. Its history stretched from the yellow fever outbreaks of the 1790s to the AIDS epidemic of recent decades, and it already contained a unit for treating critically ill patients in quarantine—mainly those with drug-resistant tuberculosis. If and when an Ebola victim turned up, most likely at Kennedy Airport, Bellevue would be the destination.

In the meantime, Americans got a tragic lesson in all that could go wrong. In late September, a Liberian national named Thomas Eric Duncan arrived in Dallas for a family visit. Feeling ill, he went to the emergency room at Texas Health Presbyterian Hospital, complaining of a headache and abdominal pain. Duncan had a slight temperature; his vital signs seemed "unremarkable." The nurse who examined him jotted down "came from Africa, 9/20/2014" on his chart, but nobody took notice—not even when his second temperature reading hit 103 before dropping two degrees with medication. The doctor who finally saw Duncan prescribed an antibiotic, which has no effect on viruses, and sent him home.

Duncan was rushed back to Presbyterian by ambulance a few days later with a high fever, vomiting, and diarrhea. This time the examining physician, noting the patient's travel history, donned protective gear and cleared the intensive care unit before admitting him. By now, however, it was too late. With virtually no preparation for Ebola, the technician charged with handling Duncan's blood work had to search the web to see if he had followed proper procedure (he hadn't), and it took four days to get back the results. The nurses caring for Duncan were unsure of what clothing to put on or how to properly dispose of it. They, too, relied on the Internet, with growing alarm. "We were looking at the pictures . . . and saying, 'We're not wearing anything like that,'" one of them recalled. Thomas Duncan died at Presbyterian on October 8; two of his nurses contracted Ebola, but survived.

Ironically, the hospital enjoyed a good reputation in Dallas. With nine hundred beds, a $600 million annual budget, and a well-respected staff, it attracted numerous celebrity patients, including former president George W. Bush. "In all fairness, critics have overlooked the role that bad luck played in Presbyterian's medical missteps," wrote a local columnist. "Duncan could have turned up in any emergency room in the country and it's disingenuous to suppose that every one of them was fully prepared for the unexpected, unprecedented arrival of the first undiagnosed Ebola patient on the continent."

This, no doubt, was true. But New York City, unlike Dallas, had anticipated the likelihood of Ebola by designating its flagship hospital to lead the fight. Drills began that August, when the World Health Organization declared an "international health emergency." Staffers trained in layers of protective gear comparable in weight and mobility to the gear they employed during earlier sarin gas attack drills—fluid-resistant gowns, knee-length booties, double gloves, and a PAPR (Powered Air-Purifying Respirator) with a face shield. Special equipment was tested, such as an electronic stethoscope that didn't expose the ears. "It's a cool gadget," said Laura Evans, Bellevue's director of critical care. "It looks like a hockey puck, but you get a nice sound quality—much better than the disposable stethoscopes we've tried."

A thirty-one-page "Ebola Response Guide" set down the rules. "Blood draws should be kept to an absolute minimum to decrease the risk of needle sticks," it stated, adding that samples "must be double-bagged in a special transportation box, which is then wiped down with bleach." To prevent the sort of mistakes that had doomed Thomas Duncan, "special shoppers" were dispatched to the ER to see how well the staff took travel histories and recognized Ebola-like symptoms. Dozens of suspicious cases were reported; none tested positive for Ebola, though a fair number were found to suffer from malaria and typhoid fever.

As a leading teaching hospital, Bellevue relied heavily on interns, residents, and even students for its medical care. The house staff at Bellevue was well known for taking "ownership" of the patient; it was one of the attractions of working there. Thus, when Ebola appeared, the house staff expected to play a major role. A petition was even circulated with the names of volunteers. Almost everybody signed.

But this time would be different. No one expected Bellevue to be flooded with Ebola patients. The virus was deadly, fast-moving, and extremely infectious. There was no time to waste training dozens of superfluous people who might contract the disease and spread it to others. The best option was to recruit a group of veterans from the relevant units—infectious disease specialists, ICU nurses, and the like. Containment was key. "Our philosophy for Ebola," said a Bellevue official, "is to have as few people as possible exposed to the patient, and that those people are at the highest level of experience and competency."

The test came in late October. "EBOLA HITS NYC," warned the *New York Post*. The news that Craig Spencer, a volunteer with Doctors Without Borders, had tested positive after returning from a field hospital in Guinea set the city on edge. Where, exactly, had Dr. Spencer been in the days before he began to show symptoms? And what threat did he pose to the people he'd come into contact with? One point was certain, though: Spencer would be spending his days at Bellevue until he fully recovered or succumbed to the disease.

His new quarters were a guarded suite in the isolation ward on the seventh floor, where patients with drug-resistant tuberculosis, an outgrowth of the AIDS epidemic, were housed in rooms with negative air pressure, ultraviolet lights to kill airborne bacteria, and HEPA (High Efficiency Particle Air) filters. With its own waste disposal systems and a laboratory for on-site testing, the ward was fully self-sufficient. Each suite contained an anteroom to "don" and "doff" protective clothing and an inner room for the patient, with extra power for lifesaving equipment. Nurses worked in pairs—a kind of buddy system to prevent careless mistakes—while a team from the CDC provided round-the-clock supervision.

When Dr. Spencer arrived at Bellevue, he was still in the early stages of the disease—similar to Thomas Duncan during Duncan's first trip to Presbyterian's emergency room. The staff kept Spencer hydrated and monitored his vital signs. (Falling blood pressure caused by fluid loss from vomiting and diarrhea is one of Ebola's great dangers.) In addition, he received experimental antiviral drugs as well as plasma from a donor who had survived Ebola while working as a missionary in Liberia—and whose blood type, fortuitously, matched his. How well these treatments worked, if at all, isn't known. But they point to the larger truth that everything possible was done to save Spencer's life during his time at Bellevue—unlike the tragedy in Dallas.

Nineteen days later, Spencer was declared "virus-free" and discharged. His ordeal demonstrated that Ebola wasn't necessarily a death sentence, that a well-prepared hospital, treating the disease early and aggressively, stood an excellent chance of saving the patient's life. Indeed, all seven victims admitted to the Ebola centers at Emory and the University of Nebraska, including the two Dallas nurses, made full recoveries. Only Thomas Duncan died.

It was a heady moment for Bellevue. "She is our flagship," said Mayor Bill de Blasio. "She serves in the toughest times and makes [us] proud." In its year-end "Reasons to Love New York" issue, *New York* magazine listed Bellevue twice in its top ten. Number 7 read: "Because Dr. Laura Evans Saved Craig Spencer's Life." And Number 8 added: "Because Dr. Laura Evans Saved Craig Spencer's Life with the Help of 119 Others"—which included snapshots of the nurses, doctors, technicians, pharmacists, waste managers, and security officers who had served on Spencer's detail.

In praising Bellevue, *New York* had inadvertently exposed the downside of the Ebola experience. Caring for Craig Spencer had taxed the institution beyond its limits. So many experienced nurses were involved that patients in the adult and pediatric ICUs had to be moved to other hospitals. Exhaustion set in, especially among those having to wear and discard the heavy protective gear. Some staffers spoke of being shunned by frightened coworkers; others, fearful of harming their families, asked to sleep in the hospital. There were rumors of "sick-outs" and high absentee rates, and the constant bedlam of roving TV crews thrusting microphones at anyone in medical scrubs.

Saving Craig Spencer's life was an extreme challenge. The cost ran into the millions; treating Spencer's medical waste alone was estimated at $100,000 a day. "We like to think of ourselves as a 'bring it on' hospital," Bellevue's chief of medical service recalled. "We're essential. We can handle just about anything." For all the fear and trouble it brought, Ebola proved him right.

EPILOGUE

Within a day or two of Craig Spencer's medical discharge, Bellevue became Bellevue again. Staffers went back to their normal posts; the ICUs returned to full capacity. The media packed up and moved on. The Great Ebola Scare of 2014—the one that barely reached American shores—is now a fading memory. Though the seventh-floor isolation ward remains "active," and the occasional "suspicious" traveler from West Africa is brought in for quarantine and testing, the urgency is gone.

It was no accident that Bellevue, a former pesthouse, took in Craig Spencer. In treating the "Ebola Doctor," Laura Evans and her team trod the path first taken by young Alexander Anderson during the yellow fever epidemics of the 1790s and followed thereafter by generations of nurses and physicians battling cholera, typhus, puerperal fever, influenza, tuberculosis, and AIDS. It's among the services long demanded of Bellevue by the nation's largest, densest, most diverse city—and one certain to continue. History assures us that Ebola will be fully tamed, but that the next "fatal strain" is also bubbling up somewhere—in a bat cave, a pig farm, an open-air poultry market. That's the nature of the war between humans and microbes. There is never a truce.

To enter Bellevue's main lobby today is to see the intersection of the present and the past. In 2005, a five-story atrium designed by Pei Cobb Freed opened to rave reviews. One side contains a sleek, glass-enclosed galleria housing the hospital's many inpatient clinics. The other side contains the brick-and-granite facade of the old administration building designed by McKim, Mead & White, with its ornate carvings and quaintly dated inscriptions. (One reads "Employes," a common usage a century ago.) The floor is polished marble, gaslight sconces are on display, and down a long corridor sits a horse-driven ambulance from 1898. There's a beefed-up security presence, and no visible signs of the damage left by Superstorm Sandy.

Yet it is in the patient areas where the past and present truly intersect. Bellevue plays many roles, as Craig Spencer's case made abundantly clear. But its primary one—to serve the poorer classes of a constantly evolving city—remains unchanged. Today, as before, its patients are overwhelmingly immigrants and their young children—no longer from Europe, but from Mexico, Central America, the Caribbean, West Africa, South Asia, and China. (Whites now rank last in the category of "patient race.") Few at Bellevue carry private or group health insurance. Indeed, the hospital receives more money from the Department of Corrections for treating prisoners than it does from Blue Cross/Blue Shield. Most patients rely on some form of Medicaid; the rest are called "self-pay," a euphemism for "no-pay," meaning the uninsured.

As a vital safety net hospital, Bellevue relies heavily on programs like the state's Indigent Care Pool and the federal government's Disproportionate Share Hospital plan to pick up what the city cannot afford. This largesse has been rapidly declining, however, and there are fears that Obamacare's restrictions on undocumented immigrants, who are ineligible for public coverage, will make things even worse. The principle of free medical care for the indigent in New York remains firm; but the implementation, excepting the Great Depression of the 1930s, has rarely been harder.

Some problems seem to defy solution. Scattered throughout Bellevue today are forty to fifty patients receiving Alternate Level of Care (ALOC). Many hospitals have them—though in smaller numbers and in much better shape. The acronym refers to someone in an acute care hospital who no longer needs acute care. But the person cannot be discharged unless he has somewhere safe to go. Some stay for two months at Bellevue, some for two years and longer. A fair number have died there. It's a staggering drain on Bellevue's limited resources, and it speaks volumes about the kind of patients it routinely admits.

There's a young man with AIDS, "very combative—sent to Bronx Lebanon and sent back same day." A "homeless female" from the Caribbean with "cognitive impairment. Sister stopped returning our calls." A seventy-seven-year-old man from Sri Lanka, "demented. No family here. Needs a walker." An "undoc. homeless man—dementia . . . cannot function in a shelter." "A middle-aged male with cog. issues— malnutrition, lice, HIV, dementia—all referrals denied."

A voluntary hospital can more easily discharge its ALOC patients because many have family attachments and private insurance. Bellevue has no such luxury. "Think of fifty valuable beds in an eight-hundred-bed hospital that never turn over," an official said. "Fifty beds! It's a sad commentary, but you just can't release vulnerable patients without considering the consequences." A physician familiar with these patients describes them as "our triple threat—undocumented, uninsured, undomiciled." In truth, he adds, "they're not so different from Bellevue's medical population. They just stay a lot longer."

More than a third of Bellevue's current inpatients fill its once notorious psychiatric wards. It is no surprise, therefore, that familiar diagnoses like "schizophrenia" and other "psychoses" are among the leading causes for admission. But today there are popular diagnoses that were barely acknowledged at Bellevue a century ago, such as "cocaine dependence," "opioid abuse," and "cellulitis and other bacterial skin infections"—the scourge of the homeless. There are few better barometers for studying a city's social needs.

Several years ago, four NYU doctors with deep ties to Bellevue wrote a stirring defense of the role of the public hospital in American medical education. Where else, they wrote, could an aspiring nurse or physician, "not yet accepting of the status quo," confront the "harsher inequities" of modern life, from AIDS and substance abuse to homelessness and prison health care? Public hospitals "embody a sense of mission. The core ethos of working in a place that exists to minister to the sick regardless of the walk of life or ability to pay is enormously influential in shaping the worldview of [those] in training."

It wasn't for everyone, they admitted. Ethos and adventure went only so far. Bellevue was frustrating and chaotic—under-budgeted, under-staffed, and crammed with patients "whose unmet psychological needs foster frequent repeat hospitalizations." Still, those who trained there got to experience "the very values that led them to the choice of medicine as a career." In treating the weak, they strengthened themselves.

That training mission remains firmly in place. What has changed at Bellevue over the years is the research component, which, while ongoing, no longer dazzles. The laboratories that nurtured the likes of William Welch and Hermann Biggs, Walter Reed and Albert Sabin, Dickinson Richards and André Cournand, are mostly gone. The patient-oriented research that once occurred in great public hospitals like Bellevue has been usurped, to a great degree, by Contract Research Organizations (CROs) that rely on subjects from the larger community for clinical trials. Hospital patients no longer dominate this process. And the research itself, based on genetically engineered animals, cells in culture, crystals, mass data collection, and a veritable army of laboratory personnel, is no longer a priority of the city's financially strapped public hospital system. It is no surprise that the locus of activity has shifted a few blocks north to the impressive facilities in and around the NYU Langone Medical Center, where competitive federal grant money pours in and top research scientists are aggressively recruited.

NYU receives close to $170 million a year from the city to provide medical services to Bellevue. It's a relationship that goes back more than a century, and in comparison to New York's other affiliation contracts, it has worked extremely well. Bellevue's emergency services are second to none. Its clinics provide first-rate primary care, and its doctors are master diagnosticians, having seen just about everything. Imagining Bellevue without NYU, or vice versa, seems an affront to history. One remains a premier teaching hospital; the other provides structure, continuity, and academic prestige.

Recently, Mayor Bill de Blasio vowed to funnel an extra $2 billion in subsidies into Health + Hospitals, which runs the city's bleeding public system. Much of the money is earmarked for neighborhood clinics—the aim being primary care over hospitalization whenever possible. But de Blasio made it clear that the public hospital system would be protected—that its centuries of service, led by Bellevue, are part of what makes New York special. "It is not for sale," he said, "and the city will not abandon it."

Lewis Thomas, the physician/essayist and National Book Award winner, liked to tell the story about a New York City street scene at the turn of the twentieth century. A woman lay on the sidewalk, the crowd around her frozen in panic. Then, from the very back, a booming voice was heard: "I am a Bellevue man. Let me through!" The sea of bodies parted. A doctor emerged, medical bag in hand, to revive the woman and bring her to her feet. The crowd burst into hearty applause.

For Dr. Thomas, Bellevue embodied the better angels of medicine, despite its many warts. His story was about respect and knowledge and helping people who are down. For millions of New Yorkers, it still rings true.

ACKNOWLEDGMENTS

This project was born, I recall, during a conversation with my good friend Dick Foley, then dean of the NYU Faculty of Arts and Sciences. I was coming to New York following a dozen glorious years at the University of Texas, and the history of iconic Bellevue, the primary teaching hospital for NYU, seemed a natural extension of my growing interest in medicine and public health.

The generosity of colleagues can hardly be overstated. Sandra Opdycke, author of *No One Was Turned Away*, a superb narrative comparing the paths of public Bellevue and private New York Hospital during the twentieth century, shared her voluminous research with me—an absolute life preserver given the impact of Superstorm Sandy upon Bellevue's spotty archive. Dr. Stanley Burns, director of the enormously rich Burns Archive, sparked my interest in medical photography, while Lynn Berger volunteered information regarding Bellevue's first photographer, O. G. Mason. Dr. Ira Rutkow, author and friend, was an insightful guide to the trajectory of American medicine. Dr. Daniel Roses, a chronicler of Bellevue's rich history, provided key insights about the hospital's past.

No one has done more to preserve that past for other researchers than Lorinda Klein, who critiqued this manuscript with a very sharp eye. Though Lorinda and I sometimes disagreed on the interpretations in this book, her comments proved a most valuable tool.

Special thanks, as well, to Dr. Doug Bails, chief of medical service at Bellevue, for his guidance in explaining both the workings of the hospital and its vital importance to the city it serves. Doug perfectly represents the spirit of medical excellence and public commitment that have marked Bellevue for close to three centuries.

Historians depend heavily on the skill and ingenuity of librarians and archivists; I was extremely fortunate to encounter some of the best, including Sushan Chin at NYU's Lapidus Health Sciences Library; Arlene Shaner at the New York Academy of Medicine; Mariam Touba at the New-York Historical Society; Stephen Novak at the Columbia Health Sciences Library; and Margorie Kehoe and Nancy McCall at the Johns Hopkins Chesney Medical Archives.

Numerous current and former colleagues at Bellevue and NYU Langone shared essential information: documents, photographs, and personal correspondence. I am deeply indebted to Robert Holzman, Elihu Sussman, Nathan Thompson, Fred Valentine, and Arthur Zitrin, among others. Many sat down with me for personal interviews and reminiscences, often more than once: Martin Blaser, Douglas Bails, Mitchell Charap, Barry Coller, Patrick Cox, Bruce Cronstein, Laura Evans, David Goldfarb, Roberta Goldring, Loren Greene, Martin Kahn, James Lebret, Jerome Lowenstein, Charles Marmar, Ruth and Victor Nussenzweig, Danielle Ofri, Dennis Popeo, David Stern, Elihu Sussman, Nathan Thompson, Fred Valentine, Jan Vilcek, Gerald Weissmann, and Arthur Zitrin.

In addition, I would like to thank Dr. Robert Grossman, dean and CEO of NYU Langone Medical Center; Dr. Steven Abramson, chief of medicine; and Katherine Wesnousky, chief of staff of the Department of Medicine, for providing a supportive environment for the writing of this book; Katie Grogan for her research assistance; Troi Santos, for his expert photographic help; Marc Triola, for explaining the mystery of numbers to a novice; Amy Lehman, for sharp analysis; and, especially, Stacy Bodziak, for simply being indispensable in all matters relating to the Division of Medical Humanities.

My friend and agent, Chris Calhoun, brought me to the ideal publishing house. At Doubleday, I had the extreme good fortune to interact with Bill Thomas, Dan Meyer, and Kris Puopolo, editor par excellence. Her enthusiasm for the book was infectious. Her patience in guiding it to completion bordered on saintly. Every author should be so fortunate. I owe Kris a debt of gratitude that grows with each reminder of her professional skill and personal kindness.

Much has changed in my life since this project began, including a new job; the loss of my beloved brother, Steve; and the birth of my amazing granddaughter, June. What has remained constant is my endless good luck in having Jane Oshinsky at my side. Her quiet strengths put my petty anxieties into perspective. Authors tend to be congenital loners; Jane is my cure.

A NOTE ON SOURCES

Much of this book is based on archival material—most coming from places beyond Bellevue Hospital, whose older records, already scattered and poorly maintained, were further damaged by Superstorm Sandy. Fortunately, records relating to admissions and patient care, as well as casebooks, correspondence, and personal papers, are available at numerous other archives, including the Sid and Ruth Lapidus Health Sciences Library at New York University, the New-York Historical Society, the New York Academy of Medicine, the Library of Congress, the National Library of Medicine, the New York City Municipal Archives, the Harry Ransom Center, the Brooklyn College Library, the Health Services Library at Columbia University, the Chesney Archives at Johns Hopkins Medical School, and the archives of the psychiatry department at Weill Cornell Medical Center. In addition, the annual reports of the various city agencies overseeing Bellevue throughout its history are publicly available and remarkably thorough.

Oral history plays a large role in the book. Dozens of current NYU/Bellevue staffers kindly sat down for interviews, as did former medical students, residents, and faculty. Each interviewee is listed in the acknowledgments. I also used archives of the Columbia Center for Oral History, the American Academy of Pediatrics, and the recently established Oral History Project at NYU Medical School.

There is a vast literature on the history of medicine, public health, and hospitals in the United States. A good place to start is Charles

Rosenberg, *The Care of Strangers,* written thirty years ago but still the gold standard in the field. Other essential works include Jerome Groopman, *How Doctors Think;* Kenneth Ludmerer, *Learning to Heal;* Regina Morantz-Sanchez, *Sympathy and Science;* Sherwin Nuland, *Doctors: The Biography of Medicine;* Paul Starr, *The Social Transformation of American Medicine;* and Rosemary Stevens, *In Sickness and in Wealth.* The literature for New York City is also quite vast. Sweeping histories of public health, the emergence of voluntary hospitals, and the confluence of immigration and disease are found in John Duffy's massive two-volume *History of Public Health in New York City;* David Rosner, *A Once Charitable Enterprise;* and Alan Kraut, *Silent Travelers.* For an indispensable general history of New York City until 1898, nothing compares to *Gotham,* by Edwin Burrows and Mike Wallace.

Certain books were especially helpful to me in providing vital insight and information about specific medical events, trends, and controversies. These include Deborah Blum, *The Poisoner's Handbook,* on the birth of forensic medicine; Sheri Fink, *Five Days at Memorial,* on the medical consequences of Hurricane Katrina; Victoria Harden, *AIDS at 30,* on the changing face of America's most feared infectious disease; Steven Johnson, *The Ghost Map,* on the birth of modern epidemiology; Gina Kolata, *Flu,* on the mysteries of the 1918–19 pandemic; Howard Markel, *An Anatomy of Addiction,* on the impact of cocaine on two towering medical figures, one a Bellevue surgeon; Candice Millard, *Destiny of the Republic,* on the link between a presidential assassination and the rise of antiseptic medicine; Jane Mottus, *New York Nightingales,* on the revolutionary Bellevue School of Nursing; Ira Rutkow, *Bleeding Blue and Gray,* on medical progress—and lack of it—during the Civil War; and Ted Steinberg, *Gotham Unbound,* on the interplay of ecology and public health in New York City.

The bookshelves groan with memoirs of patients and physicians about their experiences at Bellevue. The most recent include Eric Manheimer, *Twelve Patients,* a poignant and perceptive account of some of the cases he treated as Bellevue's former medical director; and Julie Holland, *Weekends at Bellevue,* a riveting look at the psychiatric emergency room by a physician interweaving her personal experiences with those of patients. There hasn't been a history of Bellevue per se in sixty years, but Sandra Opdycke's more recent *No One Was Turned Away,* a look at New York City medical care seen through the lens of New York Hospital and Bellevue, is a remarkably fluid and perceptive piece of writing.

NOTES

INTRODUCTION

1   "If a cop gets shot": Eric Manheimer, *Twelve Patients* (2012), 2–3.

2   "It was never the tidiest": William Nolen, "Bellevue: No One Was Ever Turned Away," *American Heritage* (February–March 1987).

2   "a staggeringly ugly experience": *New York Times*, December 3, 1945.

3   "spades": Norman Mailer, "Bellevue Diary," Norman Mailer Papers, Harry Ransom Center, Austin, Texas.

4   "When I first knew": Frederick Covan, quoted in *New York Post,* April 1, 2008.

Chapter 1: Beginnings

11   "And they took counsel": Matthew 27:7.

11   "The field lies in the neighborhood": I. N. P. Stokes, *The Iconography of Manhattan Island* (1926), vol. 5, 1340.

12   "The wheels of these chariots": *Life and Writings of Grant Thorburn Prepared by Himself* (1852), 46–50.

12   "Here lies the body of James Jackson": *New York Times,* October 28, 2009.

12   "It is important to remark": Ibid., November 12, 2009.

13   "the reception and cure": "History of Pennsylvania Hospital, *Penn Medicine,* www.uphs.upenn.edu.

13   "laid the beams and raised the roof": Claude Heaton, "The Origins and Growth of Bellevue Hospital," *The Academy Bookman* (1959), 3–10.

13   "to be Lousey": Ibid.

13   "the seed from which grew": John Starr, *Hospital City* (1957), 9.

13   "the prodigious influx": *Minutes of the Common Council of the City of New York,* September 15, 1794, 101.

14	"delightfully situated": *Memoirs of the Life and Writings of Lindley Murray* (1827), 48–49.

14	"For SALE or to be LET": *New York Daily Advertiser,* January 29, 1788.

14	"to serve as a hospital": Francis Beekman, "The Origins of Bellevue Hospital," *New-York Historical Society Quarterly* (July 1953), 214.

16	"The yellow fever will discourage the growth": Thomas Jefferson to Dr. Benjamin Rush, *The Letters of Thomas Jefferson,* September 23, 1800.

16–17	"effluvia arising directly from the body": Gary Shannon, "Disease Mapping and Early Theory of Yellow Fever," *Professional Geographer* (1981), 221–27; Bob Arnebeck, "Yellow Fever in New York City," copy in author's possession.

17	"five or six": Arnebeck, "Yellow Fever in New York City."

17	"covered with blisters": Valentine Seaman, *An Account of the Epidemic Yellow Fever as It Appeared in the City of New York in 1795* (1796), 3.

18	"Passed a restless and perturbed night": *The Diary of Elihu Hubbard Smith,* September 6, 1795 (reprinted 1973 by the American Philosophical Society).

18	"to prevent the infectious Distemper": Minutes of the New York City Health Committee, in Beekman, "The Origins of Bellevue Hospital."

18	"Dr. Smith reported": Ibid.

18	"In consequence of [this] rejection": Matthew Livingston Davis, *A Brief Account of the Epidemical Fever Which Lately Prevailed in the City of New York* (1796), 17–18.

18	"in a state of confusion": Alexander Anderson Diary, August 24, 1795, in Frederick Burr, *Life and Works of Alexander Anderson* (1893).

19	"reading all the medical books within reach": Ibid., Appendix A, 84.

19	"My present employment": Alexander Anderson Diary, October 10, 1795.

19	"[They] consist of Mr. Fisher": Ibid., August 24, 1795.

19	"We lost three patients today": Ibid., September 15, 1795.

19	"Another patient sent up in shocking condition": Ibid., August 27, 1795.

19	"She is addicted to liquor": Ibid., October 8, 1795.

20	"glory in a disregard to Feelings": Ibid., August 30, 1795.

20	"Dr. Chickering's timidity": Ibid., July 30, 1798.

20	"Nearly 750 of [our] inhabitants": "Report to the Governor," in Beekman, "The Origins of Bellevue Hospital," 226.

20	"I passed three months among yellow fever patients": Burr, *Life and Works,* Appendix A, 85.

20	"I soon discovered": Ibid., 86.

20	"I am really desperate": Ibid.

22	"apprenticed to Dr. Charlton" and others: Appendix: "List of Medical Practitioners of Eighteenth Century New York City and Long Island," in Marynita Anderson, *Physician Heal Thyself* (2004), 150–89.

22 "who had a reputation for skill with the sick": Zachary Friedenberg, *The Doctor in Colonial America* (1998), 107–10; Byron Stookey, *A History of Colonial Medical Education,* 11–18; Ira Rutkow, *Seeking the Cure* (2010), 7–27.

23 Those in medical practice routinely described themselves: List of alternate professions in *Physician Heal Thyself,* 151–89.

23 "The law makes no account": *New York Literary Gazette,* vol. 2 (1827), 21.

24 "Bloodletting was the single most": Robert Golder, "Visual and Artifactual Materials in the History of Early American Medicine," in Robert Golder and P. J. Imperato, *Early American Medicine: A Symposium* (1987), 7.

24 "a reflex for physicians": J. Worth Estes, "Patterns of Drug Use in Colonial America," in ibid., 29–37.

24 an average calendar day: New York City physician calendar contains a list of patients combined from: Dr. Samuel Seabury, "Account Book, 1780–1781," Manuscripts Division, New-York Historical Society (NYHS); and "Fees of Dr. William Lawrence," in John Bard, *The Doctor in Old New York* (1898), 310–11, copy on file in NYHS.

25 The final treatment of George Washington: Drs. James Craik and Elisha Dick, "News from 'The Times,'" reprint from *Medical Repository* (1800), 311; Peter Henriques, "The Final Struggle Between George Washington and the Grim King," *Virginia Magazine of History and Biography* (1999), 73–91.

26 His tombstone: Shearith Israel cemetery, http://www.placematters.net /node/1475.

26 "the Samson of drugs": Rutkow, *Seeking the Cure,* 38.

26 "Two young seamen": Alexander Anderson Diary, August 27, 1798.

26 "I was up all night": Ibid., July 3, 1798.

27 "The sight of [her]": Ibid., September 12, 13, 1798.

27 "I feel surpris'd": Ibid., September 14, 21, 1798.

27 "A tremendous scene have I witnessed": Ibid., December 31, 1798.

27 "Constant employment": Alexander Anderson, *Autobiography,* in Burr, *Life and Works of Alexander Anderson,* Appendix A, 90.

27 "opened only upon extraordinary occasions": Davis, *A Brief Account of the Epidemical Fever Which Lately Prevailed in the City of New York,* 16–17.

28 "So odious is the idea": Ibid.

Chapter 2: Hosack's Vision

30 "raising a considerable clamor": *New York Packet,* April 25, 1788; also Steven Wilf, "Anatomy and Punishment in Late Eighteenth Century New York," *Journal of Social History* (1989), 511–13.

30   "Through your excess": Jules Ladenheim, "The Doctors' Mob of 1788,"
     Journal of the History of Medicine (Winter 1950), 22–43.

30   "the reception of such patients": James J. Walsh, "The Doctors Riot and
     the Quest for Anatomical Material," in Walsh, *History of Medicine in
     New York,* vol. 2 (1919), 378–91.

30   "In the anatomy room": Ladenheim, "The Doctors' Mob of 1788," 23–43.

31   "seriously interrupted the cordial feeling": Ibid.

31   "to Prevent the Odious Practice": Laws of New York State, 1887, 12th
     Session, vol. 11, 5.

32   "sufferings during the whole": David Hosack to William Coleman,
     August 17, 1804, *Alexander Hamilton Papers,* Library of Congress,
     Founders Online.

33   "knocked down with a stone": "David Hosack," in Samuel Gross, *Lives of
     Eminent American Physicians* (1861), 291.

33   "the most proximate cause of the disease": A. E. Hosack, *A Memoir of the
     Late David Hosack* (1861), 293.

33   "he is liberal": Ibid., 34; Ruth Woodward, *Princetonians: 1784–1790: A
     Biographical Directory* (1991), 405.

34   "long and habitual observation": Robert W. Hoge, "A Doctor for All
     Seasons: David Hosack of New York," *American Numismatic Society
     Magazine* (Spring 2007), 46–55.

34   "He carried me to a bad [place]": *The Commissioners of the Almshouse
     vs. Alexander Whistelo . . . ,* 1808, New-York Historical Society (NYHS).
     Also, Craig S. Wilder, *Ebony and Ivy* (2013), 211–20.

34   "Why would a woman": *The Commissioners of the Almshouse vs. Whistelo.*

35   "haggard paupers": Raymond Mohl, *Poverty in New York* (1971), 84.

35   "Not half an hour before he expired": Ezra Stiles Ely, *Journal: The Second
     Journal of the Stated Preacher to the Hospital and Almshouse of the City of
     New York* (1813).

36   "six [additional] acres": *Minutes of the Common Council of the City of New
     York,* April 29, 1811.

36   "Stone Cutters, Carpenters": Ibid., November 27, 1811.

36   "Proposals Will Be Received": *New York Journal,* April 19, 1811.

37   "There is no eleemosynary establishment": Timothy Dwight, *Travels in
     New-England and New-York,* vol. 3 (1823), 440.

37   "Some of you, I am persuaded": John Sanford, "Divine Benevolence to
     the Poor on Opening the Chapel on the New Alms-House, Bellevue"
     (1816), copy on file at NYHS.

37   "The Building lately erected": *Minutes of the Common Council of the City
     of New York,* December 5, 1825.

38   "vile, offensive, and pestilential": Mohl, *Poverty in New York,* 25.

38 "Shipping and trade": Charles Bouldan, "Public Health in New York City," *Bulletin of the New York Academy of Medicine* (June 1943), 423.

39 "great depth and unusual purity": Ted Steinberg, *Gotham Unbound* (2014), 44–50.

39 "most miserable I ever beheld": Tyler Anbinder, "From Famine to Five Points," *American Historical Review* (April 2002), 360.

39 "I saw more drunk folks": Tyler Anbinder, *Five Points* (2001), 26.

39 "world of vice and misery": Ibid.

40 "so long as immense numbers": Edmund Blunt, *Stranger's Guide to the City of New York* (1817), quoted in *Eclectic Review* (January–June 1819), 274.

40 "The smoke and stench": Abel Stevens, ed., "The Five Points," *National Magazine* (1853), 267–71.

41 "well-filled stage coaches": Charles Rosenberg, *The Cholera Years* (1962), 33–34.

42 "O'Neill was seized with the malignant cholera": *Reports of Hospital Physicians and Other Documents Relating to the Cholera Epidemic of 1832* (1832).

42 "Mr. Fitzgerald was by trade a tailor": Ibid.

42 "physical stimulation": Ibid.

42 "Vomiting followed": Ibid.

43 "The patient has only then to recover": Ibid.

43 "I am already satisfied": Ibid.

43 "Tobacco has been administered": Ibid.

43 "stepping over the dead and dying": Page Cooper, *The Bellevue Story* (1948), 34.

43 "I believe it is detrimental to many persons": *Medical and Surgical Reporter* (July–December 1866), 456.

44 "Those sickened must be cured or die off": John Wilford, "How Epidemics Helped Shape the Modern Metropolis," *New York Times Learning Network* (April 16, 2008).

44 "Overcoming sometimes violent resistance": Edwin Burrows and Mike Wallace, *Gotham* (1999), 786.

45 "represented the infancy of the art": George Pierson, *Tocqueville in America* (1938), 90.

Chapter 3: The Great Epidemic

46 "a random patient, with a random disease": *New England Journal of Medicine* (1964), 449.

46 "many times greater": Eric Larrabee, *The Benevolent and Necessary Institution* (1971), 120, 215.

47 "One visited nice persons": Charles Rosenberg, "The Practice of Medicine in New York City a Century Ago," *Bulletin of the History of Medicine* (1967), 229–30.

47 "the best schools of Europe . . . the inhalation of ether . . . The treatment": Philip Van Ingen, *The First Hundred Years of the New York Medical and Surgical Society* (1946), 6–14.

47 "Doctor, I got your bill": John Starr, *Hospital City* (1957), 61.

47 "People labor under the delusion": George Rosen, *Fees and Bills* (1946), 89.

47 "a single day on the exchange": Ibid., 7.

48 "Dodge, Jonathan, M.D.": *Longworth's American Almanac: New York Registry and City Directory* (1857), 208.

48 "the rich man's friend": Robert Ernst, *Immigrant Life in New York City* (1994), 55.

48 "the honest workmen": *New York Evening Post,* December 12, 1828.

49 "a bottle or tea-cup": Charles Rosenberg, "The Rise and Fall of the Dispensary System," *Journal of the History of Medicine* (1974), 32–54.

49 "lure only the young": *New York Times,* May 28, 1855.

49 "a practical school": Rosenberg, "The Rise and Fall of the Dispensary System," 33.

49 "are nothing less than a promiscuous charity": W. Gill Wylie, *Hospitals: The History, Organization, and Construction* (1877), 4, 64.

49 "deserving American poor": Rosenberg, "The Rise and Fall of the Dispensary System," 46–47.

50 "a public receptacle for poor invalids": Larrabee, *The Benevolent and Necessary Institution,* 40.

50 "Persons [of] Decrepitude": William Russell, "The Organization and Work of Bloomingdale Hospital," *State Hospital Quarterly* (August 1919), 437.

51 "Imagine a lunatic asylum": *Report of the Special Committee . . . Relative to a New Organization of the Hospital Department of the Alms-House* (1837), 343–45.

51 "hardened infidels": Charles Rosenberg, *The Care of Strangers* (1987), 45.

52 "The opportunities for relief": Stephen Klips, "Institutionalizing the Poor: The New York City Almshouse," PhD diss., NYU (1980), 5–7.

52 "exceptionally bad habits": Alan Kraut, "Illness and Medical Care Among Irish Immigrants," in Ronald Bayor and Timothy Meagher, *The New York Irish* (1996), 159–61.

53 "The potato was the staff of life": Hasia Diner, "The Most Irish City in the Union," in ibid., 89–90.

53   "Ten deaths among one hundred passengers": Kraut, "Illness and Medical Care Among Irish Immigrants," 155.

54   "removed before ignition": Kathryn Stephenson, "The Quarantine War: The Burning of the New York Marine Hospital in 1858," *Public Health Reports* (January 2004), 79–92.

54   To scroll through the fatalities: Robert Carlisle, *An Account of Bellevue Hospital, with a Catalogue of the Medical and Surgical Staff from 1736 to 1893* (1894), 107–360.

55   "At least two-fifths of those who die": Klips, "Institutionalizing the Poor," 386–88.

56   "It is a subject worthy of congratulation": *Fourth Annual Report of the Governors of the Alms-House, New York for the Year 1852* (1852), 12.

56   "nine of twenty-two": Dr. A. L. Loomis, "The History of Typhus Fever as It Occurred in Bellevue Hospital," *Bulletin of the New York Academy of Medicine* (January 1865), 348–57.

56   "A thorough change in the mode of governing": Dr. D. R. McCready, "Remarks," *Bellevue and Charity Hospitals* (1870), v–xi.

57   "granting their services gratuitously": *Rules and Regulations for the Government of Bellevue Hospital* (1852), copy on file at New-York Historical Society.

57   "three of his students": Ibid.

57   "bleeding, cupping, leeching, and dressing wounds": Ibid.

57   "All are received upon common footing": Ibid.

57   "No person shall be admitted": Ibid.

58   "only patients who are unable to pay": Ibid.

58   "Who shall take care of our sick?": Bernadette McCauley, *Who Shall Take Care of Our Sick?* (2005), viii.

58   "Many are brought in wholly ignorant": Mary Stanley, *Hospitals and Sisterhoods* (1855), 1–2.

58   "a royal hunting ground": McCauley, *Who Shall Take Care of Our Sick?*, 9.

59   "just about the finest thing": Richard Shaw, *Dagger John* (1977), 209.

59   "board, washing, nursing": Sister Marie Walsh, *With a Great Heart* (1965), 13–22.

59   "Building in New York": McCauley, *Who Shall Take Care of Our Sick?*, 53.

59   "To clergymen and other persons": John Francis Richmond, *New York and Its Institutions* (1871), 376.

60   "serve for life": Ibid., 377–78.

61   "The institution is open every day": *Manual of the Corporation of the City of New York* (1857), 323.

61   "of the best in the city": Russel Viner, "Abraham Jacobi and German

Medical Radicalism in Antebellum New York," *Bulletin of the History of Medicine* (1992), 434–63.

62   "buried among *Yehudim* . . . *tefillin* and *zizit*": Hyman Grinstein, *The Rise of the Jewish Community in New York* (1945), 156.

62   "There were over 800 persons present": *New York Times,* February 6, 1852, May 18, 1955.

63   "whose liberal bequeath": Grinstein, *The Rise of the Jewish Community in New York,* 158–59.

63   "in cases of accident or emergency": Tina Levitan, *Islands of Compassion* (1964), 27, 30.

63   "Somewhere in a Jewish cemetery today": B. A. Botkin, *New York City Folklore* (1956), 149–50.

64   "poor Italians": McCauley, *Who Shall Take Care of Our Sick?,* 12.

64   "Here our rich men": McCready, "Remarks," vii–xv.

65   "Myriads swarm at the water side": *New York Times,* April 27, 1860.

65   "At six Monday morning": Ibid.

Chapter 4: Teaching Medicine

66   "pocketing an unlawful fee": *Boston Medical and Surgical Journal,* November 3, 1847.

66   "It is well known": Michael Sappol, *A Traffic of Dead Bodies* (2002), 127.

67   "For the sake of living humanity": "An Appeal to the State of New York," *American Lancet* (October 1853–March 1854), 109.

67   "All vagrants, dying, unclaimed": Sappol, *A Traffic of Dead Bodies,* 122–35.

67   "By offering up their bodies": "A Debt Repaid, Nativism and Dissection in New York State," unpublished paper in author's possession.

67   "whose vices have worn out": Sappol, *A Traffic of Dead Bodies,* 130.

67   "Better that the causes": *Harper's New Monthly* (April 1854), 690–94.

68   "WE PROTECT THE SICK": Sappol, *A Traffic of Dead Bodies,* 131.

68   "Thanks to the enlightened liberality": J. C. Dalton, *History of the College of Physicians and Surgeons* (1888), 84.

68   "the field is now open to all": *Boston Medical and Surgical Journal* (March 1850), 109.

70   "The boy was father to the man": S. D. Gross, *Memoirs of Valentine Mott* (1868), 5.

70   "the largest [gall] stone": "Report of Professor Mott's Surgical Cliniques in the University of New York" (1849–1850), 149.

70   "He cut firmly and boldly": James Parton, *Illustrious Men and Their Achievements* (1856), 530.

70   "Valentine Mott has performed more of the great operations": L. H.

Toledo-Payra, "Valentine Mott: American Surgeon Pioneer," *Journal of Investigative Surgery* (March 2006), 76.

70 "had been drawn up by a gradual contraction": Alfred Charles Post, *Eulogy on the Late Valentine Mott* (1866), delivered before the New York Academy of Medicine.

70 "over a bushel of testicles": "Report of Professor Mott's Surgical Cliniques," 67.

70–71 "In Mott's early Days": Samuel Francis, "Valentine Mott," in *Biographical Sketches of Distinguished Living New York Surgeons* (1866), 25.

71 "The Hercules that finally vanished the Hydra": *Diary of George Templeton Strong,* vol. 1, May 8, 1839.

71 "The scalpel slipped": Francis, "Valentine Mott," 26–27.

72 "He daily rose at 7 o'clock": Gross, *Memoirs of Valentine Mott,* 91.

72 "He is humorous only about the smell of vagrant Greeks": "Valentine Mott," *Bulletin of the New York Academy of Medicine* (August 1925), 213.

73 "this rotten and disgraceful concern": Martin Kaufman, *American Medical Education* (1976), 88–89.

73 Tuition was: Medical School fees and expenses: NYU College of Medicine, "Meeting Minutes, April 12, 1852," Ehrman Medical Archives, NYU Medical School.

73 "The treatment is blood-letting, sir": Claude Heaton, *A Historical Sketch of New York University College of Medicine* (1941), 6.

74 "a Psychological and Literary Phenomenon!": Joseph Ryan, "Doctor Gunning S. Bedford and the Search for Safe Obstetric Care," *Journal of Medical Biography* (August 2008), 134–43.

74 "As a lecturer on anatomy": F. L. M. Pattison, *Granville Sharp Pattison: Anatomist and Antagonist* (1987), 202.

74 "One professor felt for the femoral artery": *New York Herald,* July 21, 1841.

75 "When he was placed on the operating table": Ibid., September 29, 1841.

75 "the withdrawal of Dr. Valentine Mott": Walsh, "New York University Medical College," *History of Medicine in New York* (1919), 150.

75 "every disease mankind is heir to": Dr. B. W. McCready, "Introductory Address . . . Bellevue Hospital Medical College," *American Medical Times* (October 1861), 6.

76 "They galloped her out of the world": Samuel Thomson, *Narrative of the Life and Discoveries of Samuel Thomson* (1832), 68.

76 "This causes the body to lose its heat": Ibid., 19.

76 "studying patients, not books": Ibid., 262.

76 "to make every man his own physician": Michael Flannery, "The Early Botanical Medical Movement as a Reflection of Life, Liberty, and Lit-

eracy in Jacksonian America," *Journal of the Medical Library Association* (October 2002), 442–54.

77 "the radicalism of the barnyard": James Whorton, *Nature Cures: The History of Alternative Medicine in America* (2002), 68.

78 "Five of the [board members] are homeopaths": "College Hospital and Dispensary Reports," *North American Homoeopathic Journal* (1857), 275.

78 "between the two extremes": John Warner, "The Nature-Trusting Heresy," *Perspectives in American History* (1977–78), 317–18.

78 "Blood-letting, as a clinical observation": *Bellevue Medical and Surgical Reports,* November 17, 1860, 170.

78 "a well-appointed hospital crowded with grateful patients": "Majority Report of the Select Committee of the Board of Governors of the Alms-House Department, December 20, 1857," New-York Historical Society.

78 "No one who visits can fail to be struck with the throng of students": Ibid.

79 "Sir, your patient is ready": Thomas Dormandy, *The Worst of Evils: The Fight Against Pain* (2006), 219.

79 "Gentlemen, this is no humbug": Ira Rutkow, *Seeking the Cure* (2010), 55.

80 " 'Will you have your leg off?' ": Ira Rutkow, *American Surgery: An Illustrated History* (1998), 86.

80 "There is not an individual who does not shudder": Steven Lehrer, *Explorers of the* Body (2006), 83; Stephanie Snow, *Blessed Days of Anesthesia* (2008), chapters 2, 3.

80 "Better let the patient suffer a while": Harris Coulter, *Science and Ethics in American Medicine* (1973), 365.

80 "Away with the stupid fanaticism": "Remarks of the Importance of Anesthesia . . . by Valentine Mott," October 4, 1848, New York Academy of Medicine.

81 "it is better to lecture *before* or *after* cutting human flesh": Stephen Smith, "Reminiscences of Two Epochs: Anesthesia and Asepsis," *Johns Hopkins Hospital Bulletin* (1918), 274–77.

81 "the first operation I witnessed": Ibid.

81 "To behold the keen shining knife": Michael Nevins, *Still More Meanderings in Medical History* (2013), 73.

81 "The day is not far distant": "First Announcement and Circular: Bellevue Hospital Medical College," 1861, copy on file at Harry Ransom Center, Austin, Texas.

82 "in each of the departments on instruction": "Minutes of the Executive Committee of Bellevue Hospital," 1862–63, Ehrman Medical Archives, NYU Medical School.

82 *"the habitual neglect of punctuality"*: Ibid.

82   "complete our medical studies elsewhere": John Langone, *Harvard Med* (1995), 139–45; Henry Beecher, *Medicine at Harvard* (1977), 461–85.

82   "a hush fell upon the class": Regina Morantz-Sanchez, *Sympathy and Science* (1985), 48.

82   "It is much to be regretted": *Boston Medical and Surgical Journal* (February–August 1849), 58.

83   *The New York Times* published a story: *New York Times,* December 6, 11, 13, 18, 1864.

83   "Gentlemen, this is an old penis": "Bellevue Hospital," *American Eclectic Medical Review* (1872), 377.

84   "There were 500 men students": *New York Times,* April 9, 1916.

Chapter 5: A Hospital in War

85   "[Our] city belongs almost as much": Steven Jaffe, *New York at War* (2012), 145.

85   "we shall find negroes among us": Edwin Burrows and Mike Wallace, *Gotham* (1999), 865.

86   "The crucial test of this": Ernest McKay, *The Civil War and New York City* (1990), 56.

86   "Flags from almost every building": Jaffe, *New York at War,* 141.

86   "assistant surgeon of artillery": "List of internees, 1855–1864," in Robert Carlisle, *An Account of Bellevue Hospital* (1894), 148–320.

86   "surgeon of artillery": Ibid.

86   "Of medium stature": Charles A. Leale, *Eulogy of Professor Frank Hastings Hamilton* (1886), copy on file at New York Academy of Medicine.

87   "I believed the war would not last": Ibid.

87   "excited by liquor": *New York Times,* April 29, 1861.

87   "in a snug wooden house": Frank H. Hamilton, *American Medical Times* (1861), 77–79.

87   "Both of them, I confess": Ibid.

88   "I could not tell them": Ibid.

88   "A Short War Probable": *New York Times,* May 31, 1861.

88   "learned how to prosper": Jaffe, *New York at War,* 150.

89   "The major event in my world": Titus Coan to My Dear Mother, July 24, 1862, Titus Coan Papers, Box 1, New-York Historical Society (NYHS).

89   "He spoke with each man": Coan to My Dear Hattie, December 1, 1862, in ibid.

89   "I am house surgeon": December 1, 1862, in ibid.

90   "I was just in blood to my elbows": John Vance Lauderdale, November 8,

1863, in Peter Josyph, *The Wounded River: The Civil War Letters of John Vance Lauderdale, M.D.* (1993), 170.

90   "A stroll of inspection": *New York Times,* April 27, 1862.

90   "this reduction may be accounted for": Commissioners of Public Charities and Corrections, NYC, *Fourth Annual Report,* 1863.

90   "only patients who are unable to pay": "Rules and Regulations for the Government of Bellevue Hospital, 1863," Commissioners of Public Charities and Corrections, *Fifth Annual Report,* 1864; *Eighth Annual Report,* 1868, NYHS.

91   "Thomas Rigney, 36, Irish" plus all other descriptions: *Titus Coan Patient Ledger, 1862–63,* Titus Coan Papers, NYHS. Also, Ludwig Eichna, "Bellevue Hospital Patient Casebook: September 8, 1866–February 3, 1868," *Pharos* (Fall 1991), 21–26.

91   "injuries accidentally received": John Howard, *Stephen Foster: America's Troubador* (1962), 342–43.

92   "What killed Stephen Foster?": Ken Emerson, *Doo-dah! Stephen Foster and the Rise of American Popular Culture* (1997), 299.

92   "He introduced himself as Dr. John Vance Lauderdale": Josyph, *The Wounded River,* 224–25.

93   "but for one or two": Coan to My Dear Mother, July 21, 1863, Titus Coan Papers.

93–94   "a saturnalia of pillage and violence" . . . "Shame! Shame on such Irishmen": Edward Spann, "Union Green: The Irish Community and the Civil War," in Ronald Bayor and Timothy Meagher, *The New York Irish* (1996), 193–209.

94   "the lowest Irish day laborers": *Diary of George Templeton Strong,* vol. 3, July 13, 1863.

94   "New York's Civil War generated its own fratricide": Jaffe, *New York at War,* 166.

94   "Mary Williams, 24, a colored woman" and other descriptions in this paragraph: *New York Times,* July 15, 16, 17, 1863.

94   "A gong has struck again": Josyph, *The Wounded River,* 162–65.

94   Punish the violent lawbreakers: Ibid.

95   "War is the Normal condition": Frank H. Hamilton, *A Treatise on Military Surgery and Hygiene* (1865), 11–12, 66–80, 128.

96   "We operated in old-blood-stained and often pus-stained coats": National Library of Medicine, *Medicine in the Civil War* (1973), 2. Also Ira Rutkow, *Bleeding Blue and Gray* (2005) for the most thorough account of Civil War surgery.

97   "In attempting to remove a ball": Hamilton, *A Treatise on Military Surgery and Hygiene,* 175, 180–81.

97 "Civil War surgeons had to work without knowledge": Alfred Bollet, "The Truth About Civil War Surgery," *Civil War Times* (October 2004), 26–32.

97 "Surgeon Extraordinary": Elliott Hague, "Frank Hastings Hamilton: Surgeon Extraordinary of the Union Army," *New York State Medical Journal* (July 1961), 2330–36.

97 "I cannot recall learning anything": W. G. MacCallum, *William Stewart Halsted, Surgeon* (1930), 19.

98 "I was profoundly impressed": Charles A. Leale, *Lincoln's Last Hours* (1909), 2.

98 "I instantly arose": Ibid., 3–4.

98 "I grasped [her] outstretched hand in mine": Ibid., 1.

98 "I lifted his eyelids": Ibid., 5–6.

99 "the life of President Lincoln": Ibid., 7–12.

99 "in a profoundly comatose position": "Report of Dr. Charles A. Leale," April 15, 1865, *Papers of Abraham Lincoln Website*, http://www.papersofabrahamlincoln.org.

100 "The natural structure of the brain": Hamilton, *A Treatise on Military Surgery and Hygiene*, 245–47.

100 "Sometimes recognition and reason return": *Los Angeles Times,* December 27, 1977.

100 "Lincoln's death—thousands of flags": Walter Lowenfels, *Walt Whitman and the Civil War* (1961), 174–75.

101 "I am stunned": *Diary of George Templeton Strong,* April 15, 1865.

101 "In the whole of my surgical experience": James Parton, *Illustrious Men and Their Achievements* (1881), 527–30. Also, Valentine Mott, Chairman, *Narrative of Privations and Sufferings of U.S. Officers and Soldiers While Prisoners of War in the Hands of Rebel Authorities* (1864).

101 "He regarded it as an omen": S. D. Gross, *Memoir of Valentine Mott* (1869), 86–87.

101 "a victim": Ibid.

Chapter 6: "Hives of Sickness and Vice"

102 "Is war good for medicine": Christopher Connell, "Is War Good for Medicine?," *Stanford Medical Magazine* (Summer 2007).

102 "vague and confused": Bonnie Blustein, *Preserve Your Love of Science: Life of William A. Hammond, American Neurologist* (1991), 76–80.

103 "the medical middle ages": Frank Freemon, *Gangrene and Glory* (2001), 19–26.

103 "ahead of the medical care it required": Ira Rutkow, *Seeking the Cure* (2010), 62.

104   "mahogany stables trimmed in silver": Edward Ellis, *The Epic of New York City* (1966), 328.

104   "Plunder of the city treasury": James Bryce, *The American Commonwealth,* vol. 2 (1915), 389.

105   "The doors and windows were broken": Stephen Smith, *The City That Was* (1911), 35–39.

105   "In this extremity": Ibid.

106   "The country is horrified": Gert Brieger, "Sanitary Reform in New York City," *Bulletin of the History of Medicine* (1966), 419.

106   "As a body": Smith, *The City That Was,* 40–53.

106   "On a piece of ground": *Sanitary Conditions of the City: Report of the Council of Hygiene and Public Health of the Citizens of New York* (1865).

107   "The instances are many": Ibid.

107   "In a dark and damp cellar": Ibid.

107   "filth, overcrowding, excrement": Ibid.

107   "closely packed houses": Ibid.

108   "To what depth of humiliation": A transcript of Smith's testimony is in the *New York Times*, March 16, 1865.

108   "Practically, [we] are a city": Ibid.

108   "encroachment upon our right": John Duffy, *History of Public Health in New York City* (1968), 569.

109   "the most complete piece of health legislation": Smith, *The City That Was,* 158.

109   "eminently successful and always thronged": John Duffy, *A History of Public Health in New York City, 1866–1966* (1974), 44.

110   "Don't eat too much meat": *New York Times,* November 16, 1921.

Chapter 7: The Bellevue Ambulance

111   "the appearance of extreme delicacy": *Memorial of Edward Dalton* (1872), 1–12.

112   "the unwholesome exhalations": Ibid.

112   "in the history of war": William Howell Reed, *Hospital Life in the Army of the Potomac* (1866), 93.

112   "the frightful state of disorder": National Library of Medicine, *Medicine in the Civil War* (1973), 3–5.

113   "the best man in the United States": Ryan Bell, *The Ambulance* (2009), 54.

113   "He was taken to the nearest house": Page Cooper, *The Bellevue Story* (1948), 81.

114   "the Victorian equivalent": Bell, *The Ambulance,* 61.

114   "As we swept around the corners": W. H. Rideing, "Hospital Life in New York," *Harper's New Monthly Magazine* (June 1878), 173.

114 "with special reference": Francis Nichols, "The New York Ambulance Service," *The Junior Munsey* (1901), 729–32.

115 The early Bellevue ambulance cases: "Admitting Record Book: Third Surgical Division, Bellevue Hospital, 1872," Ehrman Medical Archives, NYU Medical School.

115 "a grim, black, demonic-looking craft": *New York Times,* April 7, 1872.

115 "Three Killed, Six Mortally Wounded": Ibid., July 13, 1870.

116 It took several pages of single-spaced entries: A list of the dead and wounded in the Orange Riot is found in Michael Gordon, *The Orange Riots* (1993), Appendix.

117 "That saving grace was gone": Edwin Burrows and Mike Wallace, *Gotham: A History of New York City* (1999), 1008.

117 "by law, private hospitals": *New York Herald Tribune,* February 25, 1906.

117 "Patrick Carey, a horseshoer": *New York Times,* October 13, 1888.

118 "THE PATIENT DIED": Ibid., June 29, 1896.

118 "Open your books": Emily Abel, "Patient Dumping in New York City, 1877–1917," *American Journal of Public Health* (May 2011), 789–95.

118 "sending the poor, dying patient": Ibid.

118 "helpless in the drifts": Bell, *The Ambulance,* 149.

118 "The horses, Joe and Jim": *New York Times,* March 13, 1924.

119 "nothing could exceed the fortitude": *Memorial of Edward Dalton,* 1–12.

119 "Probably no inventor": Nichols, "The New York Ambulance Service," 729.

Chapter 8: Bellevue Venus

120 "In all the large Military Hospitals": "Proposal for a Photographic Department," *Eighth Annual Report of the Commissioners of Public Charities and Corrections,* 1867.

120 "all specimens of morbid anatomy": Stanley Burns, "Civil War Medical Photography," *New York State Journal of Medicine* (August 1980), 1444–69.

121 "A stream of cold water": John McCabe, *Lights and Shadows of New York Life* (1881), 839–42.

121 "unmistakable records of this gallery": O. G. Mason, "Photographic Report, Bellevue Hospital," 1881.

121 "quietly hidden from sight": Ibid., 1879.

122 "moribund patient": Paul Schmidt, "Transfusion in America in the Eighteenth and Nineteenth Centuries," *New England Journal of Medicine* (December 12, 1968), 1319–20.

123 "There are one or two patches": "Skin Graft: Elephantiasis," in George Henry Fox, *Photographic Illustrations of Skin Diseases* (1881).

124 "a very private and select coterie": *New York News–Weekly Sunday Ledger,* December 19, 1879.

124 "several months of negotiation": Ibid.

124 "When some eight years ago": Mason, "Photographic Report, Bellevue Hospital," 1875.

125 "was finally cured": Dr. Waldron Vanderpool, "Bellevue Hospital, New York, Plastic Operation for Restoration of Nose," *Medical Gazette* (July–December 1881), 269–70.

125 "Patient suffers pain": Ibid.

125 "The nose has become firmly united": Ibid.

125 "The nose was not a great success": "Remarks by Dr. Randolph Winslow," *Transactions of the Meeting of the American Surgical Association* (1922), 668.

126 "fatty substances": Austin Flint, *A Practical Treatise on the Diagnosis, Pathology and Treatment of Diseases of the Heart* (1859).

126 "unable to walk without assistance": Jay Zampini, "Lewis A. Sayre, the First Professor of Orthopaedic Surgery in America," *Clinical Orthopaedics and Related Research* (June 2008), 226–67.

126 "Oh, doctor, be very careful": Ibid.

127 "This is almost a miracle": Lewis A. Sayre, "Lecture: Paralysis from Peripheral Irritation," *Medical and Surgical Reporter* (October 14, 1876), 305–9; Sayre, "Spinal Anemia with Partial Paralysis . . . of the Genital Organs," *Transactions of the American Medical Association* (1875), 255–74.

127 "When a man of Sayre's experience": David Gollaher, "From Ritual to Science: The Medical Transformation of Circumcision in America," *Journal of Social History* (Fall 1994), 5–36.

128 "men of well-sifted reputations": "Remarks to the Graduating Class of Bellevue Hospital College Medical School" (1872), copy on file at New York Academy of Medicine.

Chapter 9: Nightingales

129 "is principally remembered for three reasons": National Archives, "British Battles, Crimea, 1854," www.nationalarchives.gov.uk/battles/crimea.

130 "It's not worthwhile to clean him": Christopher Gill and Gillian Gill, "Nightingale in Scutari: Her Legacy Reexamined," *Clinical Infectious Diseases* (June 2005), 1800.

130 "Her interventions, considered at the time to be revolutionary": Ibid., 1801.

130 "too old, too weak": Julia Hallam, *Nursing the Image* (2000), 18.

130 "clear relationship between the diseases killing [her] patients": Gill and Gill, "Nightingale in Scutari," 1801.

130 "Recovery from sickness in the vast majority of cases": Florence Night-

ingale, "Sites and Construction of Hospitals," *Builder* (1858), 577. Also, Jeanne Kisacky, "An Architecture of Light and Air," PhD diss., Cornell University (2000), 118–31.

131   "Can you fancy half a dozen or a dozen old hags": Ira Rutkow, *Bleeding Blue and Gray* (2005), 170.

131   "uncertainty of rational judgment": Louise Knight, *Citizen: Jane Addams and the Struggle for Democracy* (2008), 78.

132   "plain almost to repulsion in dress": Thomas Brown, *Dorothea Dix: New England Reformer* (1998), 304.

132   "not to speak to those Catholic nurses": Ibid., 294.

132   "making beds, cooking food properly for the sick": Jane Mottus, *New York Nightingales* (1980), 27.

133   "philanthropy, patriotism": Ibid.

133   "I had never been": Elizabeth Hobson, *Recollections of a Happy Life* (1916), 81–84.

133   "nursing the sick, protecting the children": Mottus, *New York Nightingales,* 46.

133   "We are aware": *Third Annual Report of the Visiting Committee for Bellevue and Other Public Hospitals* (1875), 9.

134   "The nurses, or rather those employed as such": Robert Carlisle, *An Account of Bellevue Hospital* (1893), 79.

134   *"there,* and *solely there, to carry out the orders"*: Nightingale's "Advice to Bellevue Hospital" can be found in *American Journal of Nursing* (February 1911), 361–64.

134   "daughters and widows of clergymen": Mottus, *New York Nightingales,* 44–49.

134   "I do not believe in the success of a training school": Mrs. William Griffin and Mrs. William Henry Osborn, *A Short History of Bellevue Hospital and the Training Schools* (1915).

135   "slavishly afraid": David Presswick Barr interview, Columbia Oral History Project, Columbia Medical School Archives.

135   "I don't know—ask your doctor": Franklin North, "A New Profession for Women," *The Century* (November 1882), 38–47.

135   "Every effort has been made": *Annual Report of the Governors of the Almshouse* (1853), 19.

136   "His genius [had] led him to a discovery": Sherwin Nuland, *Doctors: The Biography of Medicine* (1988), 239.

136   "Case XXXII": Fordyce Barker, M.D., *The Puerperal Fevers: Clinical Lectures Delivered at Bellevue Hospital* (1874), 430–31. For a fuller listing of puerperal fever cases at Bellevue, see "First Medical Division, Cases 1866–1868, vol. 1," Columbia Medical School Archives.

136   "All admit that the saturation of the air": Barker, *The Puerperal Fevers.*

137   "Few people realize the appalling mental condition": William T. Lusk, M.D., *Clinical Report of the Lying-in Service at Bellevue Hospital* (1874), 1–9.

137   "defective ventilation [and] construction": State Charities Aid Association (Louisa Lee Schyler, President), "Report of the Special Committee Appointed to Take Active Measures in Regard to the Erection of a New Bellevue Hospital" (1874).

137   "Died on the 14th day from pyaemia": F. J. Metcalfe, "Amputations Performed at Bellevue Hospital"; D. F. Goodwillie, "Report of Cases of Anesthesia," both in *Bellevue Hospital Reports* (1869).

138   "PREPARE TO MEET YOUR GOD": *New York Times,* November 23, 1884.

138   "Everything swam in pus": Henry Dowling, *City Hospitals* (1982), 69.

138   "The best place to treat a sick or wounded man": Frank Hamilton, *A Treatise on Military Surgery* (1865).

138   "Dr. Hammond [has] been disloyal to the college": "Minutes of the College Faculty," Bellevue Hospital Medical College (1866), Ehrman Medical Archives, NYU Medical School.

139   "We give you forty-eight hours": Hobson, *Recollections of a Happy Life,* 106. Also, "Report of the Training School," in *Third Annual Report of the Visiting Committee* (1875), 27–30.

139   "I can still see the wards there": David Presswick Barr interview.

139   "The early prejudices, the opposition we had to contend with": Hobson, *Recollections of a Happy Life,* 113.

140   "an incalculable benefit to [our] hospital": Mottus, *New York Nightingales,* 53–57; Carlisle, *An Account of Bellevue Hospital,* 78–84.

140   "all-purpose female service workers": Rosemary Stevens, *In Sickness and in Wealth* (1989), 12.

140   "When my mother became a registered nurse": Lewis Thomas, *The Youngest Science: Notes of a Medicine Watcher* (1983), 61–67.

Chapter 10: Germ Theory

141   "I have little fears": Charles Rosenberg, *The Care of Strangers* (1987), 176.

142   "[You] have passed with the rank of No. 1": C. E. A. Winslow, *The Life of Hermann M. Biggs* (1929), 49.

142   "I am undecided whose course I should take": Haller Henkel to C. C. Henkel, March 5, 1878, H. H. Henkel Papers, New York Academy of Medicine.

142   "is a trick that is frequently done": Ibid., August 19, 1878. Henkel was accepted as an intern in Bellevue's First Surgical Division. See Robert J. Carlysle, *An Account of Bellevue Hospital* (1893), Appendix, 216.

142 "It is certainly the most completely appointed hospital": William Welch to father, May 1875, Box 68, William Welch Papers, Chesney Archives, Johns Hopkins University.

143 "In 1876, the year I [first] walked the wards": Walter Burket, *Surgical Papers of William Stewart Halsted,* vol. 1. (1924), xxvii. Also, "William Halsted: A Lecture by Peter Olch," *Annals of Surgery* (March 2006), 421–25.

145 "The products of the industry": Linda Gross and Theresa Snyder, *Philadelphia's 1876 Centennial Exhibition* (2005).

145 "Comparing the aggregate results": Joseph Lister, "On the Effect of the Antiseptic System of Treatment Upon the Salubrity of a Surgical Hospital," *The Lancet* (January 1870), 4–6, 40–42.

146 "a picture strong men find difficult to look at": Sheldon Nuland, "The Artist and the Doctor," *American Scholar* (Winter 2003), 121–26; Patrick Grieffenstein, "Eakins' Critics: Snapshots of Surgery on the Threshold of Modernity," *Archives of Surgery* (November 2008), 1122.

147 "A large portion of American surgeons": Remarks of Hamilton and dissenters in John Ashcroft, *Transactions of the International Medical Congress of Philadelphia* (1876), 532–34.

147 "renowned throughout the world": Lister's remarks in ibid., beginning on 535.

148 "movement of professional men": Thomas Bonner, *American Doctors and German Universities* (1963), 23.

148 "You can see the original Shylocks": William Welch to Fred Dennis, September 26, 1876, Box 12, Welch Papers.

148 "Don't be alarmed": Welch to sister, September 26, 1876, in ibid.

149 "You must go to [Leipzig]": Welch to Dennis, March 30, 1877, in ibid.

149 "We've got to get you back": Simon Flexner and Thomas Flexner, *William Henry Welch and the Age of Heroic Medicine* (1941), 116.

149 "I felt I would be a traitor": Victor Freeburg, *William Henry Welch at Eighty: A Memorial Record* (1930), 69–70.

150 "People say there are bacteria in the air": Donald Fleming, *William H. Welch and the Rise of Modern Medicine,* 72.

150 "We may summarize the conditions": Stephen Smith, "The Comparative Results of Operations in Bellevue Hospital," *Medical Record* (1885), 427–31. Also, Smith, "Reminiscences of Two Epochs—Anesthesia an Asepsis," *Bulletin of the Johns Hopkins Hospital* (1919), 273–78.

151 "There's a bacillus, catch him!": Peter Olch, "William Halsted's New York Period," *Bulletin of the History of Medicine* (1966), 503.

151 "where the numerous anti-Lister surgeons": Howard Markel, *An Anatomy of Addiction* (2012), 95.

151 "Pasteur has demonstrated that 212 degrees": H. H. Henkel, *Student Notebook,* New York Academy of Medicine.

151 "The floor was of maple": "William Halsted: A Lecture by Peter Olch." Also, Howard Markel, *An Anatomy of Addiction* (2011), 94–95.

Chapter 11: A Tale of Two Presidents

152 "Doctor, I am a dead man": Ira Rutkow, *James A. Garfield* (2006), 2–3.

153 "The President, while doing well": Telegram, Secretary of State James G. Blaine to Dr. Hamilton, July 3, 1881, Frank H. Hamilton Papers, Box 1, Library of Congress.

153 "the ball seems to have entered the liver": *New York Times,* July 13, 1881.

153 "From this moment until the death of the President": Hamilton Affidavit, Box 1, Frank H. Hamilton Papers.

153 "the country's first air conditioner": Candice Millard, *Destiny of the Republic* (2011), 178.

154 "The President is now in much greater danger": Ira Rutkow, "Dirty Nation," unpublished manuscript in author's possession.

154 "I regard his case as making good progress": *New York Times,* August 1, 2, 3, 1881.

154 "I have had a great deal of experience": Ibid., August 3, 1881.

154 "it does not give a happy impression": *New York World,* July 26, 1881.

154 "The case could not possibly be progressing more favorably": *New York Times,* July 13, 1881.

155 "The President's Best Day": Ibid., September 9, 1881.

155 "his ribs stuck out": Ira Rutkow, *Seeking the Cure* (2010), 78.

155 "between the loin muscles and the right kidney": "Official Bulletin of the Autopsy of the Body of the President," September 20, 1881.

155 "We might criticize the introduction of the finger": John Collins Warren, "The Case of President Garfield," *Boston Medical and Surgical Journal* (1881), 464.

156 "The collision of opinion": *New York Herald Tribune,* September 25, 1881.

156 "If Garfield had been a 'tough'": John Girdner, "The Death of President Garfield," *Munsey's Magazine* (October 1902), 547.

156 "Nothing could be more absurd": *Boston Medical and Surgical Journal* (February 16, 1882), 150.

156 "For professional services": All material relating to Hamilton's bill for services can be found in Box 1, Frank H. Hamilton Papers.

157 "To younger practitioners": "Eulogy Delivered Before the New York State Medical Association of Professor Frank Hastings Hamilton" (November 1886), copy on file at the National Library of Medicine.

157 "The main dish was country ham": H. L. Mencken, *Chrestomathy* (1982), 372–74.

158 "I shall make the leading features": Flexner and Flexner, *William Henry Welch,* 114–18.

158 "The [germ] theory, which has so recently occupied medical men": Ibid., 119.

158 "What are we aiming for?": "Gilman's Inaugural Address," Johns Hopkins University, https://www.jhu.edu/gilman-address; Gerald Imber, *Genius on the Edge* (2010), 59–73.

159 "Mr. Gilman is looking out for men": Welch to father, January 3, 1876, Box 57, William Welch Papers.

159 "a gentleman in every sense": John Shaw Billings to Gilman, March 1, 1884, Box 57, William Welch Papers.

159 "*You must come*": Gilman to Welch, March 15, 1884, Box 57, William Welch Papers.

159 "I do not feel as if [I'm] accomplishing what I want to do": Welch to father, March 26, 31, 1884, Box 68, William Welch Papers.

159 "the drudgery of teaching": Flexner and Flexner, *William Henry Welch and the Age of Heroic Medicine,* 130–31.

159 "Willie Welch came to see me": All correspondence between Dennis and Welch is found in William Welch Papers, Box 12.

160 "Gentlemen, Please pay drafts": Carnegie's telegram is in "Papers of Bellevue Hospital," New York Academy of Medicine.

161 "In Germany, [such] facilities are amply provided by the Government": *New York Times,* April 27, 1884.

161 "His ideas imbibed in Germany are impractical": Donald Fleming, *William H. Welch and the Rise of Modern Medicine* (1954), 68.

161 "I shall resign my position": Loomis to Welch, December 30, 1884, Loomis Folder, William Welch Papers.

162 "I am conscious that I have acted throughout in good faith": Welch to Dennis, September 27, 1884, Dennis Folder, William Welch Papers.

162 "Well, good-bye": Flexner and Flexner, *William Henry Welch and the Age of Heroic Medicine,* 134.

163 "the most vigorous period of his life": Allen Dumont, "Halsted at Bellevue, 1883–1887," *Annals of Surgery* (December 1970), 929–35.

163 "arm thoroughly cleansed and disinfected": "Record Book of Bellevue Hospital, 1883–1887," Ehrman Medical Archives, NYU Medical School.

163 "A body of gentlemen in this city": Peter Olch, "William S. Halsted's New York Period," *Bulletin of the History of Medicine* (1966), 498–510; Olch, "William Halsted and Local Anesthesia," *Anesthesiology* (1975), 479–86.

164 "from a model of patrician rectitude": Gerald Imber, *Genius on the Edge* (2010), 58.

165 "a life of controlled addiction . . . As long as he lived": Markel, *Anatomy of Addiction,* 241.

166 "The surgeon scrubs his forearms": Frederic Dennis, "Report of Two Months Service at Bellevue Hospital," *Medical and Surgical Reports of Bellevue and Allied Hospitals* (1907–8).

166 "ulcerative lesion": Dr. W. W. Keen, "The Surgical Operations on President Cleveland in 1893," *Saturday Evening Post,* September 22, 1917; Matthew Algeo, *The President Is a Sick Man* (2012), 53–88.

167 "So careful were we": *Saturday Evening Post,* September 22, 1917.

167 "Fresh, pure air, disinfected quarters": "President Cleveland's Secret Operation," *The American Surgeon* (August 1997), 758–59; Arlene Shaner, "The Secret Surgeries of Grover Cleveland," *Monthly Archive* (February 2014), New York Academy of Medicine; "Final Diagnosis of President Cleveland's Lesion," *JAMA* (December 19, 1980).

Chapter 12: The Mad-House

168 "for the poorest of the poor": W. H. Rideing, "Hospital Life in New York," *Harper's New Monthly Magazine* (June 1878), 171–89.

169 "explaining the cases and operations": Ibid.

169 "cost-per-patient-per day": Henry Dowling, *City Hospitals* (1982), 77.

169 "It is a mighty dry place": *New York Times,* May 14, 1867.

170 "The invalid, the aged, the infirm": Grand Jury Report: "An Address to the Citizens of New York: Abuses and Reforms of the Alms-House and Prison Department" (1849), New-York Historical Society (NYHS).

170 "a rapid and violent current": Blackwell Family Scrapbook, March 8, 1784; Samuel Mitchell Note on Blackwell's Island, October 20, 1796, NYHS.

170 "The moping idiot": Charles Dickens, *American Notes,* vol. 4 (1842).

171 "I had the honor of stroking the back": "A Visit to the Lunatic Asylum on Blackwell's Island," *Harper's New Monthly Magazine* (March 19, 1859). Also, "Blackwell's Island Lunatic Asylum," in ibid.; and Elizabeth Montgomery, *A Separated Place* (1988), privately published, NYHS.

171 "planting vegetables": "Report of the Resident Physician, Blackwell's Island Lunatic Asylum" (1863–73), NYHS.

171 "FRENCH SCIENTIST AND EXPLORER": Denis Brian, *Pulitzer: A Life* (2002), 67.

172 "We must raise the money": National Park Service, "Statue of Liberty: Joseph Pulitzer," www.nps.gov/joseph-pulitzer.htm.

173 "have [me] committed to one of the asylums": Brooke Kroeger, *Nellie Bly: Daredevil, Reporter, Feminist* (1995), 91–92.

173   "practicing to be a lunatic": Nellie Bly, *Ten Days in a Mad-House* (1887), 5–9.

173   "Who Is This Insane Girl?": *New York Sun,* September 26, 1887.

173   "A Mysterious Waif": *New York Times,* September 26, 1887.

173   "the third station on my way to the island . . . I began to have a smaller regard for the ability of doctors": Bly, *Ten Days in a Mad-House.*

174   "this girl of whom nothing is known": Kroeger, *Nellie Bly,* 91–92.

174   "BEHIND ASYLUM BARS": *New York World,* October 9, 16, 1887.

174   "She thoroughly understands the profession": Kroeger, *Nellie Bly,* 91–92.

175   "I had hardly expected the grand jury to sustain me": Ibid., 97–99.

175   "I have one consolation": Ibid.

176   "Imagines Himself a Mosquito" and all following headlines: "Bellevue Maniacs," Robertson Portfolio, Scrapbook Clippings (1897), New York Academy of Medicine.

176   "SHOCKING BRUTALITY OF MALE NURSES": *New York World,* December 15, 1900.

177   "No writer of fiction": *New York Times,* December 28, 1900, February 15, 19, 1901.

177   "The Case of the Garroted Frenchman": Page Cooper, *The Bellevue Story* (1948), 155.

177   "in a lunatic asylum": *New York Times,* February 16, 1901.

177   "Why did you go to Bellevue?": Ibid.

177   "That's a personal matter": Ibid.

177   "sense of chastity": Jane Mottus, *New York Nightingales* (1980), 71.

178   "too nervous": Ibid., 106–7.

178   A master of cross-examination: For the cross-examination of Minnock, see Francis Lewis Wellman, *The Art of Cross-Examination* (1903), Chapter 15.

178   "unnatural advances and acts": Sandra Opdycke, "Improper Conduct: Rumors, Accusations, and the Closing of the Bellevue Training School for Male Nurses" (n.d.), unpublished paper in author's possession.

179   "The details of the investigation": Ibid.

179   "Nursing is essentially a woman's work": Ibid.

179   "The average man does not select the profession of a nurse": Ibid.

179   "the care of alcoholics": Ibid.

Chapter 13: The New Metropolis

181   "COST OF NEW BELLEVUE": *New York Times,* April 23, 1904.

181   "surgical use": Report of the Proposed Bellevue Hospital, Box 42, Bellevue, Papers of McKim, Mead & White, New-York Historical Society (NYHS).

181　"the public inspection of the unidentified dead": Though most of the concrete plans for the new Bellevue are located in the McKim, Mead & White Papers, preliminary designs of Bellevue can also be found in the firm's collection in the Avery Architectural Library at Columbia University. See, especially, "Bellevue Hospital: New Hospital Buildings and Modernization of Existing Buildings . . . Preliminary Drawings."

181　"Dear Charlie": Stanford White to Charles McKim, May 12, 1904, McKim, Mead & White Papers, Box 147, NYHS.

181　"Dear Stanford": McKim to White, May 14, 1904, in ibid.

182　"Grand Jury Denounces Bellevue Management": *New York Times,* February 1, 1901.

183　"I think we have a conclusive responsibility": James A. Miller to George O'Hanlon, February 10, 1906, Dean's Files, Archives and Manuscripts, Health Services Library, Columbia University.

183　"I wish to cite the example": C. E. A. Winslow, *The Life of Hermann M. Biggs* (1929), 216–19.

183　"There was no attempt to give instruction": William Rom and Joan Reibner, "The History of the Bellevue Chest Service," *Annals of the American Thoracic Society* (October 2015), 1439.

184　"Doctors stripped [one] man": Edward Kohn, *Hot Time in the Old Town* (2010), 89–90.

184　"He dived overboard": *New York Times,* December 14, 1946.

184　"less pretentious": Memos in Box 147, McKim, Mead & White Papers, NYHS.

185　"OMIT DOME": "Bellevue Hospital, REDUCTIONS," May 10, 1904, in ibid.

185　"It is my opinion": George Shady, "New Bellevue Hospital Plans Filed," *Medical Record,* vol. 71, 273. Also, Arthur Dillon, "The New Bellevue Hospital," *House and Garden* (June 1904), 296–99.

185　"It seems a great deal more money": *New York Times,* November 29, 1907.

186　"fair students, better than the Irish": Kate Holliday, "The Foreign Immigrant in New York City," *Report of the Industrial Commission,* vol. 15 (1901), 465–92.

186　"show a depressing frequency of low foreheads": Alan Kraut, *Silent Travelers* (1994), 109.

186　Bellevue naturally mirrored: Bellevue nativity statistics are compiled from *Annual Report of the Commission of Public Charities* (1875–93) and *Bellevue and Annual Hospital Reports* (1902–13).

187　"mandatorily excludible": *Report of the Committee on Inquiry into the Department of Health, Charities, and Bellevue and Allied Hospitals* (1913), 22.

187 "The opinion is prevalent": *New York Times,* November 8, 1891.

187 "In the philanthropic institutions": Paul Starr, *The Transformation of American Medicine* (1982), 174.

188 The 1890s had seen a sprinkling: For Bellevue case files, see "Record Books, First Surgical Division, Bellevue Hospital, 1898"; "First Surgical Children's Division, Bellevue Hospital, 1911–1915," both in Archives and Special Collections, Health Studies Library, Columbia University.

189 "had a beneficial influence": E. H. Lewinski-Corwin, *The Hospital Situation in Greater New York* (1924), 18, 43.

189 "Today the patient approaches": Rosemary Stevens, *In Sickness and in Wealth* (1989), 30.

189 "a hotel for rich invalids": *New York Times,* January 26, 1904.

189 "we ask, 'Is it right?'": David Rosner, *A Once Charitable Enterprise* (1982), 66.

190 "Why is it that when our patients enter a hospital": Ibid., 102.

190 Among the many examples was Mount Sinai: On the drop in charity patients at Mount Sinai, see Alan Herman, "Institutional Practices in Jewish Hospitals of New York City: 1880–1930," PhD diss., NYU (1984), 72–73.

192 "FACTORIES FOR THE MAKING": *The New York Times,* July 24, 1910.

192 "The schools skate on thin ice": Abraham Flexner, *Medical Education in the United States and Canada* (1910), 275–77.

193 "On one day, 25 pounds of porterhouse steak": *Report of the Committee on Inquiry into the Department of Health, Charities, and Bellevue and Allied Hospitals,* 83.

193 "inexperienced in the diagnosing of disease": Ibid., 367.

193 "Financially the position would demand considerable sacrifice": E. H. Poole to Dr. Brewer (included in a letter to Dr. Lambert, Dean of Columbia Medical School, March 13, 1916), Dean's Files, Box 317, Health Studies Library, Columbia University.

194 "rats of heroic East River dimension": John Starr, *Hospital City* (1957), 198.

194 "My choices were extremely limited": Dr. Connie Guion Interview, Columbia Oral History Project (COHP), Health Studies Library.

194 "Her services will have no cause for regret": See, for example, letters of recommendation in Leoni Clarman Papers, Box 1, Health Services Library, Columbia University.

195 "In plain English, he was outclassed": Sandra Opdycke, *No One Was Turned Away* (1999), 67.

195 "very, very dark": May Chinn Interview, COHP.

196　"Dr. Giles is one of us": *Journal of the National Medical Association* (May 1939), 122.

196　"Days later, when I was well enough to talk": Clayborne Carson, ed., "The Autobiography of Martin Luther King, Jr." (2001), 118.

196　"We have honestly attempted to eliminate": Michael Rosenthal, *Nicholas Miraculous: The Amazing Career of the Redoubtable Nicholas Murray Butler* (2015), 343.

196　"radical": Harold Wechsler, *The Qualified Student: A History of Selective Admission in America* (1977), 161–62.

197　"Never admit more than five Jews": Gerard Burrow, *A History of Yale's School of Medicine* (2008), 107.

197　"went begging for nine years": Leon Sokoloff, "The Rise and Decline of the Jewish Quota in Medical School Admissions," *Bulletin of the New York Academy of Medicine* (November 1992), 497–518. Also, Edward Halperin, "Jews in U.S. Medical Education," *Journal of the History of Medicine* (April 2001), 140–67.

197　"the personal side of the man": John Wycoff, "Relation of Collegiate to Medical School Scholarship," *Bulletin of the Association of Medical Colleges* (January 1927), 1–16.

197　"standing in the middle third of his class": For a description of the candidates, see Charles Flood to Dr. John McCreery, "Applicants for First Surgical Division at Bellevue: Group One—Preferred," Dean's Papers, Box 247, Health Services Library, Columbia University.

198　"for a chat, during which he defended the fact": Dr. Joseph Dancis Interview, *Archives of the American Academy of Pediatrics* (1996).

198　"It gathers the dead and dying": Deborah Blum, *The Poisoner's Handbook* (2010), 17.

199　"This must be some kind of new infection": Gina Kolata, *Flu* (1999), 17.

199　"High temperature, short of breath": Dr. Connie Guion Interview, COHP.

199　"promiscuous coughing and sneezing": Francesco Aimone, "The 1918 Influenza Epidemic in New York City," *Public Health Reports* (Supplement Three, 2010), 71–79.

200　"It got to the place where I would only see the patients twice": Guion Interview.

200　"Doc, what do you think": Ibid.

201　"Our final conclusion is": Wade Oliver, *The Man Who Lived for Tomorrow* (1941), 392–99.

201　"a chastening experience": Winslow, *Hermann Biggs*, 321.

Chapter 14: Cause of Death

202   "The American does not realize": Walter George, *Hail Columbia: Random Impressions of a Conservative English Radical* (1921), 154.

203   "city on a still": Michael Lerner, *Dry Manhattan* (2007), 4

203   "favoritism, extortion, and malfeasance": Leonard Wallstein, *Report on the Special Examination of the Accounts and Methods of the Office of Coroner in the City of New York* (1915).

204   "eight undertakers, seven politicians": Ibid. Also, Deborah Blum, *The Poisoner's Handbook* (2010), 20.

204   "skilled pathologists [holding] the degree of M.D.": William Eckert, "Medicolegal Investigation in New York City," *Forensic Medicine and Pathology* (March 1983), 33–54.

204   "We have had all the reform": Francis Barry, *The Scandal of Reform* (2009), 82.

204   "the greatest activity resided": Edward Marten, *The Doctor Looks at Murder* (1940), 43–47.

204–5 "from criminal violence, or suicide": "An Act to Amend the Greater Charter of New York City," *New York State Journal of Medicine* (February 1903), 464.

205   "It would be imprecise": Blum, *The Poisoner's Handbook,* 29.

206   "All new equipment purchased in 1921": Ibid., 53.

206   "spike it with the substance involved": Henry Freimuth, "Alexander O. Gettler," *American Journal of Forensic Medicine* (December 1983), 304–5.

207   "staggered about the laboratory": Eugene Pawley, "Cause of Death: Ask Gettler," *American Mercury* (September 1954), 62–66.

207   "they oxidized it at a faster rate": Ibid.

208   "TOO OLD TO CARE FOR PETS": *New York Sun and Herald,* May 24, 1920.

208   "set forth the true facts": "Letter to the Editor," *New York Times,* June 1, 1920.

208   "Test-Tube Sleuth": *Time* (May 15, 1933), 24.

208   "The Man Who Reads Corpses": *Harper's Magazine* (February 1, 1955), 62–67.

208   "sent more criminals to the electric chair": S. K. Niyogi, "Historical Developments of Forensic Medicine in America Up to 1978," *American Journal of Forensic Medicine and Pathology* (September 1980), 255.

208   "radium girls": William Sharpe, "The New Jersey Radium Dial Painters," *Bulletin of the History of Medicine* (Winter 1978), 560–70.

209   "WILLMOTT ASHES IN POISON TEST": *New York Times,* September 13, 1934.

209 "I recall that one victim": "The Memoirs of Dr. DeWitt Stetten, Jr.," unpublished manuscript in author's possession.

210 "up slightly after a post-holiday drop": "The Liquor Market," *The New Yorker* (January 16, 1926), 7.

210 "makes men talk nutty and climb trees": Ibid.

210 "23 DEATHS HERE LAID TO HOLIDAY DRINKING": *New York Times,* December 28, 1926.

211 "The mortality rate from this cause": For a transcript of the Norris Report and a summary, see *New York Times,* February 6, 1927.

212 "No one having good wines": Ibid.

212 "It is common knowledge": Ibid.

213 "We almost never see now a pile of furniture," Philip Weiss, *Unsung Heroes: The Story of the Bellevue Hospital Social Work Department* (2005), 24.

213 "16 KILLED IN 4 DAYS": *New York Times,* July 31, 1932.

Chapter 15: The Shocking Truth

214 "seemed to be New York": Mason Williams, *City of Ambition* (2013), 81.

215 "During his first two years in office": Edward Ellis, *The Epic of New York City* (1966), 526.

215 "That's cheap!": Ibid.

215 "despairing persons of both sexes": Dr. Alexander Thomas, "History of Bellevue Psychiatric Hospital" (1982), unpublished manuscript, Lapidus Medical Library, NYU.

216 "Is it strange that the average": Menas S. Gregory, "Reception Hospitals, Psychopathic Wards, and Psychopathic Hospitals," presented to the American Medico-Psychological Association, 1907, copy in author's possession.

216 "LUNATIC WITH A PISTOL": *New York Times,* September 16, 17, 1925.

216 "I wouldn't send my dog there": Ibid., June 10, 1926.

217 "It was a big graft job": "Dr. Joseph Wortis, Recollections, told to Leo Hollister," December 14, 1994, copy in author's possession.

217 "cinquecento porticoes": Gerald Weissmann, "Bellevue: Form Follows Function," *Hospital Practice* (August 1981), 18.

218 "first-time charity recipients" . . . "the new poor": Williams, *City of Ambition,* 92.

218 "For many New Yorkers": Sandra Opdycke, *No One Was Turned Away* (1999), 73.

218 "is indeed a gigantic factory": Ibid, 77.

218 "There was a time when people": *New York Times,* September 12, 1940.

218   "They treated me first-rate": "A Reporter in Bed: Bellevue Days," *The New Yorker* (October 14, 1950), 104–5.

219   "at least 20 life-saving appointments": Gerald Weissmann, "Einstein's Letter to the Dean: Welcome to America," *Federation of American Scientists for Experimental Biology* (December 2015), 4761.

219   "overstimulation": Robert Kohn et al., "Affective Disorders Among Jews: A Historical Review and Meta-Analysis," *History of Psychiatry* (1999), 245–67.

220   "We expect a continuous growth": P. P. Yeung and S. Greenwald, "Jewish Americans and Mental Health," *Social Psychiatry and Psychiatric Epidemiology* (1992), 292–99; B. Malzberg, "Mental Illness Among Jews," *Mental Hygiene* (1930), 926–46.

220   "a niece of the former Commissioner Donahue": "Gross Defects in the Management of the Psychopathic Division of Bellevue Hospital" (1934), Box 22, Lauretta Bender Papers, Brooklyn College Archives.

220   "failure to adequately encourage": Ibid.

221   "Mean Ass Gregory": Interview with Dr. Arthur Zitrin.

221   "We rarely saw him": Arthur Zitrin, "The Greatest Little Man in the World," unpublished paper in author's possession.

221   "She was screaming": Dr. Emanuel Kotsos to Dr. Gregory, September 17, 1932 (copy in author's possession).

221   "The alliance between the director": *New York Herald Tribune,* June 27, 1934; *New York Times,* June 27, 1934.

221   "Almost overnight, residents, junior physicians": Walter Bromberg, *Psychiatry Between the Wars* (1982), 108–9.

222   "the swiftest trial of a sensational murder case": *New York Times,* May 28, 1916.

222   "Court Orders Delay": Ibid., July 20, 1933.

222   "Dr. Gregory Finds": Ibid., December 2, 1925.

222   "First I stripped her naked": Katherine Ramsland, *The Devil's Dozen* (2009), 71.

223   "Oh, you'll hear plenty about Bellevue": *New York Times,* March 12, 13, 1935.

223   "Yes, Bellevue has a lot to answer for": Ibid.

223   "not voluminous . . . not an insane person": Ibid., March 22, 1935.

223   "I always had a desire to inflict pain": Colin Wilson, *The Serial Killers* (2011), 171; *New York Times,* March 20, 22, 1935.

224   "However you define the medical and legal borders": Katherine Ramsland, *The Mind of a Murderer* (2011), 47. Also, Fredric Wertham: *The Show of Violence* (1949).

224   "a psychopathic personality without a psychosis": *New York Times,*

March 20, 22, 1935; "Albert Fish Case, 1935: The M'Naghten Rule," *Bloomberg Law* (n.d.).

224　"DR. GREGORY DIES ON GOLF LINKS": *New York Times,* November 3, 1941.

225　"It was extraordinary": Bromberg, *Psychiatry Between the Wars,* 85.

225　"with books piled to eye level": Ibid.

225　"She may not have been home": Peter Schilder, "My Family," unpublished paper, Box 22, Lauretta Bender Papers. The college professor who graded the paper gave it a C+. "I don't think you know yourself or your mother very well," he wrote.

225　"She loved her infants as infants": Lauretta Bender, "Autobiography," unpublished, Lauretta Bender Papers.

226　"I doubt that I would have graduated": Ibid.

226　"I knew immediately": Ibid.

226　"They flock to [us] by the dozen": Joseph Wortis, "Observations of a Psychiatric Intern," in Correspondence, Joseph Wortis Unit ¼112, Adolph Meyer Papers, Chesney Medical Archives, Johns Hopkins.

227　"two features which almost anyone will concede": Dennis Doyle, "Racial Differences Have to Be Considered: Lauretta Bender, Bellevue Hospital, and the African-American Psyche," *History of Psychiatry* (2010), 206–23.

227　"It was almost a pleasure": Wortis, "Observations of a Psychiatric Intern."

228　"hairline": Edward Shorter and David Healy, *Shock Therapy* (2007), 60–66.

228　"It is not simply a shock": Joseph Wortis, "Remarks Before the New York Neurological Association," Box 8, Joseph Wortis Papers, Psychiatric Archives, Cornell-Weill Medical Center, NYC.

228　"Our insulin wards now have 26 beds": Joseph Wortis to Kingsley Porter, April 20, 1937, Box 10, in ibid.

229　"I don't feel confused": Joseph Wortis, "Experience at Bellevue with Hypoglycemic Treatment of Psychosis," Adolph Meyer Papers, Wortis Unit ¼112.

229　"We can afford to wait": Ibid.

229　"[Our unit] is now pushing electro-shock": Joseph Wortis to Harold Himwich, October 21, 1940, Box 8, Joseph Wortis Papers.

230　"could damage the nervous system": Shorter and Healy, *Shock Therapy,* 32–37.

230　"Place a generous amount of electrode jelly": "Instructions for Electro-Shock Apparatus," Box 20, Joseph Wortis Papers.

231　"If you were confronted by the cross-section": Adam Feinstein, *A History of Autism: Conversations with Pioneers* (2010), 44–47.

232 "organic brain disorders": Bender, "Notes on Children's Ward," Box 22, Lauretta Bender Papers.

232 "juvenile delinquency": Jill Lepore, *The Secret History of Wonder Woman* (2014), 264–71.

232 "We have too many feeble-minded among us": Foster Kennedy, "The Problem of Social Control of the Congenital Defective," *American Journal of Psychiatry* (July 1942), 14.

233 "the essential schizophrenic process": Lauretta Bender, "One Hundred Cases of Schizophrenia Treated with Electric Shock," *Transactions of the American Neurological Society* (June 1947), 165–69.

233 "clearly related the [shocks] to sexual intercourse": Ibid. Also, Austin Des Lauriers, "Psychological Tests in Childhood Schizophrenia," *American Psychological Society, Annual Meeting* (1947), 57–67.

233 "were temporary and resulted in no sustained improvement": E. R. Clardy and Elizabeth Rumpf, "The Effect of Electric Shock Treatment on Children Having Schizophrenic Manifestations," *Psychiatric Quarterly* (1954), 616–23.

233 "all other measures have failed": Ibid.

234 "I have never seen one single instance": Feinstein, *History of Autism*, 44–47.

234 "I think they destroyed him": Barbara Seaman, *Lucky Me: The Life of Jacqueline Susann* (1996), 211–14.

234 "afraid of dying": Clardy and Rumpf, "The Effect of Electric Shock Treatment on Children Having Schizophrenic Manifestations," 621–23.

234 "I don't think they did me much good": Ibid.

234 "On the mornings when I was going to get the shock treatment": Ted Chabasinski, "A Child on the Shock Ward," *Mad in America* (July 17, 2012), http://madinamerica.com.

235 "Sometimes she would pass very close": Ibid.

235 "The little boy who had been taken": Ibid.

235 "Clearly, the warnings I had been given": Dr. Stella Chess, "Images in Psychiatry: Lauretta Bender, M.D.," *American Journal of Psychiatry* (March 1995), 436. Also, "Remembering Lauretta Bender," *Annals of Dyslexia* (1987), 1–9.

236 "we were extremely cautious": Jeff Sigafoos, "Flashback to the 1960s: LSD in the Treatment of Autism," *Developmental Neurorehabilitation* (January–March 2007), 75–81.

236 "became gay, happy, laughing frequently": Lauretta Bender, "LSD and UML Treatment of Hospitalized Disturbed Children," *Recent Advances in Biological Psychology* (1963), 84–92.

236 "beneficial results": *American Druggist* (1962), 33.

236   "the preeminent woman psychiatrist": Gwendolyn Stevens and Sheldon Garner, *The Women of Psychology* (1982).

237   "Their violent attacks and even lawsuits": Thomas, "History of Bellevue Psychiatric Hospital," 118–19.

237   "With appropriate checks and safeguards": Gary Walters, "Electroconvulsive Therapy on Young People and the Pioneering Spirit of Lauretta Bender," *Acta Neuropsychiatrica* (2010), 253–54.

237   "We consider it the treatment": Interview with Dr. Dennis Popeo.

Chapter 16: Survival

238   "Just about everything": Yale Enson and Mary Chamberlin, "Cournand and Richards at the Bellevue Cardiopulmonary Laboratory," *Columbia Magazine* (Fall 2001).

238   "Might I ask that [we] be consulted": Dean Lambert to Bellevue Board of Trustees, January 26, 1916, Dean's Files: Affiliated Hospitals, Bellevue, Box 317, Health Services Library, Columbia University.

239   "At least six clinical studies": "Plans for a Service for Chronic Lung Diseases at Bellevue Hospital," May 6, 1933, in ibid.

239   "If you succeed": André Cournand oral interview, in Allen Weisse, *Heart to Heart* (2002), 24–38.

239   "Richards introduced me": Ibid.

240   "I was convinced": Lawrence Altman, *Who Goes First* (1998), 41. Also, Werner Forssmann, *Experiments on Myself* (1974).

240   "extensive metastases": Cournand oral interview, *Heart to Heart*.

240   "Well, he did it on other people": Ibid.

240   "We had . . . a surgical resident on call": Ibid.

241   "the technique": Richards to Dean Willard Rappleye, Dean's Files, April 17, 1947.

241   "One rubbed neurons": Enson and Chamberlin, "Cournand and Richards at the Bellevue Cardiopulmonary Laboratory."

241   "I don't know if it has anything to do": Cournand oral interview, *Heart to Heart*.

242   "Women always fared better": Dr. Joseph Dancis interview; Dr. Donna O'Hare interview; both in Archives of the American Academy of Pediatrics.

242   "earned enough": Joseph Dancis interview.

242   "Well, actually I had a little lesion": Dr. Edwin Kendig interview, Archives of the American Academy of Pediatrics.

243   "the first effective antibiotic": The Nobel Prize in Physiology or Medicine, 1952, NobelPrize.org.

243   "came from low socioeconomic backgrounds": Edith Lincoln, *Tuberculosis in Children* (1963), 1–5.

244   "Word soon spread": Donna O'Hare interview.

244   "I feel obliged to complain": Richards to William Van Glahn, Dean's Files, June 20, 1947.

245   "We all wore masks": Dr. Roberta Goldring interview.

245   "Dear Dick, I will tell you": Dean Willard Rappleye to Richards, in ibid.

245   "I can win the Nobel Prize": *New York Times,* February 9, 1957.

246   "just walk in and take a look": *New York Times,* May 8, 1957.

246   "Ring Up For Down": Gerald Lowenstein, *The Midnight Meal* (2005), 114.

246   "chicken/rule out tuna": Interview with Dr. Loren Greene.

246   "If a patient needed privacy": William Nolen, "Bellevue: No One Was Ever Turned Away," *American Heritage* (February–March 1987).

247   "It seems to us a sorry reflection": Richards et al. to William Jacobs, n.d., Dean's Files, 1948–50.

247   "NOBEL WINNER SEES BELLEVUE": *New York Herald Tribune,* May 8, 1957.

247   "For the sake of decency and pride": *New York World Telegram,* May 8, 1957.

247   "Bellevue is more than a city hospital": Sandra Opdycke, *No One Was Turned Away* (1999), 129.

247   "the current uproar": Arthur and Barbara Gelb, "The Plus Side of Bellevue," *New York Times Magazine* (June 2, 1957).

248   "Contrary to popular belief": Salvatore Cutolo, *Bellevue Is My Home* (1956), 121, 128–29.

248   "referring their medical derelicts": Richards to Dean Willard Rappleye, Dean's Files, March 9, 1951.

248   "The Department of Hospitals": Elizabeth Kramer, *The New York City Health and Hospitals Corporation* (1977), 55–56.

250   "Double billing and false time sheets": Charles Morris, *The Cost of Good Intentions* (1980), 41.

250   "a few million dollars or so": Kramer, *The New York City Health and Hospitals Corporation: Issues, Problems, and Prospects,* 60.

250   "Just top of the list": Randall Woods, *LBJ: Architect of American Ambition* (2006), 569.

251   "perhaps the biggest single governmental operation": Ibid., 573.

251   "[We] cannot be restricted by decisions": Ira Rutkow, *Seeking the Cure* (2010), 259.

251   "were whatever hospitals and physicians": Woods, *LBJ,* 573.

251   "The chronic underfunding": J. B. Mitchell, "Medicaid Mills: Fact and Fiction," *Health Care Financial Review* (Summer 1980), 37–49.

252   "New York City launched a blitz": Opdycke, *No One Was Turned Away,* 141.

253   "in a bad light": Ibid., 138.

253   "was largely and traditionally populated": Lewis Thomas, *The Youngest Science* (1983), 112.

254   "What better solution": Harry Dowling, *City Hospitals* (1982), 185.

254   "The most important reason": Lawrence Hutchison, *The New York City Health and Hospitals Corporation: Panacea or Placebo?* (1970), 4.

254   "leather-lunged loner": *New York Times,* January 22, 1967.

254   "not related to their illnesses": Ibid.

255   "competent medical authority": Ibid., January 13, 1967.

256   "Hire More Workers": *New York Times,* June 6, 1971.

257   "FORD TO CITY: DROP DEAD": New York *Daily News,* October 30, 1975.

258   "I resolved that": Joseph Blumenkranz, *Bellevue Behemoth* (1984), 193.

258   "The corridors are clean": Gerald Weissmann, "Bellevue: Form Follows Function," *Hospital Practice* (August 1981), 21.

258   "a spectacular building": Thomas, *The Youngest Science,* 134–35.

258   "She resists improvements": Opdycke, *No One Was Turned Away,* 168.

Chapter 17: AIDS

259   "We were floored": Interview with Dr. Fred Valentine.

260   "I suddenly began to take sexual histories": Ronald Bayor and Gerald Oppenheimer, *AIDS Doctors: Voices from the Epidemic* (2000), 53–54.

260   "Rare Cancers Seen in 41 Homosexuals": *New York Times,* July 3, 1981.

260   "opportunistic infections": CDC, *Morbidity and Mortality Weekly Report,* July 1981, 305–8.

260   "I once caught him coming out of a gay bathhouse": Bayor and Oppenheimer, *AIDS Doctors,* 61.

261   "The variable most strongly associated": Marmor, Friedman-Kien, and Lauberstein, et al., "Risk Factors for Kaposi's Sarcoma in Homosexual Men," *The Lancet* (May 1982), 1083–87.

261   "amyl nitrate": Fred Valentine, "Surveillance Notes," copy in author's possession.

261   "Great was the reproach": Daniel Defoe, *A Journal of the Plague Year* (1722), 238.

262   "to face the danger": American Medical Association, *Code of Medical Ethics* (1847).

262   "free to choose whom to serve": AMA, *Revised Code* (1957).

262   "alternative arrangements for the care of the patient": AMA, Council on Ethical and Judicial Affairs, *Statement on AIDS* (1986).

262   "private doctors won't take people": *New York Times,* April 23, 1990.

262   "In refusing to deal with such patients": B. Friedman, "Health Profes-

sions, Codes, and the Right to Refuse HIV Infectious Patients," *Hastings Center Report* (April–May 1988), 20.

263 "It had no name": Abigail Zuger, "AIDS on the Wards: A Residency in Medical Ethics," *Hastings Center Report* (June 1987), 16.

263 "They'd say, 'You're going to get AIDS'": Seymour Shubin, "Caring for AIDS Patients: The Stress Will Be on You," *Nursing* (October 1989), 44.

264 "JUNKIE AIDS VICTIM WAS HOUSEKEEPER": *New York Post,* June 14, 1983.

264 "In an instant, all I could feel": *New York Times,* December 23, 1985.

264 "By the speed of the buzz": Richard Ostreicher, "On Medical Residents," Laubenstein, *Tales of Linda* (2013), 54.

265 "She took wonderful care of her patients": Bayor and Oppenheimer, *AIDS Doctors,* 121.

265 "Someone suggested it might be because": Laubenstein, *Tales of Linda,* 10.

265 "She'd better clip her damn nails": Ibid., 33.

265 "the part of Dr. Emma Brookner": Ibid., 10.

266 "Over and over [they] mentioned to me": Zuger, "AIDS on the Wards," 19.

266 "a substantial degree of concern": Nathan Link, "Concerns of Medical and Pediatric House Officers About Acquiring AIDS from Their Patients," *American Journal of Public Health* (April 1988), 455–59.

267 "There was a lot of talk going around": Interview with Dr. David Goldfarb.

267 "I've never seen this before": *Newsday,* September 15, 1985.

267 "The AIDS patient who never quite gets visited": Zuger, "AIDS on the Wards," 19.

267 "I mean this is a place": *Newsday,* September 15, 1985.

267 "Every third admission seemed to be a patient": *New York Times,* July 27, 2012.

267–68 "AIDS is so very complicated": *New York Times,* December 23, 1985.

268 "One woman has rampant diabetes": Michael Pillinger, "The Bellevue Experience," *NYU Physician* (Spring 1985), 33.

268 "They all die on you": *New York Times,* December 23, 1985.

268 "AIDS had saturated our training": Danielle Ofri, "Pas De Deux," in Lee Gutkind, ed., *Becoming a Doctor* (2010), 10. Also, "The Impact of AIDS on Medical Residency Training," *New England Journal of Medicine* (1986), 177–80.

269 "Thank you for this very nice lecture": Bayor and Oppenheimer, *AIDS Doctors,* 96.

269 "We know how involved and dedicated you are": Ibid.

269 "Almost everything in San Francisco": Interview with Dr. Robert Holzman.

270 "We came in about 47th out of 50": *New York Times,* May 31, 1988.

270 "no AIDS crisis": Charles Perrow and Mauro Guillen, *The AIDS Disaster* (1990), 35.

271 "single men without dependents": *New York Times,* August 7, 1989.

271 "Over 60 percent of our [AIDS] patients are drug abusers": R. Holzman et al., "Bellevue Hospital's Administrative Response to the AIDS Epidemic," copy in author's possession.

271 "It wasn't just a 'better safe than sorry thing'": Holzman interview.

272 "Imagine sombody completely miserable": Source wished to remain anonymous.

272 "I can't blame her": Edward Ziegler and Lewis Goldfrank, *Emergency Doctor* (1987), 247.

272 "a nurse's disease": Shubin, "Caring for AIDS Patients," 44.

273 "THE ONLY THING BETWEEN THIS PLACE": *New York Times,* December 23, 1985.

273 "It's different from other diseases": *New York Times,* October 4, 1987.

273 "The situation could resolve itself": *Evans v. Bellevue, New York Law Journal,* decision rendered July 28, 1987.

274 "He wanted to die with dignity": *New York Times,* July 16, 17, 28, 1987.

274 "reasonable expectation of recovery": Ibid., July 17, 1987.

274 "There is nothing more precious than human life": *Evans v. Bellevue.* Also, Anthony Di Somma, "Evans v. Bellevue," *Library Law Journal: Issues in Law and Medicine* (1988), 235–38.

274 "living will": Governor's Task Force on Life and Law, *Life Sustaining Treatment: Making Decisions and Appointing a Health Care Agent* (1987).

275 "Airway Team": Interview with Dr. Nathan Thompson.

275 "This wasn't cowboy medicine": Source wishes to remain anonymous.

276 "Man of the Year": *Time* (December 30, 1996).

276 "I have begun to believe": Andrew Sullivan, "When Plagues End," *New York Times Magazine* (November 10, 1996).

276 "all dying, some rapidly, most slowly": "Saying Goodbye to Bellevue Virology," *Infection Disease Division Newsletter* (2012), NYU Langone Medical Center, 1.

Chapter 18: Rock Bottom

277 "A GREAT HOSPITAL IN CRISIS": *New York Times,* February 21, 1988.

278 "She was tough": Ibid., January 23, 1989.

278 "thin needle biopsy": Ibid., April 5, 1988.

278 "There ain't nobody there": Ibid., January 9, 1989; New York *Daily News,* January 9, 10, 1989.

279 "Ratman": *Newsday,* February 6, 1989.

279   "He took great joy": *New York Times*, January 10, 1989.

280   "Can I talk to you for a minute?" *New York Times,* January 13, 1989;
       Walt Bogdanich, *The Great White Lie* (1991), 12–30.

280   "On a typical day in 1989": New York *Daily News,* January 27, 1989.

280   "The Beast of Bellevue": Bogdanich, *The Great White Lie,* 20.

281   "at least three reports": *Johnson v. New York City HHC* (June 1998).

281   "hopeless paralytic": *New York Times,* May 28, 1919.

281   "taking a banana": Dr. Alexander Thomas, "History of Bellevue
       Psychiatric Hospital" (1982), unpublished manuscript in author's pos-
       session. Thomas was the longtime chief of psychiatry at NYU Medical
       School.

282   William Morales: For information on the Morales case, see Bryan Bur-
       rough, *Days of Rage* (2015), 471–75; *New York Times,* September 16,
       1984; Susan Reverby, "Enemy of the People," *Bulletin of the History of
       Medicine* (2014), 403–30.

283   "She was so loved": *Newsday,* February 9, 1989.

283   "We thought he was faking": *New York Times,* October 31, 1989.

283   "not require a hospital security system to be flawless": *People v. Smith*
       (N.P. App. Div. 1994); *Johnson v. New York City HHC.*

284   "toy cops": *New York Times,* March 27, 1989.

284   "Bellevue security sucks": Bogdanich, *The Great White Lie,* 20.

284   "Clusters of men": *New York Times,* February 3, 1971.

285   "cold weather alert": Ibid., September 14, October 30, 1987, April 11,
       1988.

285   "With our traditional sensitivity": Thomas, "History of Bellevue Psy-
       chiatric Hospital"; H. Richard Lamb, *A Report on the Task Force of the
       Homeless Mentally Ill* (1992).

286   "after some cajoling": Jennifer Toth, *Mole People,* 56–57.

286   "These people": Ibid., 155.

286   "Noises arise in the darkness": *New York Times,* January 12, 1992.

286   "Wintertime was the worst": Danielle Ofri, "Pas de Deux," in Lee Gut-
       kind, *Becoming a Doctor* (2010), 10.

286   "An acrid smell of cheese": Michael Pillinger, "The Bellevue Experience,"
       NYU Physician (Spring 1985), 34.

287   "scabrous and pocked": Ibid.

287   Social work studies in Philip Weiss, "The Story of Bellevue Hospital and
       Bellevue Social Workers" (2005), unpublished manuscript in author's
       possession.

287   "[We've] changed from a receiving hospital": Thomas, "History of Belle-
       vue Psychiatric Hospital."

287   "I hate to put it this way": *New York Times,* September 20, 1983.

287   "the choo-choo train of drunks": "Bellevue's Emergency," *New York Times Sunday Magazine,* February 11, 1996.

288   "We treat all the problems of society": *New York Times,* November 24, 1992.

288   "Our security stinks": *Newsday,* February 26, 1989.

288   "The risk of working in a place": Ibid., February 6, 1989. Also, *New York Times,* January 13, 1989.

288   "an unshaven derelict": Gerald Weissmann, *Darwin's Audubon* (2001), 265.

Chapter 19: Sandy

290   "It's hard for me to believe": "The Bellevue Murder: Could It Happen in Your Hospital?" *Hospital Security and Safety Management* (May 1989).

290   "large numbers of homeless": Ibid.

291   "We work hard": *Newsday,* March 6, 1989.

291   "the flagship of public hospital care": "Privatizing HHC," *City Journal* (Spring 1993).

291   "[We're] a big institution": *New York Times,* March 7, 1995.

291   "I can't tell you now with a straight face": Ibid.

292   "little to do with the needs": Ibid.

292   "who are sicker, more difficult to manage": United Hospital Fund, *The State of New York City's Municipal Hospital System* (1989).

292   "We've had more Bellevue heads": *New York Amsterdam News,* June 21, 1997.

292   "I will only run a hospital": *New York Times,* May 31, 1988.

292   "I don't need to subject myself": Ibid., December 6, 1988. Also, Walt Bogdanich, *The Great White Lie* (1991), 15.

293   "the city should remain": Jeremiah Barondess, "Municipal Hospitals in New York City—A Review of the Report of the Commission to Review the Health and Hospitals Corporation," *Bulletin of the New York Academy of Medicine* (Summer 1993), 15.

293   "a nice thing, a good thing": Sandra Opdycke, *No One Was Turned Away* (1999), 184.

294   "This is war zone medicine": *New York Times,* November 4, 1990.

294   "She was in a state of profound shock": Salvatore Cutolo, *Bellevue Is My Home* (1955), 123. Also, New York *Daily News,* July 25, 1945.

295   "put back together": Cutolo, *Bellevue Is My Home,* 125.

295   "Oxygen tanks were piled": Katherine Finkelstein, "Bellevue's Emergency," *New York Times Sunday Magazine,* February 11, 1996.

295   "It's gonna be a big one": *Los Angeles Times,* September 5, 2011.

295   "the hospital shifted gears": Ibid.

295 "The second tower falls": Mack Lipkin, "Medical Ground Zero," *Annals of Internal Medicine* (May 2002), 704–7.

295 "I've been thinking about something like this": *New York Times,* September 18, 2001; *Boston Globe,* September 14, 2001.

296 "Thousands of medical workers": *Los Angeles Times,* September 5, 2011.

296 "The center zone is death on impact": Ibid.

296 "Police cars barreled up": Tony Dejer, "Lessons Learned: New York Downtown Hospital and 9/11," *Health Leaders Magazine* (October 5, 2006).

296 "We took heads, arms, legs": Marilyn Larkin, "New York Physicians Respond to the Terror, Tragedy, and Trauma," *The Lancet* (September 22, 2001), 940.

297 "Initially, I thought I had died": "Last Man Out," *Sixty Minutes II,* November 4, 2004.

297 "So many lives were lost that day": Stuart Marcus, "Remembering 9/11: Reflections from Bellevue Hospital and New York University Medical Center," *Surgery* (2002), 502–5.

297 "Has anyone seen Richard": *New York Times,* September 29, 2001. Also, Victor Seidler, *Remembering 9/11: Terror, Trauma and Social Theory* (2013), 39.

298 "I would look down during nights on call": Russell Saunders, "Never Forget," *The Daily Beast,* September 10, 2015.

299 "Often, the capacity of emergency generators": J. David Roccaforte, "The World Trade Center Attack: Observations from New York's Bellevue Hospital," *Critical Care* (2001), 307–9.

299 "disasters outside their walls": *Insurance Journal,* November 6, 2012.

302 "We were told it would take ten seconds": Interview with Dr. Doug Bails.

302 "There was no electricity": *Insurance Journal,* November 6, 2012.

303 "The patients started arriving at around 1:00 a.m.": Phyllis Maguire, "New York Hospitals and the Hurricane," *Today's Hospitalist* (December 2012).

303 "Do you think they'd have kept me in there": David Remnick, "Leaving Langone: One Story," *The New Yorker* (October 30, 2012).

304 "In the event of total power loss": Interview with Dr. Laura Evans; Laura Evans et al., "In Search of the Silver Lining: The Impact of Superstorm Sandy on Bellevue Hospital," *Annals of the American Thoracic Society* (April 2013), 135–42.

305 "There was no division of labor": "The Night of the Hurricane," *Bellevue Literary Review* (Spring 2013).

305 "This being Manhattan": Danielle Ofri, "Bellevue and the Hurricane," *New England Journal of Medicine* (December 13, 2012), 2265–67.

305 "19 S East Stairwell": The whiteboard still hangs in 17 West as a reminder of Sandy.

305 "I am caught behind a team": Kelsey Frohman, "Bellevue Hospital: Sandy Recap," Ravenscroftschool.com, October 30, 2012.

306 "I have to pee": Ibid.

306 "All hospitals are required to do disaster planning": *New York Times,* November 2, 2012.

306 "It's Bellevue, we're used to crisis": Erin Haggerty, "When Bellevue Had to Evacuate Its Criminally Insane," *Bedford + Bowery,* October 29, 2013.

307 "I can recall the patient monitor going black": "Alumni Share Stories from Hurricane Sandy," University of Wisconsin–Madison School of Medicine, March 12, 2013.

307 "The amount of heroism that arises": Sheri Fink, "Beyond Hurricane Heroics—What Sandy Should Teach Us About Preparedness," *Stanford Magazine* (Summer 2013).

Chapter 20: Rebirth

309 "Most of our knockout mice": Interview with Dr. Bruce Cronstein.

309 "I felt an awful sense of despair": Gordon Fishell, "After the Deluge," *Nature* (April 25, 2013), 421.

309 "We made a dash to retrieve": Interview with Dr. Martin Blaser. Also, Martin Blaser, *Missing Microbes* (2014), 258.

309 "It was like Sophie's Choice": Apoorva Mandavilli, "One Year After Sandy, Uneven Recovery at New York University's Labs," *Scientific American* (October 29, 2013).

309 "We began packing up": "ACTG Still Struggles in Sandy's Aftermath," *ACTG AIDS Clinical Trials Group* (December 2012).

310 "We knew that a hurricane was coming": Fishell, "After the Deluge," 421.

310 "If you were one of the mice": "Sandy and the Laboratory Mice," *Earth in Transition* (October 2012).

310 "We will never place animals": Daniel Engber, "Sandy's Toll on Medical Research," *Slate* (November 1, 2012).

310 "People don't pick hospitals": Reuters, November 4, 2012.

311 "[Our] centers are the site of massive rodent slaughter": Engber, "Sandy's Toll on Medical Research."

311 "I talk about disasters": Ibid.

311 "Hand-scrawled messages were taped to our cubicle": *New York Times,* November 26, 2012.

312 "using vast sums of money": Chris Glorioso, "I-Team: Two Years After Sandy, FEMA Aid to Hospitals Questioned," NBC News, New York.

313 "When NYU has an army of wealthy donors": Louis Flores, "Criticisms

over Obscene NYU Sandy Grant," www.progressivequeens, November 7, 2014.

314 "came from Africa": *Dallas Morning News,* September 25, 2014.

314 "We were looking at the pictures": *New York Times,* October 25, 2014.

315 "In all fairness": *Dallas Morning News,* October 12, 2014.

315 "It's a cool gadget": *New York Times,* February 10, 2015.

315 "Blood draws should be kept to an absolute minimum": Bellevue Hospital Center, *Ebola Virus Disease Response Guide,* 2014.

316 "Our philosophy for Ebola": Nicholas St. Fleur, "What Makes a Hospital 'Ebola Ready'?," *Scientific American* (October 23, 2014).

316 "EBOLA HITS NYC": *New York Post,* October 23, 2014.

317 "She is our flagship": Transcript: Mayor de Blasio at Bellevue Hospital on the Discharge of Dr. Craig Spencer, November 11, 2014.

317 "Reasons to Love New York": *New York,* December 14, 2014.

317 "We like to think of ourselves": Interview with Dr. Doug Bails.

Epilogue

320 "very combative": "Active ALC cases for January 13, 2016" (copy in author's possession).

320 "Think of fifty valuable beds": Interview with Dr. Doug Bails.

320 "our triple threat": Interview with Dr. James Lebret.

320 "not yet accepting the status quo": Marc Gourevitch et al., "The Public Hospital in American Education," *Journal of Urban Health* (September 2008), 779–86.

322 "It is not for sale": *New York Times,* April 25, 2016.

ILLUSTRATION CREDITS

Insert A

Page 1, top left and bottom: Courtesy of the Lillian and Clarence de la Chapelle Medical Archives at NYU; **top right:** Old Paper Studios / Alamy

Page 2, top left: Library of Congress Prints and Photographs Division; **top right:** Courtesy of the Lillian and Clarence de la Chapelle Medical Archives at NYU; **bottom:** The Granger Collection, New York

Page 3, top: U.S. National Library of Medicine; **bottom:** Courtesy of the Lillian and Clarence de la Chapelle Medical Archives at NYU

Page 4, top: Courtesy of the Lillian and Clarence de la Chapelle Medical Archives at NYU; **bottom:** Courtesy of Bellevue Hospital Center Archive

Page 5, top: The Granger Collection, New York; **center and bottom:** Courtesy of the Lillian and Clarence de la Chapelle Medical Archives at NYU

Page 6, top: U.S. National Library of Medicine; **bottom left and right:** Courtesy of Bellevue Hospital Center Archive

Page 7, top left and bottom: Courtesy of the Lillian and Clarence de la Chapelle Medical Archives at NYU; **top right:** Class album—Manuscripts & Archives, Yale University

Page 8: Philadelphia Museum of Art, gift of the Alumni Association to Jefferson Medical College in 1878 and purchased by the Pennsylvania Academy of the Fine Arts and the Philadelphia Museum of Art in 2007 with the generous support of more than 3,600 donors. Object number: 2007-1-1

Insert B

Page 1, top: Library of Congress Prints and Photographs Division; **bottom:** Courtesy NYC Municipal Archives

Page 2, top: Courtesy of Bellevue Hospital Center Archive; **center:** Courtesy of the Lillian and Clarence de la Chapelle Medical Archives at NYU; **bottom:** Courtesy NYC Municipal Archives

Page 3, top: © Carl Mikoy; **center:** Courtesy of the Lillian and Clarence de la Chapelle Medical Archives at NYU; **bottom:** Courtesy of Bellevue Hospital Center Archive

Page 4, top: Courtesy of the Lillian and Clarence de la Chapelle Medical Archives at NYU; **center:** Jim Henderson; **bottom:** Courtesy of Dr. Fred T. Valentine

Page 5, top: NYU School of Medicine; **bottom:** Jose Jimenez / Primera Hora / Getty Images

Page 6, top: Anatoly Kashlevskiy; **center and bottom:** Courtesy of Dr. Douglas Bails

Page 7, top: Karsten Moran / *The New York Times;* **center:** Courtesy of Dr. Douglas Bails; **bottom:** REUTERS / Adrees Latif

Page 8, top: © Troi Santos; **bottom:** © Bruce R. Jaffe

INDEX

ABOUT THE AUTHOR

David Oshinsky, Ph.D., is a professor in the NYU Department of History and director of the Division of Medical Humanities at the NYU Langone Medical Center. In 2006, he won the Pulitzer Prize in History for *Polio: An American Story*. His other books include the D. B. Hardeman Prize–winning *A Conspiracy So Immense: The World of Joe McCarthy*, and the Robert Kennedy Prize–winning *Worse Than Slavery: Parchman Farm and the Ordeal of Jim Crow Justice*. His articles and reviews appear regularly in *The New York Times* and *The Wall Street Journal*.